LANGUAGE SAMPLING
With Children and Adolescents

Implications for Intervention

Third Edition

LANGUAGE SAMPLING

With Children and Adolescents

Implications for Intervention

Third Edition

Marilyn A. Nippold, PhD, CCC-SLP

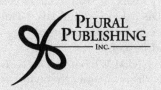

PLURAL
PUBLISHING
INC.

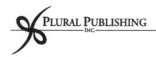

5521 Ruffin Road
San Diego, CA 92123

e-mail: information@pluralpublishing.com
Website: https://www.pluralpublishing.com

Typeset in 11/13 Garamond by Flanagan's Publishing Services, Inc.
Printed in the United States of America by Integrated Books International
24 23 22 21   2 3 4 5

Library of Congress Cataloging-in-Publication Data

Names: Nippold, Marilyn A., 1951– author.
Title: Language sampling with children and adolescents : implications for
    intervention / Marilyn A. Nippold.
Other titles: Language sampling with adolescents
Description: Third edition. | San Diego, CA : Plural Publishing, Inc.,
    [2021] | Preceded by Language sampling with adolescents : implications
    for intervention / Marilyn A. Nippold. Second edition. 2014. | Includes
    bibliographical references and index.
Identifiers: LCCN 2020046928 | ISBN 9781635502763 (paperback) | ISBN
    1635502764 (paperback) | ISBN 9781635502695 (ebook)
Subjects: MESH: Language Disorders—diagnosis | Language Tests | Language
    Disorders—therapy | Speech-Language Pathology—methods | Language
    Development | Child | Adolescent
Classification: LCC RJ496.S7 | NLM WL 340.2 | DDC 618.92/85506—dc23
LC record available at https://lccn.loc.gov/2020046928

Contents

Preface

This is the third edition of *Language Sampling With Adolescents*, first published in 2010 and then revised in 2014 as a second edition. Whereas the first two editions focused solely on adolescents, this third edition has expanded to include preschool and school-age children, in addition to adolescents. Hence, the book now covers ages 3 through 18 years. Another change is that each discourse genre (conversation, narration, exposition, and persuasion) now has its own chapter, with implications for intervention. This change reflects the expanding knowledge base in spoken and written language development and disorders, thanks to the many tireless researchers throughout the world who have been publishing their work in scholarly journals. It also reflects the growing awareness that each genre is unique in that it calls upon different sets of cognitive, linguistic, social, and emotional resources. For example, a speaker's true language competence may not be revealed unless the topic is relatively complex and the individual is knowledgeable about it and motivated to share that insight. In other words, when a language sampling task "stresses the system" (Lahey, 1990), we are more likely to gain an accurate picture of the speaker's ability to communicate in naturalistic, real-world contexts. It is in this way that language sampling can be one of the most valuable assessment tools available to clinicians.

A NOTE TO INSTRUCTORS

When this book is used as a text for university courses in language development or language disorders in children and adolescents, I suggest that students be assigned to read chapters from Part II: Grammar Review and Exercises, while they are reading chapters from Part I: Working With Children and Adolescents. This would provide students the opportunity to review grammar in manageable chunks before they apply the information to analyze language samples. Note that the chapters in Part I build on each other by explaining why language sampling is important to speech-language pathologists (Chapter 1), how it has evolved throughout the years (Chapter 2), and how it can be carried out successfully (Chapter 3). Then, in Chapters 4 through 7, Part I discusses the unique aspects of the different genres—conversational, narrative, expository, and persuasive—followed by a discussion of how language sampling can be employed with students who have autism spectrum disorders (Chapter 8). The chapters in Part II also build on each other. For example, by covering different types of words and phrases in Chapter 9 before different types of clauses in Chapter 10, students will understand how certain types of words and phrases are similar to certain types of clauses (e.g., nouns and nominal clauses; adjectives and relative clauses; adverbs and adverbial clauses). Moreover, by covering clause types before sentence types (e.g., simple, compound, complex) in Chapter 11, they will understand how the type of sentence is determined by the type(s) of clause(s) it contains. Finally, by covering sentence types before units of measurement (Chapter 12), students will be able to distinguish between complete and incomplete C-units and T-units and determine whether a "run on" sentence is actually one, two, or three C-units or T-units. The final chapters on analyzing conversational (Chapter 13) and narrative, expository, and persuasive (Chapter 14) language samples offer students the opportunity to apply the information they have learned from all previous chapters.

Hence, it is suggested that during the first half of a semester, students be assigned to read the chapters in this sequence: 1, 9, 2, 10, 3, 11, and 12. It is also recommended that class time be spent discussing students' answers to the grammar review exercises as they compare their own answers to those contained in Appendices A, B, C, and D. Then, during the second half of the semester, students could read Chapters 4, 5, 6, 7, and 8, complete the exercises in Chapters 13 and 14, and compare their answers to those contained in Appendices E and F. By following this sequence, students would be well prepared to elicit, transcribe, and analyze language samples from children and adolescents with typical or disordered language development during the final weeks of the course. The experience of conducting their own language samples with speakers of different ages will assist students to apply the information they have learned from this book.

—Marilyn A. Nippold

Acknowledgments

Some of the writing of this book was supported financially by the University of Oregon through the HEDCO Foundation, a Hope Baney Faculty Award, and a Summer Faculty Award. Funding for some research projects was provided by the National Institute on Deafness and Other Communication Disorders (NIH), Grant 2P50DC02746-06A1; and the US–Israel Binational Science Foundation. All financial support is gratefully acknowledged. In addition, a special note of appreciation is expressed to the Systematic Analysis of Language Transcripts (SALT) software company, particularly to Jon Miller, Karen Andriacchi, and Ann Nockerts, and to the Child Language Data Exchange System (CHILDES), particularly to Brian MacWhinney and Paul Fletcher, for providing some of the language samples that were included. Sincere appreciation is also expressed to the many children and adolescents whose spoken or written language samples were included. Without their cooperation, this book could not have been written.

*This book is dedicated to Jordan Marie,
Jackson James, and Jenna Grace.*

PART I

Working With Children and Adolescents

CHAPTER 1

Why Language Sampling?

anguage sampling is one of the most valuable assessment tools available to speech-language pathologists (SLPs) who work with children and adolescents who experience language disorders. Moreover, it is especially relevant in the era of social distancing and telepractice, in which the in-person administration of norm-referenced, standardized language tests can be challenging (Kester, 2020). In contrast, language samples can be elicited via Zoom or other cloud platforms for video and audio conferencing, with the assistance and coaching of a child's parent, older sibling, or caregiver. Yet language sampling is not a simple process that anyone can carry out successfully. On the contrary, it requires a detailed understanding of language development and language disorders; a curious mind that relishes problem-solving; strong interpersonal skills; ample motivation; and generous amounts of patience, practice, and persistence. Nevertheless, most SLPs are up to the job, and when they do embrace the challenge of learning how to elicit, transcribe, and analyze language samples, they are demonstrating their professionalism by *practicing at the top of their license.* In other words, they are maximizing "time spent delivering services [they] are uniquely qualified to provide" (McNeilly, 2018).

As SLPs, we are in this profession because we understand and value the human ability to communicate in real-world settings, and we wish to ameliorate the dire consequences for individuals and for society when this ability is compromised. Furthermore, we appreciate the fact that expertise in spoken language disorders is *our* domain and one that takes us firmly back to our roots when, in 1925, the American Academy of Speech Correction (predecessor of the American Speech-Language-Hearing Association) was formed in New York City for the purpose of ameliorating speech disorders (https://ashaarchives.omeka.net/exhibits/show/founding/item/8; retrieved June 12, 2020). Although the field has expanded greatly since those early days, no other profession can claim this legacy of advocacy for individuals with communication disorders.

It is essential to remember also that the ability to use language to express oneself with accuracy, clarity, and efficiency in social, academic, and vocational settings is a basic human right. In our modern, information-driven world in which effective and effortless communication is the standard expectation for all citizens, children and adolescents who experience difficulties with spoken or written language—during formal or informal situations—are seriously hampered in their social, academic, and vocational endeavors. So let's take a moment to applaud all SLPs who are dedicated to improving the communication skills of children and adolescents!

So why is language sampling an excellent way to evaluate a child or adolescent who has a language disorder? The primary reason is that language sampling focuses on *how* the individual communicates in the real world, under natural conditions (Costanza-Smith, 2010). For this reason, the information gained from a language sample will enable the SLP to design an intervention plan to improve the client's ability to communicate more effectively in everyday situations. Depending on the age of the client, those situations may include, for example, the home, school, or job site when speaking with parents, classmates, teachers, or coworkers.

DO ALL SLPS EMPLOY LANGUAGE SAMPLING?

Unfortunately, many SLPs do not employ language sampling as part of their regular clinical practice, primarily because they believe it takes too much time (Pavelko, Owens, Ireland, & Hahs-Vaughn, 2016). In addition, if they do elicit language samples, they do not necessarily transcribe or analyze them formally (Westerveld & Claessen, 2014). Factors contributing to these patterns include having had little training in language sampling in their graduate education programs, especially for use with older students; having limited knowledge of later language development, especially of complex syntax; and having limited access to computer technology.

In this book, each of these concerns is addressed. For example, regarding the claim that language sampling takes too much time, one must weigh that concern, on the one hand, with the wealth of information, on the other hand, that one can obtain about a child's ability to communicate, even from a short language sample. This point was demonstrated by Scott Prath (2018), a bilingual SLP, who provided the following excerpt from a child's narrative sample and listed some key aspects of language competence that each utterances reveals, shown in brackets:

C = child

C "There once was a boy and a frog" [story initiation / character identification]

C "Then, he jumped inside the box" [cohesive element / past tense marker / preposition use / object name]

C "They ran behind the trees" [pronoun / past tense irregular verb / preposition / article / plural marker]

Mean length of utterance (MLU) = 6.3 words

In addition to obtaining this "immediate snapshot" (Prath, 2018) of the child's language competence, by transcribing and analyzing the full sample, the SLP would be able to document specific strengths and weaknesses in oral expression—information that could be used to formulate and defend any clinical decisions or recommendations being made about the need for services.

Regarding the broader topic of the SLP's knowledge base, there is no longer a shortage of information concerning language sampling techniques for use with school-age children and adolescents or of information on later language development. During the past 40 years, these have become topics of expanding international interest, and many studies have been conducted to examine the development of spoken and written language production in school-age children and adolescents, often using language sampling as the primary method of data collection (e.g., Berman & Nir-Sagiv, 2007; Berman & Slobin, 1994; Berman & Verhoeven, 2002; Frizelle, Thompson, McDonald, & Bishop, 2018; Klecan-Aker & Hedrick, 1985; Nippold, Hesketh, Duthie, & Mansfield, 2005; Nippold, Ward-Lonergan, & Fanning, 2005; Ravid & Berman, 2006; Verhoeven et al., 2002). As a result, many language sampling tasks have been created that can be used by SLPs to elicit and analyze conversational, narrative, expository, and persuasive discourse, and much has been learned about the development of syntax and other aspects of language during the school-age and adolescent years (Berman, 2004; Nippold, 2016; Scott, 1988). In addition, audio recording devices have improved substantially in terms of their sound quality, transportability, and storage capacity, and computer programs such as Systematic Analysis of Language Transcripts (SALT; Miller, Andriacchi, & Nockerts, 2019) have continuously been updated, making it faster and easier to elicit, transcribe, and analyze language samples. Moreover, the process of interpreting the results of a language sample has improved with the establishment or expansion of databases of typical children and adolescents speaking in different genres (e.g., Bishop, 2004; Leadholm & Miller, 1992; Miller et al., 2019).

HOW CAN LANGUAGE SAMPLING BE HELPFUL TO CLINICIANS?

Knowing how to elicit, transcribe, and analyze language samples is critical to understanding and improving the communication skills of our clients, especially in view of the fact that at least 10% of school-age children and adolescents have language disorders that restrict their ability to express themselves effectively. This includes, for example, students with specific language impairment (SLI), nonspecific language impairment (NLI), learning disabilities, autism spectrum disorders, and traumatic brain injury (e.g., Bishop & Donlan, 2005; Landa & Goldberg, 2005; Lewis, Murdoch, & Woodyatt, 2007; Marinellie, 2004; Moran & Gillon, 2010; Moran, Kirk, & Powell, 2012; Nippold & Hesketh, 2009; Nippold, Mansfield, Billow, & Tomblin, 2008, 2009; Scott & Windsor, 2000; Ward-Lonergan, 2010; Ward-Lonergan, Liles, & Anderson, 1999). Frequently, students with these conditions exhibit limitations in their use of complex syntax, literate vocabulary, pragmatics, and in their overall language productivity. Regarding syntax, children and adolescents with developmental language disorders (DLDs) such as SLI or NLI often produce shorter and simpler utterances than their peers with typical language development (TLD). Moreover, preschool (ages 3 and 4 years) and younger school-age children (ages 5–9 years) with DLDs often struggle with grammatical morphemes, making errors on verb tenses, plurals, and pronouns (Leonard, 2014). As they grow older and move into the later school years, children with DLDs make fewer errors on grammatical morphemes but struggle to produce complex sentences with adequate subordination (Nippold et al., 2008, 2009). Regarding lexical development, many school-age children and adolescents have difficulty using literate vocabulary such as abstract nouns, morphologically complex words, metacognitive verbs, and figurative expressions. During social situations, pragmatic issues may arise where they struggle to answer questions, stay on topic, speak coherently, and add relevant information to a conversation (Timler, 2018). They also may be less attentive to others' perspectives and less productive as speakers and writers compared to their peers with TLD (Paul & Norbury, 2012).

In summary, much has been learned about typical language development during the preschool, school-age, and adolescent years and about the nature of expressive language deficits experienced by children and adolescents (Berman, 2004, 2008; Berman & Nir, 2010; Miller et al., 2019; Nippold, 2007; Paul & Norbury, 2012). Armed with a clear understanding of typical language development during these years, SLPs can examine the ability of children and adolescents to communicate in natural settings by eliciting and analyzing spoken and written language samples and using the results to establish appropriate intervention goals. Standardized language tests such as the Clinical Evaluation of Language Fundamentals–Fifth Edition (CELF-5; Wiig, Semel, & Secord, 2013) are helpful in identifying language deficits (Tomblin & Nippold, 2014) in students who speak Standard American English. However, those tests sample language out of context and do not provide the type of rich, naturalistic information that is required to formulate relevant intervention goals. In contrast, language sampling can assist the SLP to obtain this information by focusing on the language needed to succeed in social, academic, and vocational settings and to identify weaknesses in key areas such as the use of complex syntax, the literate lexicon, and pragmatics. In other words, language sampling offers greater ecological validity than norm-referenced standardized language testing (Costanza-Smith, 2010; Hewitt, Hammer, Yont, & Tomblin, 2005). Moreover, unlike norm-referenced standardized language tests, language samples can be elicited, transcribed, and analyzed as often as is necessary. Therefore, they can be used to monitor a client's progress during intervention and after it, whether the clinical activities are carried out in person or via telepractice. Some of the many benefits of language sampling with children and adolescents are listed in Table 1–1.

Table 1–1. Some Benefits of Language Sampling With Children and Adolescents

The results of a language sample can indicate how well the child or adolescent communicates in "real-world" settings:

- Talking with parents or siblings while playing a game
- Telling a parent what happened at school
- Telling a teacher the details of a playground conflict
- Conversing with others in person or on the phone
- Giving an oral report in history class
- Explaining to a peer how to play a game or sport
- Convincing a senior citizen to vote for a school bond

continues

Table 1–1. *continued*

When assessing children and adolescents who are culturally and linguistically diverse, language sampling can be used instead of standardized tests and interpreted informally to determine how well the child speaks or writes, given his/her age or grade level.

Language samples can be used to establish functional goals and monitor progress during intervention.

During cognitively challenging speaking tasks, a language sample can reveal weaknesses in the use of complex syntax and the literate lexicon.

- Frequent use of simple or incomplete sentences with little subordination:
  - "You deal the cards. Take your turn. Pay a fine."
  - "You throw it to first base. Get the guy out."
  - "It's about two guys. One's bad."
- Frequent use of imprecise, vague, or concrete words:
  - "You play the song with this guitar-type thing."
  - "I don't know what it's called, but it's small and round."
  - "Our team needs stuff. We don't got enough."

Difficulties with pragmatics can be observed, especially during conversations.

- Frequent interruptions and overlaps
- Off-topic comments
- Lack of empathy, sensitivity, awareness
- Failure to consider others' perspectives

Language productivity may be low in spoken or written language.

- Speaker produces fewer words and utterances.
- Content is inaccurate, limited, or otherwise impoverished.

The results can supplement the findings of a standardized test.

- Speaker uses short, simple utterances.
- Speaker produces grammatical errors.
- Speaker uses imprecise words (vague).

The results can offer direction for intervention, focusing on:

- Language needed to succeed socially, in school, and on the job
- Appropriate pragmatic behaviors
- Use of complex syntax and literate vocabulary
  - Subordinate clauses (relative, adverbial, nominal)
  - Subordinate clauses embedded within other subordinate clauses
  - Abstract nouns (e.g., ambition, strategy, expectation)
  - Morphologically complex words (e.g., availability, philanthropic)
  - Metacognitive verbs (e.g., determine, surmise, perceive)
  - Figurative expressions (metaphors, similes, idioms, proverbs)

WORKING WITH CULTURALLY AND LINGUISTICALLY DIVERSE CLIENTS

Language sampling is especially helpful when assessing children and adolescents who come from culturally or linguistically diverse backgrounds (e.g., Ebert, 2020; Heilmann & Malone, 2014; Heilmann, Rojas, Iglesias, & Miller, 2016; Prath, 2018; Roseberry-McKibbin & O'Hanlon, 2005). For example, if a child speaks African American English or is an English Language Learner (ELL), norm-referenced standardized tests that emphasize Standard American English and mainstream culture should be avoided, and language sampling should be the primary method of assessment. Thus, it is imperative that SLPs familiarize themselves with a child's dialect or native language to avoid falsely assuming that any differences observed in a language sample reflect a language disorder (Horton & Apel, 2014; Johnson & Koonce, 2018; Paul & Norbury, 2012; Rojas & Iglesias, 2019; Washington, 2019). For a recent review of research on language sampling with bilingual children and discussion of clinical implications, the reader is referred to Ebert (2020).

Regarding students from culturally and linguistically diverse backgrounds, an especially encouraging application of language sampling is in the context of dynamic assessment (DA) as a strategy for determining the presence or absence of a language disorder (Gillam & Peña, 2004; Peña, Gillam, & Bedore, 2014; Petersen, Chanthongthip, Ukrainetz, Spencer, & Steeve, 2017). The purpose of DA is to determine how well a child can learn language when provided with optimal instruction; those who learn quickly and easily are considered to have stronger language learning ability—and hence typical language development—than those who struggle to learn despite optimal instruction, evidencing poor language learning ability and hence a language disorder. To investigate this phenomenon in school-age children, Petersen et al. (2017) conducted a study with 42 Spanish–English bilingual children aged 6 through 9 years. Of this group, 10 children had previously been identified as having a language disorder and were receiving intervention in the schools; the remaining 32 children had demonstrated typical language development and hence were not receiving intervention. Each child participated in a "test–teach–test" activity in English, in which both test sessions (25 minutes each) involved the elicitation of a narrative retell language sample. Following the first test session, an examiner provided individualized instruction (teach session) to improve the child's use of story grammar elements and subordinate clauses. The child's ability to learn language (modifiability rating) was determined by comparing performance on the second test to that on the first test in terms of story grammar elements and subordinate clauses; children who showed greater gains were deemed to have typical language development, whereas those with fewer gains were deemed to have a language disorder. Results confirmed that children with lower modifiability ratings were more likely to have been diagnosed with a language disorder compared to those with higher ratings, indicating that DA can be helpful in identifying language disorders in bilingual children.

Although additional research on DA is needed with other groups of children and adolescents from culturally and linguistically diverse backgrounds, this strategy is a laudable effort to evaluate language-learning ability when norm-referenced standardized language tests are not an option. As explained by Roseberry-McKibbin and O'Hanlon (2005), when SLPs are serving students who are ELLs, it is inappropriate to administer norm-referenced, standardized language tests if those measures were developed for and normed on native English-speaking students; to do so would violate federal guidelines established to avoid biased and discriminatory assessment practices. In contrast, those authors recommended that a language sample be elicited in the child's native language while interacting with a parent, sibling, or classmate who speaks that language. Then, with the help of a skilled interpreter, the SLP could compare the results against major milestones in development that cut across languages and cultures.

For example, the language sample could be used to examine MLU and the presence of main and subordinate clauses because these features reflect development across languages (Berman & Verhoeven, 2002; Verhoeven et al., 2002). The extent to which the utterances in a sample are grammatically correct, given the child's age, language, and dialect, is also an important consideration (Ebert, 2020; Ivy & Masterson, 2011). In addition, the SLP could investigate how well the child uses spoken language to perform basic pragmatic functions such as initiating conversations, making requests, asking and answering questions, taking turns, staying organized, and attending to the perspectives of others. For case studies of children and adolescents, including those from diverse backgrounds, and for additional information on the benefits of language sampling, the reader is referred to Paul and Norbury (2012), Prath (2018), Rojas and Iglesias (2019), and DiVall-Rayan and Miller (2019).

SCOPE OF THIS BOOK: AGES AND GENRES

This book addresses language sampling in preschool children (3 and 4 years), school-age children (5–11 years), and adolescents (12–18 years). For all three age groups, it covers language sampling in conversation, and for school-age children and adolescents, it also covers narrative, expository, and persuasive discourse. A *conversation* is a dialogue in which people take turns expressing their ideas, making comments, and asking questions in a spontaneous fashion. Because the goal of a conversation is often to establish, build, or maintain a relationship, speakers tend to support each other by acting as scaffolds, helping expand or clarify what is being said. Conversations are therefore important for people of all ages, including children, adolescents, and adults. The interactive nature of conversations makes them more supportive than other genres such as narrative, expository, or persuasive discourse in which the speaker is engaged in more of a monologue and bears most of the responsibility for communicating in an accurate, clear, and efficient manner. Nevertheless, these other genres are also critical for social development, as when a child or adolescent tells stories to entertain a peer (narrative), explains to a classmate how to complete an assignment (expository), or tries to convince a friend to assist with a community project (persuasive). Beyond the social uses of language, students attending elementary, middle, or high schools in the United States are expected to use spoken and written language to meet state-mandated educational standards or benchmarks and to excel in the classroom.

Speech-language pathologists who work in elementary, middle, or high schools are frequently called upon to address students' spoken and written language skills. Working collaboratively with classroom teachers, many SLPs tailor their assessment and intervention activities to help students meet specific Common Core State Standards (CCSS) for English Language Arts (National Governors Association Center for Best Practices and Council of Chief State School Officers, 2010; https://www.corestandards .org). According to the CCSS, beginning in kindergarten and continuing through grade 12, students are expected to demonstrate increasing levels of spoken and written language proficiency. Regarding spoken language, CCSS expectations for grade 6, for example, include the ability to "participate effectively in a range of conversations and collaborations with diverse partners, building on others' ideas and expressing their own clearly and persuasively" (p. 48). Students are also expected to "present information, findings, and supporting evidence such that listeners can follow the line of reasoning" (p. 48). Similarly, regarding written language, standards in middle school and high school include the ability to produce persuasive and expository essays that are clear, coherent, organized, logical, and supported by evidence and to produce narrative essays that convey real or imaginary events with proper sequencing, structure, and detail. Given the key role that language plays in school success, it is critical that SLPs have the knowledge and tools needed to assess and intervene effectively in all four genres: conversational, narrative, expository, and persuasive discourse.

In addition to CCSS in speaking and writing, teachers place their own high expectations on students in the classroom on a daily basis. For example, regarding *narrative* discourse, the language of storytelling, a 5th-grade teacher may ask the class to read, retell, and discuss (orally or in writing) a folk tale such as *The Baker's Neighbor*, which concerns a conflict between an angry shopkeeper and a cheerful customer (Afflerbach, Beers, Blachowicz, Boyd, & Diffily, 2000). The story contains many abstract words (e.g., "disbelief," "fragrance," "pleasures," "privilege"), and the characters express contrasting values and personality traits (e.g., greed, selfishness, contentment, honesty). To perform these activities, students must understand the story and its characters, including their actions, perspectives, and motivations. This requires that students listen, read, speak, and write proficiently. As students progress through the grade levels, teachers' classroom expectations become even higher. In high school, for example, English teachers may require students to read, retell, and discuss the fable by Jean de La Fontaine, *The Value of Knowledge* (McDougal Littell, 2006). This story, a comment on pretentious and excessive wealth, concerns two citizens who represent contrasting values—one who is wealthy but rude and arrogant (the boor) and another who is poor but witty and humble (the bookman/wit). The fable concludes with the following literate lines:

> Our bookman doesn't deign respond: There's much too much that he might say. But still, revenge is his, and far beyond mere satire's meager means. For war breaks out and Mars wreaks havoc round about. Homeless, our vagabonds must beg their bread. Scorned everywhere, the boor meets glare and glower; welcomed, the wit is plied with board and bed. So ends their quarrel. Fools take heed: Knowledge is power! (p. 543)

Students with language disorders are likely to be challenged mightily by this literate language assignment of reading, retelling, and discussing this fable. Why? Because to be successful, they must interpret low-frequency words (e.g., "deign," "revenge," "satire," "meager," "plied"), figurative expressions (e.g., "beg their bread," "knowledge is power"), and uncommon syntactic structures (e.g., "revenge is his, "and far beyond mere satire's meager means," "Mars wreaks havoc," "plied with board and bed"). In addition, in order to discuss the story, students would need to use complex syntax and literate terms, as in the following sentence of 26 words and four clauses:

> Although one of the characters in the story, the boor, is wealthy, people do not enjoy spending time with him because he is rude and arrogant.

Expository discourse, the use of language to convey information, is the most common genre used in the upper grades of elementary school, continuing into middle school and high school. Although narrative discourse predominates during the early grades, when students reach the 4th grade, a transition occurs in which expository discourse becomes the standard genre of the classroom (Nippold & Scott, 2010). At that time, teachers begin lecturing in class about complex topics in areas such as science, social studies, geography, mathematics, and history, and students' textbooks are written primarily in a direct, informative manner. In turn, students must display their knowledge of this newly acquired information through oral reports, group presentations, formal essays, and other assignments in which expository discourse is the expected genre. For example, consider the following excerpt from a 5th-grade science textbook:

> Scientists have classified plants into two main groups. Vascular plants, such as ferns and trees, have tubes. Because they have tubes to carry water, nutrients, and food, vascular plants can grow quite tall. Nonvascular plants, such as mosses, do not have tubes. So water must move from cell to cell. These plants need to live in a moist place, and they do not grow to be very large. (Jones et al., 2002, p. A53)

After reading about different classifications of plants and listening to their teachers' lectures, students are asked to write an expository essay in which they do the following:

> Gather several types of plants, and examine their characteristics. Write clues describing each plant. Your clues can be about color, smell, height, size, or the plant's use, or they may tell where it was found. Read your clues to your classmates, and see if they can guess your plant. (Jones et al., 2002, p. A53)

As students progress through middle school and high school, the complexity of their reading and writing assignments becomes even greater, as illustrated by the following excerpt from a textbook used to teach American government in high school:

> John Marshall (Chief Justice of the United States) set precedents that established important powers of the federal courts. Marshall served as Chief Justice of the United States from 1801 until 1835. As a Federalist, he established the independence of the judicial branch. In *Marbury v. Madison*, Marshall claimed for the Supreme Court the power to declare a law unconstitutional, and he affirmed the superiority of federal authority under the Constitution in *McCulloch v. Maryland* and *Gibbons v. Ogden*. In *McCulloch v. Maryland*, he wrote:
>
> > This provision is made in a constitution, intended to endure for ages to come, and consequently, to be adapted to the various crises of human affairs. (McClenaghan, 2005, p. 81)

After learning about this American statesman, students are asked to do the following:

> Write a paragraph explaining the meaning of Marshall's words in this quotation. Use information from your reading of the text to support your answer. (McClenaghan, 2005, p. 81)

Although both of these expository examples call upon the ability to use and understand complex syntax and challenging vocabulary, the high school example is more difficult because the sentences are longer, contain greater amounts of subordination, and employ a greater number of low-frequency words that express numerous complex and abstract concepts (e.g., precedents, independence, branch, superiority, authority, provision, ages, crises, affairs).

Persuasive discourse, the use of language to convince other people to perform some action or to adopt a certain belief, is another prominent genre in US public elementary, middle, and high school classrooms. To illustrate, 5th-grade students learning about nutrition in science class may be asked to debate the issue of eating only plants versus eating both plants and animals. In debating this issue, they may be asked to offer reasons for and against both types of diets—vegetarian and omnivorous—before drawing their own conclusions (Jones et al., 2002, p. A113). To perform this activity successfully, students may need to gather information not only from their textbooks but also from library books, science journals, newspapers, the Internet, and knowledgeable adults such as organic farmers, biologists, chemists, and nutritionists.

BEYOND THE CLASSROOM

Beyond the classroom, proficiency with each of the genres—narrative, expository, and persuasive—is often called upon in the workplace where, in today's world, many adolescents have part-time jobs after school, on weekends, or during the summer months that require the ability to speak proficiently. For example, an adolescent who works at a daycare center may be asked to tell entertaining stories to young children (narrative discourse); one who works at a recreation center may be asked to explain how to play an unfamiliar game (expository discourse); one who volunteers for a political party may be expected to convince fellow citizens to vote for a bond measure supporting education (persuasive discourse); and one who works in a veterinarian's office may be asked to explain an important health care procedure to a pet owner over the telephone (expository discourse), speaking in the following authoritative manner:

> Dr. Jones will be able to examine Zoe at six o'clock this evening. In the meantime, please keep her calm and comfortable, remove all food and water, and wrap her leg in a clean, dry towel before bringing her into the clinic.

Examples of other jobs that would require an older student to use complex spoken language include explaining to a customer why the brakes on her road bike need to be replaced (expository) while working as a bicycle mechanic, or describing the highlights of a historic town to a group of senior citizens (expository and narrative) while working as a tour guide. Young people who can rise to the occasion during such speaking tasks are more likely to perform their jobs successfully and be rehired or promoted to the next level of responsibility. Hence, those who possess strong language skills will have an advantage over their peers who do not.

MOVING BEYOND THE PRESCHOOL YEARS

Although language sampling as a formal activity has enjoyed a long history in our field (see Chapter 2), it has traditionally been used with preschool children, focusing on a child's use of complete and intelligible utterances, and appropriate words and grammatical morphemes, and measuring growth with common metrics such as mean length of utterance in words or morphemes. Although language sampling has been used less frequently with school-age children and adolescents, this situation has improved in recent years as more information has become available about the detailed and continuous nature of later language development (e.g., Lundine, 2020; Nippold, 2016; Nippold, LaFavre, & Shinham, 2020). In addition, numerous studies of school-age children and adolescents have demonstrated how the SLP can elicit, transcribe, and analyze spoken or written language samples with older students (e.g., Heilmann, Malone, & Westerveld, 2020; Lundine & McCauley, 2016)—samples that can yield appropriate goals for language intervention. Hence, this book also discusses intervention goals and activities, based on the results of a language sample. For preschool children with language disorders, intervention often emphasizes instruction in morphosyntax, the lexicon, and pragmatic skills in conversations. In contrast, for older students, intervention should address not only conversational skills but also narrative, expository, and persuasive discourse, with the goal of improving a student's chances for success in social, academic, and vocational endeavors. This can best be accomplished when the intervention activities are cognitively stimulating, motivating, and relevant to the students' daily lives. When intervention focuses on the use of complex syntax and literate vocabulary, students become able to communicate with greater accuracy, clarity, and efficiency, using appropriate words, phrases, and clauses. When intervention also addresses pragmatic skills, they will be able to communicate with greater confidence and poise.

Although few SLPs would disagree with these goals, we often have to "make the case" with administrators and policymakers as to why older students—particularly adolescents—should receive speech-language services. After all, those professionals often argue, if adolescents are continuing to struggle with language disorders, isn't it too late to intervene? The resolute answer is, "No, it is not too late to help these young people!" (Nippold, 2010b). They are in a critical period of human development, transitioning from childhood to adulthood, moving from concrete to abstract thought, and preparing for the complexities of life in the 21st century as self-sufficient, competent, and contributing members of society. What happens now can "make or break" them, and fortunately, the knowledgeable SLP, collaborating with classroom teachers, can assist school-age children and adolescents who have language disorders to begin to gain traction and to move forward in building their spoken and written language skills.

WHY THE FOCUS ON COMPLEX SYNTAX?

Throughout this book, the use of complex syntax for children and adolescents is emphasized in assessment and intervention. The reason for this emphasis is that syntax is the structural foundation of language (Crystal, 1996). As such, it enables an individual to express an infinite number of ideas. In particular, complex thought requires the use of complex syntax for efficient communication, evidenced by the following 21-word sentence, which contains two relative [REL] clauses, one adverbial [ADV] clause, and one main clause [MC]:

> Athletes who train [REL] in weather that is [REL] unusually warm need [MC] extra fluids throughout the day so that they will avoid [ADV] hyperthermia.

An emphasis on syntax also reflects the perspective of this author that language proficiency is a basic human right. Given that we live in an information-driven world in which accurate, clear, and efficient communication is the standard expectation for all citizens, any difficulties with spoken or written language can hamper the pursuit of independent living, economic prosperity, and personal satisfaction. In addition, poor communication skills are a major source of strife and turmoil in the world today and are a substantial barrier to harmonious relationships. What better reasons can there be to support our efforts to promote spoken and written language development in all children and adolescents who are in our care today?

To convince any remaining skeptics of the importance of providing effective language intervention to all students—and of the benefits of eliciting language samples—the final section of this chapter presents excerpts from samples that were elicited from adolescents with typical and impaired language development (Tomblin & Nippold, 2014). Each adolescent was asked to perform the same task—to explain some key strategies needed to succeed at football. Each excerpt is coded for all main and subordinate clauses, and the results are discussed in order to illustrate how language sampling with students can reveal individual strengths and weaknesses.

The first speaker is a 14-year-old boy with TLD (Tomblin & Nippold, 2014, p. 103):

> Make [MC] sure your teammates know [NOM] the play.
>
> And don't argue [MC] with your teammates because if you're arguing [ADV] with a lineman, the lineman could let [ADV] the guy get [INF] by and you could get [ADV] drilled.
>
> So your linemen are [MC] a big part of the game.
>
> You want [MC] your linemen in all of your plays.
>
> You want [MC] your linemen to feel [INF] good about themselves and their job because it doesn't seem [ADV] like they do [NOM] a lot.
>
> They just block [MC] the guy.
>
> But if nobody was [ADV] there, the running backs would get [MC] nowhere.
>
> And it helps [MC] to have [INF] a good lineman, and a good running back that can block [REL], and a halfback that can block [REL], and receivers that can catch [REL] and know [REL] their routes well, and just a team that doesn't fight [REL] and argue [REL] about everything. (44 words)
>
> If you mess [ADV] up, then just do [MC] better next time or try [MC] harder.

This excerpt contains 9 utterances and 149 words, and it has an MLU of 16.56 words. With 10 main clauses and 17 subordinate clauses, its clausal density (CD) is 3.0 clauses. Informal analysis suggests that the speaker has a strong knowledge base, reflected in his appropriate use of football terminology (e.g., "lineman," "halfback," "running back," "receiver") and relevant figurative expressions (e.g., "get drilled," "mess up"). Syntactically, many of his sentences are complex, and the longest one, at 44 words, contains 7 subordinate clauses. In addition to these lexical and syntactic strengths, pragmatic strengths include an awareness of the thoughts, feelings, and roles of the different players and of the negative consequences when team members cannot work together harmoniously.

The next speaker is a 14-year-old boy with SLI (Tomblin & Nippold, 2014, p. 103):

> You have [MC] to wear [INF] pads because when you're hit [ADV], it hurts [ADV].
>
> They have [MC] to work [INF] together and get [INF] the ball down the field.

You pass [MC] the ball.

And you run [MC] the ball so you can get [ADV] to the end zone to score [INF].

You have [MC] to know [INF] how to kick [INF].

Because if you get [ADV] to the fourth down, you have [MC] to punt [INF] the ball away if you're [ADV] not ready to make [INF] it.

With six utterances and 73 words, this excerpt has an MLU of 12.17 words. It also contains 6 main clauses and 13 subordinate clauses, giving it a CD of 3.17 clauses. These numbers indicate that the production of complex sentences is a relative strength for this adolescent. He also uses a number of football terms and expressions (e.g., end zone, fourth down, run the ball) appropriately and shows an awareness of the need for team members to work together. However, in contrast with his peer with TLD (Speaker #1), his sample is sparser in terms of the amount of information it conveys, possibly reflecting a more limited knowledge of football. There is also less variety in the types of nouns, verbs, and subordinate clauses that he employs.

The third speaker is a 13-year-old boy with NLI (Tomblin & Nippold, 2014, p. 103):

You should be [MC] a team player.

Like motivate [MC] your team to win [INF], not to fight [INF].

Have [MC] good sportsmanship.

Don't criticize [MC] or put [MC] down other teammates.

Be [MC] kind to other teammates.

Work [MC] as a team.

Encourage [MC] other people.

Be [MC] kind to your coaches.

This speaker's excerpt is much sparser than the other two, and with its eight utterances and 43 words, it has an MLU of only 5.38 words. Although it contains 9 main clauses, there are only 2 subordinate clauses, reflecting a preponderance of simple sentences and a CD of only 1.38 clauses. The speaker therefore shows significant limitations in the use of complex syntax. Nevertheless, some strengths include the use of metalinguistic verbs ("motivate," "criticize," "encourage") and an abstract noun ("sportsmanship"), and an awareness of the importance of working with teammates and coaches in a cooperative and friendly manner.

In summary, these three excerpts demonstrate how the SLP can gain insight into the unique strengths and weaknesses that individual speakers display in their production of spoken language—information that can be used to plan meaningful and relevant intervention activities for children and adolescents. This is especially true when the SLP has a strong background in the nature and course of language development; is familiar with the spoken and written language demands of real-world situations, including contemporary classrooms; and is able to work intensely with students and collaboratively with teachers and other school professionals.

Embracing the challenge of eliciting, transcribing, and analyzing language samples appropriately and using the information to plan meaningful intervention is extremely rewarding. Not only does it allow SLPs to practice at the top of their license but also language sampling helps ensure that clients with language disorders receive the most effective services possible.

CHAPTER 2

History of Language Sampling

L anguage sampling has a long tradition in the field of speech-language pathology. Table 2–1 highlights certain events in the history of language sampling. Modern language sampling can be traced back to the late 19th century with the publication of the first diary studies. These were longitudinal studies conducted by parents—often linguists, psychologists, or other scientists—who carefully observed and described their own children's language development, beginning in infancy and continuing into childhood. The data typically consisted of handwritten notes and direct quotations of the child, playing alone or interacting with family members in everyday situations. Hippolyte Taine (1877) published one of the earliest studies of this type, describing his daughter's early development. Charles Darwin (1877), Milton Humphreys (1880), and William Preyer (1889) soon followed with similar reports of their own children's development.

Diary studies continued into the 20th century. For example, Werner Leopold, a professor of English at Northwestern University, wrote a four-volume series (Leopold, 1939–1949) on the language development of his daughter Hildegard, who was acquiring both English and German. Although most diary studies have focused on the first few years of life, the account of Hildegard's development covered the years from birth through adolescence, and it is one of the most detailed and well-known studies ever reported. However, in the absence of audio recorders, diary studies were limited in the amount of language that could be recorded, particularly after the child had moved beyond the single-word stage and was speaking rapidly and in multiword utterances. Thus, the reports of Hildegard's language, for example, consisted mainly of summaries of her behavior (e.g., at age 10 years: "Hildegard finds difficulty in telling me

Table 2–1. History of Language Sampling

- 19th century
  - Diary studies begin, with focus on early development of typical children.
    - Taine (1877)
    - Darwin (1877)
    - Humphreys (1880)
    - Preyer (1889)
- 20th century
  - Diary studies continue, e.g., Leopold (1939–1949).
  - Formal language sampling begins.
    - M. Smith (1926)
    - McCarthy (1930)
    - Templin (1957)
  - Invention of the tape recorder (Wikipedia, 2009)
    - "Blattnerphone" (L. Blattner, Germany, 1929)
    - "K1" (F. Matthias, Germany, 1935)
    - Both had poor sound quality
    - Ampex Electronics Company of California developed high-quality tape recorder for singer Bing Crosby (1947).
  - Chomsky's influential books are published: *Syntactic Structures* (1957) and *Aspects of the Theory of Syntax* (1965).
  - Researchers use tape recorders to collect language samples longitudinally.
  - Emphasis is placed on the development of syntax in young children.
  - Interest in determining underlying linguistic rules or "competence."
    - Braine (1963)
    - W. Miller & Ervin (1964)
    - Bloom (1970)
    - Brown (1973)
    - de Villiers & de Villiers (1973)
  - Formal language sampling programs are published.
    - Developmental Sentence Scoring (DSS; Lee, 1974)
    - Language Sampling, Analysis, & Training (LSAT; Tyack & Gottsleben, 1974)
    - Language Assessment, Remediation, and Screening Procedures (LARSP; Crystal, Fletcher, & Garman, 1976)
    - Assessing Language Production in Children (Miller, 1981)
    - Language Sample Analysis: The Wisconsin Guide (Leadholm & Miller, 1992)
    - Guide to Analysis of Language Transcripts (Retherford, 1993)
    - Strong Narrative Assessment Procedure (SNAP; Strong, Mayer, & Mayer, 1998)
  - Developmental studies include older children and adolescents (e.g., Hunt, 1970; Loban, 1976).

Table 2–1. *continued*

- ○ Developmental studies examine written language as well as spoken language (Hunt, 1970; Loban, 1976).
- ○ Interest in persuasive discourse emerges and expands.
  - Spoken persuasion
    - Wood, Weinstein, & Parker (1967)
    - Flavell, Botkin, Fry, Wright, & Jarvis (1968)
    - Bragg, Ostrowski, & Finley (1973)
    - Finley & Humphreys (1974)
    - Clark & Delia (1976)
    - Piche, Rubin, & Michlin (1978)
    - Bearison & Gass (1979)
    - Delia, Kline, & Burleson (1979)
    - Ritter (1979)
    - D. Jones (1985)
    - Erftmier & Dyson (1986)
  - Written persuasion
    - Crowhurst & Piche (1979)
    - Rubin & Piche (1979)
    - Crowhurst (1980, 1987, 1990)
    - Kroll (1984)
    - McCann (1989)
    - Knudsen (1992)
    - Wong, Butler, Ficzere, & Kuperis (1996)
- ○ Interest in narrative discourse emerges and expands.
  - Botvin & Sutton-Smith (1977)
  - Kernan (1977)
  - Stein & Glenn (1979)
  - Roth & Spekman (1986)
  - Liles (1985, 1987, 1993)
  - Merritt & Liles (1987, 1989)
  - Scott (1988)
  - Bamberg & Damrad-Frye (1991)
  - Liles, Duffy, Merritt, & Purcell (1995)
- ○ Computer programs designed to analyze language samples.
  - Systematic Analysis of Language Transcripts (SALT; Miller & Chapman, 1983)
  - Child Language Analysis Program (CLAN; MacWhinney, 1988)
  - Computerized Profiling (Long & Fey, 1993)
- 21st century
  - ○ Widespread use of digital recorders and microcassettes.
  - ○ Interest in narrative discourse continues to expand.
    - Scott & Windsor (2000)

continues

Table 2–1. *continued*

- Windsor, Scott, & Street (2000)
- Berman & Verhoeven (2002)
- Verhoeven et al. (2002)
- Justice et al. (2006)
- Wetherell, Botting, & Conti-Ramsden (2007)
- McCabe, Bliss, Barra, & Bennett, (2008)
- Ukrainetz & Gillam (2009)
- Heilmann, Miller, Nockerts, & Dunaway (2010)
- Sun & Nippold (2012)
- Ebert & Scott (2014)
- Peña, Gillam, & Bedore (2014)
- Guo & Schneider (2016)
- Channell, Loveall, Conners, Harvey, & Abbeduto (2018)
- Guo, Eisenberg, Schneider, & Spencer (2020)

○ Interest in adolescent language expands (Berman, 2004; Nippold, 2016).

○ Research in language sampling with adolescents continues.
- Wetherell et al. (2007)
- Nippold, Frantz-Kaspar, et al. (2014, 2015)
- Nippold, LaFavre, & Shinham (2020)
- Nippold, Vigeland, Frantz-Kaspar, & Ward-Lonergan (2017)
- Miller, Andriacchi, & Nockerts (2016)
- Nippold & Hayward (2018)

○ Normative databases expand (e.g., Miller et al., 2019; Westerveld & Vidler, 2016).

○ New language sampling programs are published for school-age children, emphasizing narrative discourse.
- Expression, Reception and Recall of Narrative Instrument (ERRNI; Bishop, 2004)
- Edmonton Narrative Norms Instrument (ENNI; Schneider, Dubé, & Hayward, 2005)

○ Persuasive discourse is examined in children, adolescents, and adults.
- Felton & Kuhn (2001)
- Nippold, Ward-Lonergan, & Fanning (2005)
- Nippold & Ward-Lonergan (2010)
- Heilmann, Malone, & Westerveld (2020)

○ New and expanded focus on examining expository discourse in children and adolescents.
- Scott & Windsor (2000)
- Berman & Verhoeven (2002)
- Verhoeven et al. (2002)
- Nippold, Hesketh, Duthie, & Mansfield (2005)
- Nippold, Mansfield, & Billow (2007)

Table 2–1. *continued*

- Nippold, Mansfield, Billow, & Tomblin (2008, 2009)
- Nippold (2009)
- Nippold & Scott (2010)
- Westerveld & Moran (2011, 2013)
- Heilmann & Malone (2014)
- Lundine & McCauley (2016)
- Lundine (2020)

○ Renewed advocacy of language sampling as a clinical tool.
  - Costanza-Smith (2010)
  - Heilmann (2010)
  - Heilmann, Miller, & Nockerts (2010)
  - Price, Hendricks, & Cook (2010)
  - Heilmann, DeBrock, & Riley-Tillman (2013)
  - Westerveld & Claessen (2014)
  - Pavelko, Owens, Ireland, & Hahs-Vaughn (2016)
  - Timler (2018)
  - Eisenberg (2020)
  - Pezold, Imgrund, & Storkel (2020)
  - Scott (2020)

○ Research in language sampling with culturally and linguistically diverse students expands.
  - Gutiérrez-Clellen, Restrepo, Bedore, Peña, & Anderson (2000)
  - Craig & Washington (2002, 2004)
  - Gillam & Peña (2004)
  - Thompson, Craig, & Washington (2004)
  - Washington & Craig (2004)
  - Miller et al. (2006)
  - Horton-Ikard & Pittman (2010)
  - Ivy & Masterson (2011)
  - Mills, Watkins, & Washington (2013)
  - Horton & Apel (2014)
  - Pearson, Jackson, & Wu (2014)
  - Peña et al. (2014)
  - Boerma, Leseman, Timmermeister, Wijnen, & Blom (2016)
  - Heilmann, Rojas, Iglesias, & Miller (2016)
  - Ebert & Pham (2017)
  - Perry (2017)
  - Kapantzoglou, Fergadiotis, & Restrepo (2017)
  - Petersen, Chanthongthip, Ukrainetz, Spencer, & Steeve (2017)
  - Johnson & Koonce (2018)
  - Graham-Bethea & Kamhi (2019)
  - Ebert (2020)

about her experiences in coherent German narration," Vol. 4, p. 148) and isolated quotations (e.g., at age 14 years: "Oh Papa, don't speak German in the street," Vol. 4, p. 153). Despite their limitations, diary studies offered insights into the complex and creative nature of language development in children, sparking broad interest in it as a serious topic of scientific investigation. Further information on diary studies is available in Ingram (1989) and Behrens (2008).

During the 1920s, researchers began to conduct cross-sectional studies of language development by examining large numbers of children at different ages (Ingram, 1989). For example, M. Smith (1926) studied 124 children (ages 2–5 years), McCarthy (1930) studied 140 children (ages 1–4 years), and Templin (1957) studied 430 children (ages 3–8 years). In those studies, samples of conversational speech were elicited from each child and often analyzed for the mean number of words per utterance. However, rather than using audio recorders to collect the samples, researchers wrote down the children's utterances as they were speaking (Ingram, 1989). Given the large number of utterances that even young children can produce, the validity of their findings was questionable. Nevertheless, those early studies paved the way for later research that examined language development in greater detail, and Chomsky's (1957, 1965) work on transformational grammar prompted even more sophisticated studies (e.g., Bloom, 1970; Braine, 1963; Brown, 1973; de Villiers & de Villiers, 1973; Miller & Ervin, 1964).

INVENTION OF THE AUDIO RECORDER

It is intriguing to consider how the invention of the audio recorder helped revolutionize the study of language development. In 1929, Ludwig Blattner, a German scientist, developed the "Blattnerphone" for recording human speech. Then, in 1935, Frederick Matthias developed the "K1," also in Germany. The sound quality of those early recorders was quite poor, and it was not until 1947 that Ampex Electronics Company of California developed a high-quality audio recorder for the American singer Bing Crosby. A perfectionist, Crosby wished to prerecord the songs that would be played on his radio shows. A shrewd businessman, Crosby invested in the company for large-scale commercial production of audio recorders (Wikipedia, 2009).

Eventually, audio recorders became available to the general public, including researchers and clinicians. This made it possible to establish valid databases of spoken language development in young children (e.g., Miller, 1981) and to study older children and adolescents (e.g., Loban, 1976), who present even greater challenges because of the amount and complexity of spoken language they produce. Figure 2–1 shows an excerpt from a language sample elicited from a toddler. Without being able to audio record this child's speech, one could probably write down most of her single-word utterances. However, even an expert transcriber would have difficulty keeping up with her when she begins to produce successive multiword utterances. Now consider the adolescent in Figure 2–2.

Girl—Age 17 Months

- juice juice
- allgone
- gimme wawa
- pwease!
- whatdat?
- doggie!
- kitty go!

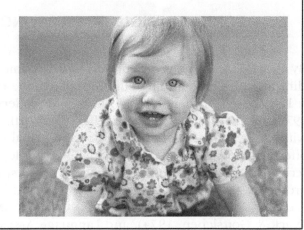

Figure 2–1. Early utterances, relatively easy to transcribe by hand. (Camille Tokerud/Photographer's Choice RF/Getty Images)

Girl—Age 17 Years

Q: Why is track and field your favorite sport?

A: Well I had a knee injury my freshman year playing volleyball. And I couldn't do a lot of running. And in track and field, I can be a thrower, which is in the field events, and not have to do a lot of running, and work at my own pace, and not have to compete with other students, just competing to better yourself. So you don't have to say, "Oh well, they're better than me so I can't be as good as them."

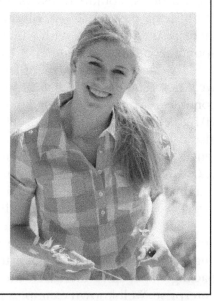

Figure 2–2. Adolescent talk, impossible to analyze without an audio recorder. (PT Images/Getty Images)

Given the sophisticated nature of her oral language, it would be virtually impossible to transcribe her speech without a reliable audio recorder! For superior sound quality, most clinicians today use digital voice recorders for language samples, which are available as separate electronic devices or as apps downloadable for their iPhones.

FORMAL LANGUAGE SAMPLING PROGRAMS

By the 1970s, language sampling had become a widely recommended clinical tool for examining children's language development (e.g., Bloom & Lahey, 1978; Lynch, 1978; Trantham & Pedersen, 1976; Wiig & Semel, 1976; also see Launer & Lahey, 1981, for further discussion). Consistent with this recommendation, a number of formal programs were published, offering guidelines for speech-language pathologists on how to elicit, transcribe, and analyze samples of conversational speech. Several well-known programs are listed in Table 2–1. They include Developmental Sentence Scoring (DSS; Lee, 1974), Language Sampling, Analysis, & Training (LSAT; Tyack & Gottsleben, 1974), and Language Assessment, Remediation, and Screening Procedures (LARSP; Crystal, Fletcher, & Garman, 1976). Additional programs were developed in the 1980s and 1990s, including those by Miller (1981), Leadholm and Miller (1992), and Retherford (1993). Those programs were designed to identify a young child's linguistic weaknesses, thereby providing direction for intervention. For example, if a language sample showed that a 4-year-old child omitted certain grammatical classes (e.g., articles, conjunctions) or used grammatical morphemes inconsistently (e.g., past tense -ed, plural -s), intervention would be designed to increase the frequency with which the child used those forms correctly in spontaneous speech (Launer & Lahey, 1981).

The strategy of analyzing language samples to identify grammatical weaknesses and to use that information to develop goals for intervention continues to be recommended (e.g., Costanza-Smith, 2010; Paul & Norbury, 2012; Pezold, Imgrund, & Storkel, 2020). Currently, language samples are also used to develop goals for increasing the production of complex sentences, even in preschool children (Barako Arndt & Schuele, 2013; Curran & Owen Van Horne, 2019; Eisenberg, 2020). They are also used to identify pragmatic deficits in children and adolescents, leading to intervention that targets social communication skills (Timler, 2018).

Since the 1980s, researchers and clinicians who have studied language development or those who have designed or used clinical tools for language sampling have been assisted greatly by the invention of software packages that have increased the speed, accuracy, and efficiency of this enterprise. Well-known examples include Systematic Analysis of Language Transcripts (SALT; Miller, Andriacchi, & Nockerts, 2019), Child Language

Analysis Program (CLAN; MacWhinney, 1988), and Computerized Profiling (Long & Fey, 1993). Without those computer-assisted programs, we still might be analyzing language samples by hand! SALT has been especially helpful to the field because it has been updated continuously since its beginning and now includes a bilingual Spanish/English version (http://www.languageanalysislab.com).

BEYOND CONVERSATION

In the field of speech-language pathology, there is a strong tradition of eliciting language samples in conversational discourse for individuals of all ages (e.g., Larson & McKinley, 2003; Lee, 1974; Loban, 1976; Nelson, 1998; Nippold, Frantz-Kaspar, & Vigeland, 2017; Paul, 2007; Templin, 1957; Tyack & Gottsleben, 1974). However, during the 1970s, interest in studying children's ability to tell stories—to employ narrative discourse—began. Given the complex nature of narratives, those early studies often included older children and young adolescents (e.g., Botvin & Sutton-Smith, 1977; Kernan, 1977; Stein & Glenn, 1979).

Interest in studying narrative discourse continued during the 1980s and 1990s (e.g., Berman & Slobin, 1994; Eder, 1988; Hadley, 1998; Klecan Aker & Caraway, 1997; Leadholm & Miller, 1992; Liles, 1985, 1987, 1993; Liles, Duffy, Merritt, & Purcell, 1995; Merritt & Liles, 1987, 1989; Roth & Spekman, 1986; Scott, 1988) and has remained strong during the 21st century (e.g., Berman & Verhoeven, 2002; Justice et al., 2006; McCabe, Bliss, Barra, & Bennett, 2008; Nippold, Frantz-Kaspar, et al., 2014, 2015; Nippold & Hayward, 2018; Nippold, Vigeland, Frantz-Kaspar, & Ward-Lonergan, 2017; Scott & Windsor, 2000; Sun & Nippold, 2012; Ukrainetz & Gillam, 2009; Windsor, Scott, & Street, 2000). It has been particularly heartening in recent years to witness an increasing number of studies examining narrative discourse in children from culturally and linguistically diverse backgrounds, including those who speak African American English (e.g., Mills, Watkins, & Washington, 2013) and those who are bilingual (e.g., Boerma, Leseman, Timmermeister, Wijnen, & Blom, 2016; Kapantzoglou, Fergadiotis, & Restrepo, 2017; Peña, Gillam, & Bedore, 2014; Petersen, Chanthongthip, Ukrainetz, Spencer, & Steeve, 2017).

Given the growing interest in narrative discourse, researchers were prompted to design language sampling programs specifically to elicit narrative discourse, such as the Strong Narrative Assessment Procedure (SNAP; Strong, Mayer, & Mayer, 1998). More recent tools have been published by Bishop (2004) and by Schneider, Dubé, and Hayward (2005). However, because none of the available tools were designed specifically to examine narrative ability in adolescents, Nippold, Frantz-Kaspar, et al. (2014, 2015, 2017) created tasks for adolescents focusing on fables (see Chapter 5).

It was important to examine narrative speaking in adolescents because storytelling is often used in social, academic, and vocational contexts during this stage of development. In addition, language samples that involve narrative speaking tend to elicit greater syntactic complexity than samples of conversational speech in children, adolescents, and adults (Leadholm & Miller, 1992; Nippold, Frantz-Kaspar, et al., 2014, 2015, 2017) and are therefore more likely to reveal a speaker's linguistic competence.

During the past 20 years, interest in examining other genres besides conversational and narrative discourse has grown. In particular, the importance of expository and persuasive discourse has been recognized (e.g., Heilmann & Malone, 2014; Heilmann, Malone, & Westerveld, 2020; Lundine, 2020; Lundine & McCauley, 2016; Nippold & Scott, 2010; Nippold & Ward-Lonergan, 2010; Nippold, Ward-Lonergan, & Fanning, 2005; Scott & Windsor, 2000; Westerveld & Moran, 2011, 2013), and research has demonstrated that genre makes a substantial difference in the complexity of language that a speaker or writer produces. Just as samples of narrative discourse can elicit greater syntactic complexity than samples of conversational discourse (Leadholm & Miller, 1992; Nippold, Frantz-Kaspar, et al., 2014), samples of expository and persuasive discourse can elicit greater syntactic complexity than samples of conversational and narrative discourse in speakers of all ages (Berman & Verhoeven, 2002; Crowhurst, 1980; Crowhurst & Piche, 1979; Heilmann et al., 2020; Nippold, Cramond, & Hayward-Mayhew, 2014; Nippold, Hesketh, Duthie, & Mansfield, 2005; Scott & Windsor, 2000; Verhoeven et al., 2002).

The importance of expository discourse is underscored by the finding that samples elicited in this genre are more likely to reveal both strengths and weaknesses in syntactic development compared with samples of conversational discourse (e.g., Nippold, Hesketh, et al., 2005; Nippold, Mansfield, & Billow, 2007; Nippold, Mansfield, Billow, & Tomblin, 2008, 2009; Nippold & Sun, 2010). To illustrate this point, Table 2–2 contains excerpts from the conversational samples of two adolescents. Speaker #1 is a 15-year-old boy with typical language development, and Speaker #2 is a 14-year-old boy with autism spectrum disorder. For Speaker #1, the mean length of C-unit (MLCU) for his entire conversation was only 5.38 words. Although he responded politely to the interviewer's questions, his sentences were short, with little elaboration. Speaker #2 produced an MLCU of 7.17, slightly higher than that of Speaker #1. However, many of his utterances were fragments and did not meet criteria for a C-unit, which consists of a main clause and any subordinate clauses attached to it. Then, during an expository task in which each speaker talked with an interviewer about the game of chess, each boy's level of syntactic complexity increased dramatically, illustrated by the excerpts contained in Table 2–3. For example, when Speaker #1 explained to an adult how various chess pieces move, the MLCU for his entire sample was 19.83. Similarly, when Speaker #2 explained to an adult some key strategies needed to win a

Table 2–2. Excerpts from the Conversational Samples of Two Adolescents (from the Author's Files)

Speaker #1, a 15-year-old boy with typical language development (MLCU = 5.83 words)

Q: Do you have any brothers or sisters?

A: Yes, I have two brothers.

Q: What are their names?

A: My older brother is named Andrew. And my younger brother is named Ross.

Q: How old are they?

A: Andrew is 19. Ross is 9.

Q: What else can you tell me about them?

A: Well, Ross is hyperactive. And Andrew lives on his own now. And he doesn't return calls very often.

Speaker #2, a 14-year-old boy with autism spectrum disorder (MLCU = 7.17 words)

Q: Do you have a favorite TV show or movie?

A: Not really. I don't really watch TV much. I mostly play video games rather than watch TV or movies.

Q: What kind of video games do you play?

A: Um, usually Black Saturday games. It's like strategy type games.

Q: Do you like to read books or magazines?

A: Books, not magazines. Books just like the adventure types. Like not mysteries but just like adventure.

---

game of chess, the MLCU for his entire sample was 10.39. Had the speech-language pathologist not elicited the expository samples in addition to the conversational samples, the syntactic competence of these boys would not have been revealed.

Like expository discourse, persuasive discourse offers the potential to reveal linguistic competence when, for example, students are asked to take a position about a controversy (e.g., "Should animals be trained to perform in circuses?") and to produce a speech or write an essay in which they describe and defend their views. During such tasks, age-related developmental gains in syntax, semantics, and pragmatics can be documented (e.g., Nippold, Ward-Lonergan, et al., 2005). Examples include increases in mean length of utterance; the use of relative clauses, abstract nouns, and metacognitive and metalinguistic verbs; and an expanding ability to view a controversy from diverse perspectives and to offer multiple reasons to support an argument.

Table 2–3. Excerpts from the Expository Samples of the Same Adolescents Mentioned in Table 2–2 (from the Author's Files)

Speaker #1, a 15-year-old boy with typical language development (MLCU = 19.83)

And then there is the knight, which moves in an "L" shape, which is really good at forking pieces, like attacking two different pieces at the same time so that they have to lose one of them. Because its movement is so irregular, nothing but another knight can really stop it. Then there is the rook, which can move horizontally or vertically. And they tend to be really useful because you can put a rook behind a pawn and march the pawn down the board to try to get a queen. And the rook will be defending it the entire time.

Speaker #2, a 14-year-old boy with autism spectrum disorder (MLCU = 10.39)

It's good to learn some defensive strategies to try to arrange your pieces in ways that they are hard to crack, like hard to get through and break through. Then you have to always stay on the offensive because other people will play off of you. And just keep advancing over and over and over. And offensive, you have to be kind of defensive. And the same time, you study your moves and try thinking several moves ahead.

Nevertheless, as discussed throughout this book, it is important to elicit samples of conversational, narrative, and expository discourse in school-age children and adolescents and samples of persuasive discourse in adolescents. This is because all four genres can provide useful information to a speech-language pathologist. For example, conversational samples can reveal limitations in pragmatics, the social use of language. Narrative, expository, and persuasive samples can reveal limitations in the use of complex syntax—weaknesses that may not be apparent in general conversation (Nippold et al., 2008).

Hence, it is expected that in the years ahead, researchers and clinicians will continue to investigate discourse development and to design innovative techniques for eliciting, transcribing, and analyzing language samples in all four genres. The goal will be to utilize the expanding databases to design new methods of evaluating and enhancing the ability of children and adolescents to communicate with accuracy, clarity, and efficiency in spoken and written language.

CHAPTER 3

General Procedures

When evaluating the language skills of a preschool child, school-age child, or adolescent, one or more norm-referenced standardized language tests should be administered to identify the presence of a language disorder. This assumes, of course, that the normative data provided by the standardized language test reflects the cultural and linguistic background of the child or adolescent who is being evaluated. Examples of frequently administered tests include the Clinical Evaluation of Language Fundamentals–Fifth Edition (Wiig, Semel, & Secord, 2013), the Clinical Evaluation of Language Fundamentals Preschool–Third Edition (Wiig, Secord, & Semel, 2020), and the Test of Language Development–Primary: Fifth Edition (Newcomer & Hammill, 2019). For many children and adolescents, tests such as these are often more effective than language samples in documenting the presence of a developmental language disorder.

However, such tests provide little information that can be used to plan language intervention (Heilmann & Malone, 2014). In contrast, a language sample can provide this type of information because it reflects how the child actually communicates in the real world, thereby offering greater ecological validity than norm-referenced standardized language tests (Hewitt, Hammer, Yont, & Tomblin, 2005). For this reason, after a developmental language disorder has been documented using norm-referenced tests, language sampling should be used to determine how well the child speaks or writes in everyday situations so that appropriate and individualized goals for language intervention can be established. Another advantage of language samples is that, unlike norm-referenced tests, they can be elicited repeatedly without having a test–retest effect and can therefore be used to monitor a child's progress during language intervention.

This chapter focuses on techniques that can be used to maximize the extent to which a language sample is representative of a speaker's best performance. With this goal in mind, it offers guidelines for working with preschool children, school-age children, and adolescents.

PRESCHOOL CHILDREN (AGES 3–4 YEARS)

Eliciting a Representative Sample

When working with preschool children, it is often best to elicit a language sample in the context of spontaneous play. When young children are relaxed and playing with a set of attractive toys, they are more likely to talk freely and naturally than if they are being asked questions during a formal interview or asked to tell a story while looking at pictures. Thus, rather than attempting to elicit narrative, expository, or persuasive language samples with preschool children, play-based conversational samples are often the most appropriate choice.

Table 3–1 provides a list of activities that could be used with preschool children, along with some suggestions for eliciting a representative language sample—one that reflects the child's best performance. It is emphasized that the manner in which the examiner behaves and talks will influence the child's performance in terms of language productivity and complexity. For example, if the examiner says very little, acts bored, and does not smile or make eye contact, the child may simply play with the toys alone and in silence. In addition, if the examiner dominates the conversation, talking rapidly and asking numerous closed-ended questions (e.g., "What is your favorite color?" "How old are you?" "Where do you live?"), the child may be overwhelmed or intimidated by the perceived need to keep up with the examiner, leading the child to shut down or produce only single-word responses. On the other hand, if the examiner is patient, relaxed, kind, shows interest in the child, and tries to have fun by laughing or making silly comments (e.g., "Oh no! I just burned the soup! Looks like we'll have to order take-out tonight! I'll call *Pizza Man*"), the child may warm to the situation and speak more naturally.

Another point to remember is that preschool children can become overstimulated if too many toys are introduced at once. Under those conditions, rather than talking about the toys with the examiner, the child may decide to explore all of them at once. Thus, it is often better to introduce just a few toys at first, adding items as they are needed to maintain the child's interest.

In my experience eliciting language samples with preschool children, it has been helpful to set up a doll house, farm set, parking structure, or other similar item. A small number of thematic toys (e.g., miniature furniture, animals, or vehicles) can be introduced, along with a few toy people who live or work there and some special items they may need (e.g., food, gardening tools, crow bar). Together, the child and examiner can pretend to cook dinner, milk the cow, or change a truck's tire. During these activities, it is especially helpful if the speech-language pathologist (SLP) models sentences that are clear, complete, grammatically correct, relevant, and

Table 3–1. Guidelines for Eliciting Play-Based Conversational Language Samples With Preschool Children

- Elicit the sample in an environment that is comfortable, quiet, safe, and free of distractions.
- Set up a doll house, farm set, parking garage, or outdoor scene (e.g., beach, park, playground, campground).
- Arrange the toys with the child (e.g., people, animals, food, furniture, vehicles, sand bucket, shovel, swing set, slide, lake, sailboats, etc.).
- Talk about the toys, modeling sentences that are clear, complete, grammatically correct, relevant to the situation, and potentially of interest to the child (e.g., "This man wants to park his motorcycle in the garage. But all the parking spaces are taken. He will have to wait until a car pulls out.").
- Make open-ended comments that might prompt the child to formulate a response—for example, "I wonder if the man will have to wait a long time for a parking space to open up."
- After making such statements, insert a long pause, allowing the child time to comment.
- Avoid overlaps and interruptions of the child's speech by attending closely to the child's body language and facial expressions.
- Smile and make eye contact with the child frequently during the session.
- Show you are interested in what the child says by nodding, smiling, saying "yes," "hmm," repeating the child's utterances, or commenting on what the child has said.
- Expand on the child's utterances, using correct grammar and appropriate words—for example,
  - Child: "Him wanna park him bicycle."
  - Examiner: "Yes, he wants to park his motorcycle so he can shop at the mall."
- Remember that expansions show the child that you are interested in his or her ideas, which may encourage the child to talk more.
- Remember that expansions provide a model of longer, more complex utterances, which may prompt the child to produce more complicated utterances.
- Remain patient if the child is quiet; refrain from trying to force the child to talk.
- Refrain from asking closed-ended questions (e.g., "Do you have a dog? What's his name?") because these tend to elicit single-word responses (e.g., "yes," "Sidney").
- Introduce new toys or activities only as needed to maintain the child's interest in talking.
- Use humor directed at the toys or the examiner, but not at the child—for example, "This little dog stole the boy's favorite rubber duck. Then, she hid under the bed when the boy came home! Now I wonder what that little dog will do with the boy's favorite toy!"

potentially of interest to the child (e.g., "This little dog likes to sleep on the couch during the day. But the mom wants him to sleep on the floor."). Following a long pause that would allow—but not force—the child to talk, the examiner could make additional comments, such as "I have a poodle at home. . . . He sleeps on my bed when I'm at work!" By modeling these sorts of sentences, inserting some pauses, and then asking some open-ended questions (e.g., "I wonder what that little dog will do when the mom goes to work!" . . .), the child may start talking in a similar fashion, expressing his or her own ideas about what might be happening or what the characters might be thinking or feeling, producing a language sample that represents the child's best performance.

When eliciting a play-based language sample, it is wise to remember that no matter how exciting or engaging we believe an activity will be, the child may not share that belief. Thus, we need to be flexible and willing to modify our carefully designed plans. In other words, we need to follow the child's lead by allowing the child to direct the activities as much as possible. For example, if the child begins to make pancakes out of Play-Doh, the examiner should not attempt to redirect the child but, rather, should join in and make supportive comments (rather than ask questions) followed by extended pauses (e.g., "OK, I will look for some maple syrup . . . I like lots of syrup on my pancakes. . . . Wonder what else we need. . . . Maybe some plates and . . . ").

As examiners, we also need to recognize those conditions in which the SLP is not necessarily the best person to elicit the language sample. Sometimes we need to allow others to perform the job, such as a parent, teacher, or older sibling. I recall a situation many years ago when I was working as an SLP with Joey (not his real name), a 4-year-old boy who had specific language impairment (SLI). Despite my best efforts to elicit a representative language sample from him on several occasions, Joey said very little other than a few words and short phrases. One day, however, Joey's parents and older brother Gordon (not his real name) came to the clinic. Gordon took Joey outside to play while the parents and I met to discuss Joey's progress. The windows of the clinic room were open and we could all hear Joey and Gordon playing in the garden. What struck me was how "talkative" Joey had become when interacting with Gordon. Even more amazing was how freely Joey produced some long utterances that, although somewhat unintelligible, contained grammatical errors, confirming his SLI. Oh how I wished I could have recorded the language sample of Joey interacting with Gordon! This experience taught me that even young children know that SLPs are listening to them, ready to take note of their errors, in contrast to a trusted sibling. It also taught me to believe in the potential of every child to become a strong communicator and to realize that children will reveal their best language skills when they feel relaxed, accepted, and comfortable with their surroundings.

Transcribing and Analyzing the Sample

Once a language sample has been elicited from a preschool child, the SLP will need to transcribe the recording as accurately as possible, including all utterances produced by the child and the examiner. Because Systematic Analysis of Language Transcripts (SALT; Miller, Andriacchi, & Nockerts, 2019) has long been used to successfully analyze language samples with preschool children, it is important to follow SALT's conventions. For example, SALT offers guidelines for segmenting and punctuating utterances, parenthesizing maze behavior, flagging errors in word use, and identifying bound morphemes. A free tutorial for learning these features is available through SALT's website (https://www.saltsoftware.com).

Once these conventions have been followed, the SLP will be able to use SALT's databases for preschool children of different ages. Key measures of syntactic development to examine include mean length of utterance in words (MLU-w), mean length of utterance in morphemes (MLU-m), and the subordination index (SI) composite score. Key measures of verbal productivity include the total number of words produced (TWD) and the total number of utterances or communication units (C-units) produced (TCU). In preschool children who speak Standard American English (SAE), their use of grammatical morphemes should be examined, including the past tense -*ed* (She jump *ed*), plural -*s* (two cup*s*), possessive -*s* (Mom'*s* cat), third person singular -*s* (He walk*s*), and the copula (she *is* here) and auxiliary (she *is* running) verbs. By age 5 years, children with typical language development have mastered these morphemes, but those with developmental language disorders often omit them, even into the school years.

However, if a child speaks a dialect such as African American English (AAE), it is imperative that the SLP become familiar with the grammatical patterns unique to that dialect to avoid erroneously assuming that the child's grammatical patterns reflect a language disorder. For detailed information on AAE, and guidelines for analyzing language samples from children who speak AAE, the reader is referred to Craig, Washington, and Thompson-Porter (1998); Craig and Washington (2002, 2004); Craig, Washington, and Thompson (2005); Johnson and Koonce (2018); Mills, Watkins, and Washington (2013); and Washington (2019). In addition, Table 3–2 contains a list of morphosyntactic features that some speakers of AAE may use. Gaining familiarity with these features can assist the SLP to avoid diagnosing a language disorder in a child who speaks AAE and is simply using the dialect of his or her home or community. As explained by Hamilton, Mont, and McLain (2018), morphosyntactic patterns of AAE are just as rich, complex, and systematic as patterns of SAE and are just as effective in communication. Therefore, they should not be labelled "grammatical errors," viewed as inferior to SAE, or considered to be symptomatic of a language deficit or language weakness of any kind.

Table 3–2. Common morphosyntactic features of African American English (AAE) contrasted with Standard American English (SAE).

Morphosyntactic features with examples:

1. Deletion of copula *be* verbs (e.g., is, am, was, were, are) in a systematic fashion

    AAE: This a cookie; I happy; he here yesterday; we hungry last night; we tired today

    SAE: This is a cookie; I am happy; he was here yesterday; we were hungry last night; we are tired today

2. Deletion of auxiliary *be* verbs (e.g., is, am, was, were, are) in a systematic fashion

    AAE: He throwing a ball; I eatin' lunch now; they playin' baseball yesterday; they dancing at the party

    SAE: He is throwing a ball; I am eating lunch now; they were playing baseball yesterday; they are dancing at the party

3. Deletion of present tense third-person singular marker *–s*; same verb form used in person and number (e.g., I like X, you like X, he like X)

    AAE: He *eat* breakfast; she *play* volleyball; it *run* fast; she *go* to school; he *like* applesauce; he *do* the work; she *don't* see it

    SAE: He eats breakfast; she plays volleyball; it runs fast; she goes to school; he likes applesauce; he does the work; she doesn't see it

4. Subject-verb agreement difference; same verb form used in person and number (e.g., I was X-ing, you was X-ing, he/she/it was X-ing)

    AAE: *They was* kickin' a ball; *we was* eatin' soup

    SAE: They were kicking a ball; we were eating soup

5. Fitna/sposeta/bouta—indicates that something is about to happen: fitna = "fixin to"; sposeta = "supposed to"; bouta = "about to"

    AAE: She is *fitna* go to school; he is *sposeta* go home; she was *bouta* cook dinner

    SAE: She is going to go to school; he is supposed to go home; she was about to cook dinner

6. Undifferentiated pronoun case—subject, object, possessive pronouns used interchangeably

    AAE: My sister forgot *she* lunch; *him* cut the rope; *them* bakin' bread

    SAE: My sister forgot her lunch; he cut the rope; they are baking bread

7. Multiple negation—multiple negative markers used for emphasis; conveys intensity

    AAE: I do*n't* want *nobody* to give me *none* of that cough syrup

    SAE: I don't want anyone to give me any cough syrup

Table 3–2. *continued*

8. Zero possessive—the possessive marker -*s* is not attached to a noun; instead, the owner's name is placed immediately before the noun, or a non-possessive pronoun (e.g., they, he, she) is used rather than a possessive pronoun (their, his, her)

   AAE: They goin' to *John* house; they ridin' *Jane* horse; that the *dog* bed; this *Tommy* truck; she eat *she* dessert last night; Jason take *she* doll last week

   SAE: They are going to John's house; they are riding Jane's horse; that is the dog's bed; this is Tommy's truck; she ate her dessert last night; Jason took her doll last week

9. Deletion of past tense -*ed* marker; instead, past tense is indicated by other words in the sentence (e.g., yesterday, last night) or in the larger context (e.g., telling about an event that already happened)

   AAE: She *rip* open the box yesterday; she *cook* oatmeal this morning; he *look* up the field and *grab* the ball; she *ski* last winter; he *try* last night to read a book

   SAE: She ripped open the box yesterday; she cooked oatmeal this morning; he looked up the field and grabbed the ball; she skied last winter; he tried last night to read a book

10. Use of present tense verb form in place of past irregular verb form; instead, past tense is indicated by other words in the sentence (e.g., last week, last night, yesterday)

    AAE: The dog *dig* a hole under the fence last week; she *say* a prayer last night

    SAE: The dog dug a hole under the fence last week; she said a prayer last night

11. Invariant *be*—using the infinitive form of the verb "to be" (unconjugated)

    AAE: She *be* runnin' fast; he *be* goin' home; they *be* sittin' down; we *be* laughin' at him

    SAE: She is running fast; he is going home; they are sitting down; we are laughing at him

12. Zero *to*—the word "to" is deleted before an infinitive verb

    AAE: She hopin' for she sister *come* home soon; he want the teacher *ring* the bell

    SAE: She is hoping for her sister to come home soon; he wants the teacher to ring the bell

13. Zero plural—the plural marker -*s* is deleted from a noun; instead, plurality is expressed by a number or quantifier (e.g., one, five, some) placed before the noun

    AAE: She be cuttin' some *flower*; He buy two *shirt* yesterday; he run five *mile* everyday

    SAE: She is cutting some flowers; He bought two shirts yesterday; he runs five miles everyday

continues

Table 3–2. *continued*

14. Double modal (modal stacking)—two modal auxiliary verbs (e.g., might, could, should) are used together in one sentence, e.g., might could

    AAE: I *might could* fix the door; I *might should* find the cat

    SAE: I might be able to fix the door; maybe I should find the cat

15. Regularized reflexive—reflexive pronouns (e.g., himself, themselves) used in a consistent form (e.g., hisself, theyself)

    AAE: He eats by *hisself*; they taught *theyself*

    SAE: He eats by himself; they taught themselves

16. Indefinite article "a" rather than "an" before a word that begins with a vowel

    AAE: He ate *a* apple; they hear *a* owl hootin'; they go to *a* island

    SAE: He ate an apple; they heard an owl hooting; they went to an island

17. Appositive pronoun—one pronoun and a noun or two pronouns are used together

    AAE: My *daddy he* bought me a donut; the older *ones them* want a donut too

    SAE: My daddy bought me a donut; the older ones want a donut too

18. Remote past *been*—something that occurred in the past continues to the present; used to emphasize that an event that happened in the remote past continues

    AAE: I *been knowin'* how to play flute; I *been livin'* on Walnut Street

    SAE: I have known how to play flute for a long time; I have lived on Walnut Street for many years

19. Preterite *had*—use of auxiliary verb *had* followed by a past regular or irregular verb to express the simple past tense

    AAE: I *had tripped* over the rope; she *had went* to school; they *had got* lost

    SAE: I tripped over the rope; she went to school; they got lost

20. Completive *done*—something is completely finished and over with; used for emphasis

    AAE: We *done* said enough; this party *done* finished; I *done* told you that

    SAE: We've said enough; this party is finished; I told you that

21. Existential *it*—The pronoun *it* is used in place of the pronoun *there*

    AAE: *It* more to say about that; *it* a big dog in the park; *it* a lot of people in town

    SAE: There's more to say about that; there's a big dog in the park; there's a lot of people in town

22. Resultative *be done*—the consequences of doing something negative

    AAE: We *be done* got sick if we eat them apples; we *be done* lost all our money if we keep bettin' on the horses

    SAE: We will get sick if we eat those apples; we will lose all our money if we keep betting on the horses

Table 3–2. *continued*

23. Double marked possessive -*s* on a word that is already possessive, e.g., mine, your

    AAE: That dog like *mines*; that *yours* new car

    SAE: That dog is like mine; that is your new car

24. Double marked plural -*s* on a word that is already plural, e.g., children, women

    AAE: Those three *childrens* live here; four *womens* come to the door

    SAE: Those three children live here; four women came to the door

25. Non-inverted question—making a statement with rising intonation rather than asking a yes/no, wh-question, or how-question

    AAE: She goin' to school? She doin' something? That how you write it?

    SAE: Is she going to school? What is she doing? How do you write it?

Source: List and examples adapted from Hamilton, Mont, & McLain (2018, p. 114), Ivy & Masterson (2011, p. 40), and Washington (2019, pp. 133-139).

SCHOOL-AGE CHILDREN (AGES 5–11 YEARS) AND ADOLESCENTS (AGES 12–18 YEARS)

Eliciting a Representative Sample

Unlike preschool children, most school-age children and adolescents do not require a play-based conversational language sample to elicit their best performance. Rather, for conversational discourse, these students are capable of individual face-to-face interviews during which they are asked to talk about their family, friends, school, hobbies, holidays, or other topics of interest. Although most school-age children are also capable of engaging in narrative and expository discourse, the more difficult persuasive discourse should be saved for adolescents.

Listed in Table 3–3 are a number of challenges associated with language sampling in school-age children and adolescents. One issue is that a speaker's performance is influenced heavily by psychosocial factors. These include the speaker's knowledge of the topic, motivation to talk about it, and the degree to which the examiner's questions and comments stimulate complex thought. When speakers are well informed about the topic, interested in discussing it, and presented with stimulating prompts, their performance is likely to be quite strong. Genre is another factor that influences performance, with numerous studies showing that greater syntactic complexity often occurs during expository and narrative discourse compared with conversational discourse (Nippold, 2009; Nippold, Frantz-

Table 3–3. Some Challenges Associated With Language Sampling in School-Age Children and Adolescents

---

- Performance is influenced by psychosocial factors.
  - Is the child or adolescent knowledgeable of the topic?
  - Is the child or adolescent motivated to talk?
  - Do the interviewer's questions and comments stimulate complex thought?
- Performance varies with genre, with greater syntactic complexity occurring in
  - expository than in conversational discourse; and
  - narrative than in conversational discourse.

Kaspar, & Vigeland, 2017; Nippold, Hesketh, Duthie, & Mansfield, 2005). Thus, in addition to conversation, language samples should also be elicited in narrative and expository discourse, as discussed in Chapters 5 and 6.

In the past, another concern was the paucity of normative data for language sampling tasks with school-age children and adolescents. However, this situation has improved markedly in recent years due to the establishment and expansion of databases of spoken language samples elicited in various genres with speakers of different ages. For example, for speakers of American English, SALT has a conversational database for ages 3 to 13 years (n = 584), multiple narrative databases for ages 4 to 13 years (n = 830), an expository database for ages 10 to 18 years (n = 354), and a persuasive database for ages 14 to 18 years (n = 113) (Miller et al., 2019). SALT also provides details concerning the specific tasks that were used in establishing those databases along with helpful suggestions for eliciting representative samples and analyzing them appropriately. Given the availability of these databases through SALT, SLPs no longer need to worry about the absence of "normative data" for interpreting language samples elicited from English-speaking children and adolescents.

However, it is emphasized that in addition to using formal language sampling tasks for which normative databases are available, language samples can and should be elicited in social and academic contexts in which there is a genuine need to communicate with accuracy, clarity, and efficiency, as for example when a child is telling a folk tale drawn from his or her native culture (narrative discourse), explaining how to cook a special dinner using Grandmother's old recipes (expository discourse), or arguing with classmates about why the school's dress code should be changed (persuasive). Because there are an infinite number of real-world situations such as these, it would be impossible to establish normative databases for individuals of all ages speaking in all genres. Yet to ignore the manner in which children and adolescents speak in these natural contexts would be to lose sight of one of the foremost advantages that language sampling offers over other methods of assessment—the ability to evaluate how the individual actually communicates. Thus, if we wish to make language intervention maximally relevant to the client's life, language samples should be elicited in these situations and analyzed beyond the norms, falling back on our knowledge of typical language development to guide intervention.

In view of this information, key factors that are important to analyze with school-age children and adolescents are listed in Table 3–4. Language productivity and syntactic complexity are emphasized because these factors are often problematic for children and adolescents with developmental language disorders. During the language sampling interview, the SLP should encourage the speaker's best performance in order to reveal both strengths and weaknesses. This can be accomplished by treating the child

Table 3–4. Key Factors to Analyze in Language Samples of Children and Adolescents

---

- Total utterances produced, a measure of language productivity

- Total words produced, a measure of language productivity

- Mean length of C-unit/T-unit, a measure of syntactic complexity

- Clausal density, a measure of syntactic complexity

- Specific types of subordinate clauses produced
  - Nominal [NOM]
    Capture the King is *where you don't have to say "check."*
    I believe *Topalov will win the tournament.*
  - Relative [REL]
    He just beat Topalov, *who was the best in the world.*
    The rider *who won the Tour de France that year* was from Italy.
  - Adverbial [ADV]
    I learned chess *when I was three years old.*
    The rook can move horizontally or vertically *as much as it wants.*
  - Gerundive [GER]
    Swimming in the ocean can be lots of fun.
    My cousin's favorite activity is *baking cakes and pies for parties.*
  - Infinitive [INF]
    We wanted *to go to the beach* but forgot our sunscreen.
    We plan *to eat our sandwiches* at a picnic table by the lake.
  - Participial [PRT]
    Soaring across the river, the blue heron searched for fish.
    We crossed the rushing stream, *placing our feet carefully* on the flat rocks.

---

or adolescent speaker with respect, communicating clearly and honestly, and establishing and maintaining a positive interaction style—guidelines listed in Table 3–5.

Regarding the issue of respect, the SLP should explain that the purpose of the activity is to learn about the child or adolescent in order to obtain information that will be helpful in planning language intervention. The SLP should obtain the student's written permission to conduct the session and to audio-record the interview, asking the child or adolescent to sign an assent form. Questions should be encouraged and answered honestly.

During the interview, the importance of the SLP's *interaction style* cannot be overemphasized. To reveal strengths in the school-age child or adolescent, the SLP must show genuine regard for the individual and his

Table 3–5. Guidelines for Eliciting Spoken Language Samples With School-Age Children and Adolescents

Respect

- Conduct the interview in a quiet area, free of distractions.
- Explain the purpose of the activity.
- Explain how the information will be used.
- Obtain permission from the child or adolescent (in writing):
  - To be interviewed and audio-recorded
- Encourage questions from the child or adolescent.
- Answer questions honestly.

Interaction style

- Convey respect and genuine interest in the child or adolescent.
- Listen patiently through lengthy or confusing discourse.
- Remain calm, attentive, and upbeat.
- Avoid arguments with the child or adolescent.
- Avoid interruptions and overlaps of speech.
- Use appropriate eye contact and body language.
- Make supportive and positive comments.
- Ask open-ended questions.
- Ask one question at a time.
- Pause after asking a question (count to four silently).
- Repeat or rephrase a question, as necessary.
- Feel free to "go with the flow" to encourage spontaneity.
- Use humor, as appropriate (good-natured, kind, not offensive).

or her feelings, attitudes, and beliefs. This can be accomplished by taking time to listen patiently; to remain calm, attentive, and upbeat; to avoid arguments, interruptions, and overlaps of speech; and to show interest through appropriate eye contact, body language (e.g., smiling, nodding), and supportive comments (e.g., "Uh-huh," "I know what you mean," "Tell me more"). It is critical also to pause (e.g., count to four silently) after asking a question to allow the speaker time to formulate a coherent reply. Although verbal interaction in today's world is often fast-paced and competitive, with speakers and listeners quick to fill the silence, SLPs need to use a more relaxed style of interaction with children and adolescents—one that is kind, accepting, and shows that the speaker's comments matter. Interjecting a bit of humor into the session by sharing a comic strip, riddle, or nondeprecating joke may also help the child or adolescent feel more comfortable talking with the examiner.

Regarding the interaction, it is important that the SLP follows a structured protocol that includes questions or prompts that were designed to elicit certain types of information in a particular genre (e.g., conversational or expository). However, in addition to following the protocol, the SLP should feel free to "go with the flow" and to make comments and ask follow-up questions that will encourage the child or adolescent to continue speaking, to elaborate on an idea, and to communicate freely and confidently. In other words, the examiner should attempt to promote a naturalistic interaction style with the speaker.

Speech-language pathologists frequently ask how many utterances they should attempt to elicit when interviewing a school-age child or adolescent. Research has not yet determined an ideal number of utterances (Heilmann, Miller, & Nockerts, 2010). The best rule of thumb may be "the more the better" in order to obtain a representative sample. Realistically, however, this is not always practical, and meaningful results can be obtained with fewer than the standard 50 to 100 utterances that are often recommended (e.g., Miller et al., 2019). Rather than attempting to reach a certain minimum number of utterances, it is more important to encourage the child or adolescent to talk by bringing up stimulating topics, making open-ended comments (e.g., "I wonder why he did that"), commenting positively on what the speaker has said, trying to learn from the speaker, and following the other suggestions for eliciting language samples, as described previously.

Using Technology

Issues regarding technology also must be addressed in order to make language sampling maximally productive. Some key points are listed in Table 3–6. Although these points may seem obvious, too often they are forgotten, leading to frustration and wasted time and effort.

Table 3–6. Key Points Regarding the Spoken Language Sampling Session

---

Using Technology

- Ensure that the environment is quiet and free of distractions.
- Use a good quality audio recorder (digital or analog).
- If using an analog tape recorder, employ a high-quality audiotape.
- Adjust the volume of the audio recorder before starting the interview.
- Turn on the recorder and ask the speaker to count to 10.
- Immediately replay the recorder to ensure proper volume and clarity.
- If necessary, adjust the distance between the speaker's mouth and the microphone.
- Restart the audio recorder before beginning the formal interview.

Transcribing the Sample

- Transcribe the sample as soon as possible after eliciting it. When the sample is fresh in mind, it is easier to transcribe accurately.
- If using SALT, enter each new utterance on its own line.
- Transcribe the sample verbatim, with all mazes and errors included.
- Put parentheses around all mazes (false starts, hesitations, revisions).
- Allow the speaker's final reformulation to stand by parenthesizing what comes before it.

  For example, maze behavior has been properly parenthesized in the following utterance:

  > (Whenever I um we I mean) when I go to Grandma's, I (take um uh) take my backpack.

- If using SALT, all mazes will automatically be disregarded when parenthesized.
- Run-on sentences should be broken up so that main clauses linked by coordinate conjunctions, such as *and, but,* and *or,* each begin a new utterance. The following utterance, even though spoken continuously, would be broken at the slashes:

  > My parents went to Portland for the weekend / but I stayed with my cousin in Creswell / and my brother went camping with a friend.

  Two or more main clauses spoken continuously without a pause and without a conjunction (e.g., "I don't know how to braid hair my friend did this," "It's a potluck bring your favorite dish") are broken into multiple utterances as follows:

  > I don't know how to braid hair.
  > My friend did this.
  > It's a potluck.
  > Bring your favorite dish.

Table 3–6. *continued*

Using SALT

- To code clause types, place the code type in brackets, one space after its verb, using codes such as MC (main clause), ADV (adverbial clause), REL (relative clause), NOM (nominal clause), INF (infinitive clause), PRT (participial clause), or GER (gerundive clause).

- To code word types, place the code in brackets with no space after the word, using codes such as [ABN] (abstract noun), [MCV] (metacognitive verb), or AC (adverbial conjunct).

- Following these procedures will enable SALT to create separate lists for clauses and words.

For example, the SLP should practice using the recording equipment in advance and ensure that everything is working properly before eliciting a language sample with a child or adolescent. To illustrate this point, I share the following story. One day, a graduate student in speech-language pathology had arranged an interview with an adolescent at his high school, after having gone through a lengthy process of gaining permission from the school district, the boy's parents, and the boy himself in order to obtain a language sample for a research project. She arrived at the school well before the appointment, checked in with the head secretary, and set up the audio recorder in a quiet room near the main office. The interview with the adolescent went extremely well, with the graduate student eliciting a lively, detailed, and intriguing sample of expository discourse. However, upon returning home and attempting to transcribe the sample, she discovered that she had pushed the wrong button on the audio recorder and that nothing had been recorded, to her great dismay! Unfortunately, it was impossible to return to the school and redo the interview. I share this sad story, hoping it will help others attend to the important details of language sampling, knowing that it is often the little things in life that make a big difference.

Transcribing the Sample and Using SALT

Language samples with school-age children and adolescents can be analyzed after they have been transcribed and entered into SALT. Some relevant points are listed in Table 3–6. As with preschool children, all utterances of both the speaker and the examiner should be transcribed. Then, SALT can be adapted so that the speaker's utterances can be coded for various types of clauses (e.g., main and subordinate). In addition, SALT will automatically calculate mean length of C-unit (MLCU), mean length of T-unit (MLTU), or mean length of utterance (MLU), metrics that are discussed in Chapter 12. Regarding the transcription, it is important to listen to the recording carefully and to type the speaker's utterances exactly as they were produced, with all mazes (i.e., false starts, repetitions, and revisions) included. Parentheses should be placed around mazes, allowing the final reformulation to stand. Any words within parentheses will not be counted when SALT calculates the mean number of words per utterance (C-unit/T-unit). With practice, the SLP will be able to transcribe directly into SALT, placing each new utterance on its own line. Some clinicians prefer initially to transcribe the sample into Microsoft Word and copy and paste it into SALT later. However, this is an extra step that can be avoided once the SLP has had more practice transcribing the sample directly into SALT.

After entering a sample into SALT, the SLP can go back over it and identify instances of main and subordinate clauses, using codes such as [MC] (main clause), [ADV] (adverbial clause), and [NOM] (nominal clause). All codes should be enclosed in brackets. When clauses are coded, the code should immediately follow the verb and be separated by one space, as in the following examples:

> If a piece takes [ADV] out the piece that has [REL] the king in check, I can take [MC] out that piece.

> So if I had [ADV] like a castle and a bishop up here, which is [REL] the one that can move [REL] on a diagonal, I can kind of like protect [MC] it.

When coding words, such as abstract nouns or metacognitive verbs, the code (e.g., [ABN], [MCV]) should immediately follow the word, with no space, as in these examples:

> Sometimes that bird thinks[MCV] I am a giant.

> I remember[MCV] the big word for happiness[ABN]. It's exuberance[ABN]!

By using these conventions, SALT will automatically tabulate the number of times that each type of clause or word occurred in the sample and will create separate lists of clause types (e.g., MC, REL, ADV, NOM) and word types (e.g., ABN, MCV). In addition, SALT can be adapted to perform any type of coding function, depending on the interests of the SLP. The codes discussed in this book are those that were used in numerous research projects. Chapters 9 and 10 contain exercises for identifying different types of words, phrases, and clauses that are important for analyzing language samples in children and adolescents.

IMPLICATIONS FOR INTERVENTION

The ultimate goal of language intervention with children and adolescents is to improve their ability to communicate in meaningful contexts beyond the therapy room. This includes, for example, the diverse social, academic, and vocational settings they encounter today as children or adolescents and will encounter tomorrow as adults. Given these expectations, it is reasonable to focus on intervention activities that will generalize to real-world settings—such as the home, school, or job site—emphasizing the need for children and adolescents to use spoken or written language in a way that is accurate, clear, and efficient. By eliciting, transcribing, and analyzing language samples, SLPs can gain insight into the unique strengths and weaknesses that an individual child or adolescent brings to the different situations. Although language sampling is not a perfect process, the information gained from it can be used to establish relevant goals for intervention and to monitor change as the individual achieves greater accuracy, clarity, and efficiency when communicating with others for genuine purposes.

For example, suppose a 7-year-old boy shows limited use of complex syntax. To examine this pattern in detail, the SLP could elicit and transcribe a narrative language sample using one of the Frog stories (e.g., *Frog Goes to Dinner*; Mayer, 1974). Based on the results of the sample, analyzed in SALT, the SLP may decide to target the use of complex syntax by having the child retell stories from the classroom during language intervention, focusing on the production of complex sentences that contain different types of subordinate clauses. These might include, for example, sentences with relative clauses (e.g., The boy chased the puppy *who stole his favorite dinosaur*) or nominal clauses (e.g., The boy hoped *the puppy would bring back his dinosaur*), using a variety of evidence-based intervention techniques (e.g., focused stimulation, modeling, imitation, sentence recasting, sentence combining, sentence completion). After several months of regular and intense intervention, the SLP could elicit another narrative sample using a different Frog story (e.g., *Frog, Where Are You?* Mayer, 1969), using SALT to analyze the sample, and noting standard metrics of syntactic development (e.g., MLCU, CD) and the use of different types of subordinate clauses. Because the Frog stories were not used during intervention, the SLP could objectively measure the amount of progress that has occurred by comparing the child's performance pre- and post-intervention using similar but not identical Frog stories. In this way, narrative language samples can be used to monitor a child's progress in acquiring the ability to use complex syntax as a result of participating in individualized language intervention.

CHAPTER 4

Conversational Discourse

conversation is a dialogue in which people are speaking informally, helping establish, extend, or otherwise modify their relationship by sharing thoughts, feelings, and beliefs and by exchanging information and experiences. Unlike the monologic nature of narrative or expository discourse in which one speaker dominates, conversation is more of a balanced interaction in which participants take turns serving as speakers and listeners, supporting each other by asking and answering questions, making comments, and showing interest in the topic. The ability to engage successfully in conversations contributes to an individual's social and emotional well-being.

PRESCHOOL CHILDREN (AGES 3–4 YEARS)

During the preschool years, children's conversational skills gradually improve in conjunction with the development of pragmatics. For example, they learn to ask and answer questions, listen carefully, add information to an exchange, stay on topic for longer periods of time, and attend more closely to the needs and perspectives of their conversational partners. They also acquire the ability to make indirect requests and to adjust the content and tone of their discourse to the age and status of the listener by, for example, expressing themselves less directly and more politely with older and less familiar individuals (Hulit, Howard, & Fahey, 2011). In addition, as their lexical, syntactic, and morphological development continues, children are able to use language with greater accuracy, clarity, and efficiency during conversations.

When eliciting language samples with 3- and 4-year-old children, speech-language pathologists (SLPs) may be more successful if they use play-based conversational interactions. This approach offers an opportunity to obtain a sample that reflects the child's best spontaneous language production. Guidelines for successfully carrying out this type of language sampling activity are discussed in Chapter 3. Highlights of this approach include the use of age-appropriate toys, following the child's lead, making supportive comments, avoiding closed-ended questions, and modeling the production of longer and more complex utterances.

Analysis of Play-Based Conversational Language Samples

Reports have indicated that one of the most valid and reliable measures of spoken language development in 3- and 4-year-old children is mean length of utterance (MLU), which is the average number of words (MLU-w) or morphemes (MLU-m) produced per utterance (Rice et al., 2010). It is useful to know that once a language sample has been entered into Systematic Analysis of Language Transcripts (SALT), the program will automatically calculate MLU.

In a study of spoken language development in children using play-based conversational language samples, Rice et al. (2010) reported that MLU gradually increased during the preschool years but that children with specific language impairment (SLI) consistently lagged behind their age-matched peers with typical language development (TLD) on both MLU-w and MLU-m. A child's MLU in conversation is therefore considered to be a valuable index for identifying language impairment, especially up to approximately age 5 years. At age 5 years and older, other types of speaking tasks, such as structured interviews, should be used to elicit language samples unless children have obvious or severe language deficits. This is because play-based tasks no longer stress the older child's cognitive–linguistic systems sufficiently to reveal language deficits.

Table 4–1 contains data from Rice et al. (2010, p. 344) for MLU-w and MLU-m based on the play-based conversational language samples of children with TLD, ages 2;6 through 8;11. These data may serve as a point of reference for children who speak Standard American English (SAE). If a child speaks another dialect such as African American English (AAE) or is a bilingual Spanish–English speaker, caution is advised when consulting this database, especially in relation to MLU-m. This is because morphosyntactic rules will differ across dialects and languages, and the means and standard deviations for children speaking SAE may not apply to those who speak another dialect or are learning English as a second language. However, for children who speak AAE and therefore use some of the morphosyntactic features listed in Table 3–2, MLU-w is a more reasonable metric than MLU-m because it is calculated on the basis of the number of words – not morphemes – the child produces per utterance (Ivy & Masterson, 2011).

Table 4–1. Data Collected by Rice et al. (2010, p. 344) for Children Ages 3 to 9 Years, Reporting MLU-w and MLU-m (in 6-Month Intervals) from Play-Based Conversational Language Samples

Age Range	n	MLU-w		MLU-m	
		Mean	SD	Mean	SD
2;6–2;11	17	2.91	0.58	3.23	0.71
3;0–3;5	29	3.43	0.61	3.81	0.69
3;6–3;11	38	3.71	0.58	4.09	0.67
4;0–4;5	49	4.10	0.65	4.57	0.76
4;6–4;11	74	4.28	0.72	4.75	0.79
5;0–5;5	78	4.38	0.63	4.88	0.72
5;6–5;11	77	4.47	0.61	4.96	0.70
6;0–6;5	70	4.57	0.66	5.07	0.75
6;6–6;11	63	4.70	0.66	5.22	0.71
7;0–7;5	51	4.72	0.83	5.22	0.91
7;6–7;11	47	4.92	1.03	5.45	1.13
8;0–8;5	41	5.08	0.84	5.67	0.97
8;6–8;11	18	4.99	0.71	5.51	0.79

MLU-m, mean length of utterance, average number of morphemes; MLU-w, mean length of utterance, average number of words.

In addition to reporting MLU, the presence of grammatical morphemes should be examined in the conversational language samples of preschool children who speak SAE. By age 5 years or earlier, most children have mastered the use of common grammatical morphemes such as past tense -*ed* (He walk*ed*), third person singular -*s* (She sing*s*), plural -*s* (two cat*s*), the possessive -*s* (Mom'*s* cat), copula and auxiliary verbs (Tim *is* a teacher; Mom *is* going to the store), the articles *a* and *the* (*a* book versus *the* book), possessive pronouns (*his, her, their, my* cat), and pronouns in subject (*He* like pancakes) and object (He gave the ball to *her*) position in obligatory contexts. However, children with language impairments such as SLI often make errors on these morphemes (Leonard, 2014), even into the school years (Guo, Eisenberg, Schneider, & Spencer, 2020; Scott & Windsor, 2000), producing utterances such as "Him walk to school today," "Mom drive Bob car home," "That him dog," "Them cook eggs yesterday," and "Me have two dog." Using SALT, these and other grammatical errors can be flagged and counted in a conversational language sample and appropriate goals for intervention can be established for preschool and young school-age children who struggle with morphosyntactic development.

To measure grammatical errors in the language samples of preschool children, and to monitor children's progress over time as a result of language intervention, the SLP could focus on the most common errors by calculating the finite verb morphology composite (FVMC), as described in Chapter 12. In addition to MLU and FVMC, another useful metric for preschool children is the percentage grammatical utterances (PGU), also described in Chapter 12. However, the PGU uses picture prompts to elicit a descriptive language sample rather than a play-based conversational language sample.

In analyzing language samples from preschool children, clausal density (CD), the average number of clauses produced per utterance or C-unit, should also be noted. By the time most children are 5 years old, they regularly produce complex sentences that contain multiple clauses—for example, "I wanna go to the park and play with Henry." With SALT, it is easy to determine CD for an entire sample by counting the number of verbs in each utterance (because each verb represents a clause), accessing the subordination index (SI) identifier, and choosing the appropriate code (e.g., SI-1, -2, -3) from the drop-down window. For example, the code of SI-1 indicates one verb/clause, the code of SI-2 indicates two verbs/clauses, and so on. Once all utterances have been coded, SALT will automatically calculate and report the SI code composite. If a preschool child with a language disorder has a CD or SI code composite of 1 or less, this indicates that the child is producing only simple sentences. Thus, the SLP may wish to encourage the child to begin using some early developing complex sentences such as those containing catenatives (e.g., gonna, wanna) and infinitive verbs (e.g., to go, to play) in order to produce sentences such as "I wanna go to the park" or "He's gonna play with his new truck." Activities in which preschool children with language disorders receive numerous exposures to these grammatical structures through focused stimulation, prompted imitation, and utterance recasting, along with frequent opportunities to use those structures in their own speech, can be effective in facilitating the development of complex syntax.

Table 4–2 contains an example of a play-based conversational language sample that was elicited from a 3-year-old child with typical language development (Fletcher & Garman, 1988) and made available through the CHILDES database. Once entered into SALT by this author, the sample was segmented into C-units and formatted using SALT conventions. For example, bound morphemes were separated from the root word with a slash (/), unintelligible elements were marked with xxx, mazes were parenthesized, nonverbal behaviors were placed within braces, and the SI code was inserted at the end of each utterance. In addition, contracted words were separated by one space in order to credit them as separate words.

Table 4–2. Excerpt from a Play-Based Conversational Language Sample with a 3-Year-Old Girl, Sally (Not Her Real Name)

The sample was adapted from Fletcher and Garman (1988) and coded using SALT conventions. See text for explanation. E, Examiner; C, Child

MLU-w = 3.89

MLU-m = 4.42

SI composite score = 1.08

TWD = 214

TCU = 55

E What is this? {E picks up toy windmill}

C It's go round and round [SI-1].

E It goes round and round.

E That's right.

E Do you know what it's called, Sally?

E It's called a windmill.

C Shall we put it there [SI-1]?

E We put it there, right.

C Can I sit on this chair [SI-1]?

E You sit on the little red chair.

C And I wonder what this is [SI-2].

E I think it's a water pump.

C Yes, it/'s a water pump [SI-1].

E It's a water pump, isn't it?

C Shall we put it there [SI-1]?

E Yes, put it there.

E And there are some logs of wood, aren't they?

C That/'s a garden [SI-1].

E Look, what is this? {E points to toy Christmas tree}

C That/'s the Christmas tree [SI-1]!

E That's a Christmas tree, isn't it.

C A Christmas tree [SI-0].

E Did you have a Christmas tree at home for Christmas?

C Yes [SI-X].

E Was it a big one?

C Uhhuh, xxx a big one xxx [SI-X].

E And were there lots of presents underneath it?

C Uhhuh [SI-X]. {C nods}

E What is this? {E points to toy duck}

C That/'s a quack_quack [SI-1].

continues

Table 4–2. *continued*

E That's a quack_quack, isn't it?

C Uhhuh [SI-X]. {C nods}

C I wonder what they/'re do/ing with that thing [SI-2].

C I can/'t do anymore [SI-1].

E You can't put it off?

E It's a bit difficult sometimes.

E They're in the tree now.

C I wanna get it on my own [SI-2].

C There, a mmmooo [SI-0].

E It's a cow, isn't it?

C Is a mmmooo [SI-1].

C Thing/s to put on [SI-1].

E Have you seen some cows somewhere?

C I seen the mmmooo [SI-1].

E You've seen moos.

C That/'s a horse [SI-1].

E That's a horse and that's another horse.

C It/'s a mmmooo [SI-1].

E Uhhuh, it's a cow, isn't it?

C That/'s a man [SI-1].

E Where does the man go?

E Is he driving the tractor?

C He/'s ly/ing down [SI-1].

E He's lying down in front of the tractor.

C It is be/ing funny [SI-1].

E It's being funny.

E And that's another horse.

C Ran down the garden [SI-1].

E He ran down the garden?

E To get where?

C In the house [SI-0].

E He wants to get in the house?

C Uhhuh, cause he/'s cold [SI-1].

E It's cold outside, isn't it?

C And that/'s a xxx [SI-X].

E That's a?

C Is a mmmooo [SI-1].

C (It) it can/'t move [SI-1].

E What do you do at home?

Table 4–2. *continued*

E What do you play with?

C (Um) I play with toy/s like that [SI-1].

E You play with toys like that.

C (I I they are) I got some book/s at home [SI-1].

E Uhhuh.

C And you can read them to me [SI-1].

E I can read them to you?

C When xxx at nursery you can read them [SI-X].

E Look, I've got some puppets here.

C (Um) I want to put them on [SI-2].

E You can put them on.

C What color are they [SI-1]?

E That's orange.

E The nose is orange and this is orange and this is yellow.

C And this is grey [SI-1].

C What color is it [SI-1]?

E It's yellow and this is pink.

C Yes [SI-X].

C And what color/'s that teeth [SI-1]?

C White [SI-X].

E The teeth are white.

E That's right.

C And what color is that [SI-1]?

E That's grey.

C What color is that [SI-1]?

E Black.

C That/'s black [SI-1].

E Now look, Sally.

C Yes [SI-X].

E Horsie and tiger, they often fight with each other.

C Do they [SI-1]?

E If horsie says "tiger is naughty," then tiger says, "No, tiger is not naughty."

C No, tiger is not naughty he say/3s [SI-2].

E If horsie says "tiger likes school," then tiger says, "No, tiger doesn't like school."

C No, they doe/sn't like school, say/3s the tiger [SI-2].

E You be tiger now.

E What does tiger say?

C Tiger go/3es to bed early [SI-1].

continues

Table 4–2. *continued*

E Horsie's going to get a Smartie now.

E Ask tiger if he's got a Smartie.

C You got a Smartie [SI-1]?

E Ask him if it's tasty.

C It/'s tasty [SI-1]?

E Ask him if you can have it.

C You can have it [SI-1].

E Ask him if he likes Smarties.

C You like Smartie/s [SI-1]?

E OK, you can have the Smartie now.

C He think/3s he want/3s one [SI-2].

E Watch what horse and tiger are doing and listen to what they say (takes both puppets).

E Horsie says something and tiger says the last part.

E If horsie says "tiger is hungry," then tiger says "isn't he?"

C Is/n"t he [SI-1]?

E If horse says "tiger likes school," then tiger says "doesn't he?"

C Does/n't he [SI-1]?

Next, the child's MLU-w, MLU-m, and SI composite score were calculated automatically by SALT and are reported in Table 4–2. Upon referencing SALT's play-based conversational database for the child's chronological age, and the data from Rice et al. (2010) reported in Table 4–1, the results confirmed typical language development, as all key metrics were within the expected range.

SCHOOL-AGE CHILDREN (AGES 5–11 YEARS) AND ADOLESCENTS (AGES 12–18 YEARS)

For children aged 5 years or older, conversational language samples can usually be elicited in structured, face-to-face interviews. Beyond the preschool years, structured interviews are usually preferable to play-based conversational language samples because the latter are no longer as engaging to these older students. In addition, because play-based samples provide less cognitive stimulation, they are less likely to prompt the use of complex language.

However, it is important to acknowledge that during conversations, school-age children and adolescents with typical and impaired language development tend to produce utterances that are shorter and less complex than those they produce during other genres such as narrative or expository discourse (Nippold, 2009; Nippold, Frantz-Kaspar, & Vigeland, 2017; Nippold, Hesketh, Duthie, & Mansfield, 2005; Nippold, Mansfield, Billow, & Tomblin, 2008). Although samples of conversational discourse are less likely to reveal deficits in syntactic development compared with samples of expository discourse (e.g., Nippold et al., 2008), it is still useful to elicit conversations because those sessions can help build rapport with the school-age child or adolescent and can reveal relevant information about the student's attitudes, interests, and concerns. Moreover, during a conversation, the SLP will have the opportunity to observe any pragmatic issues that might be challenging to the student (e.g., difficulty answering questions, staying on topic, adding relevant information, making eye contact). Finally, some school-age children and adolescents with language impairments, such as those with more severe ASD, will show deficits in the use of complex syntax during conversations, as discussed in Chapter 8.

To elicit a conversational language sample with a school-age child or adolescent, it is recommended that the SLP follow a structured protocol, such as the one shown in Table 4–3, which is called the General Conversation task. After asking a question, the SLP should pause and allow the child or adolescent time to formulate a reply. When it appears that the student has finished talking, the SLP should feel free to comment on the student's response and to ask additional questions to encourage elaboration, promoting a more natural interaction. Table 4–4 contains an excerpt from a conversation that took place between an SLP and a 13-year-old girl with typical language development. It illustrates how the SLP encouraged conversation by showing interest in what the girl said, asking topic-relevant questions, and making supportive comments. The sample has been coded for main and subordinate clauses.

Table 4–3. General Conversation Task (Nippold, 2009, p. 860)

Interviewer: First of all, I'd like to learn something about you. I'm going to ask you a few general questions. Then you can ask me some questions, too. OK?

  A. Do you have any brothers or sisters? (if yes) What are their names? How old are they? What else can you tell me about them?

  B. Do you have any pets at home? (if yes) Tell me about your pets.

  C. Do you have a favorite TV show or movie? (if yes) Tell me about it.

  D. Do you like to read books or magazines? (if yes) Which ones?

  E. Now do you want to ask me anything? (Allow 1–2 quick questions.)

Table 4–4. General Conversation Between 13-Year-Old Girl with TLD (C) and Examiner (E) (from the Author's Files)

The sample has been coded for clause types: MC = main clause; ADV = adverbial clause; NOM = nominal clause; REL = relative clause; INF = infinitive clause; PRT = participial clause; GER = gerundive clause.

Girl, Age 13, Conversing About General Topics of Interest (TCU = 30; MLCU = 8.77; CD = 1.37)

E What would you like to tell me about yourself?

E For example, school, family, friends, pets, or your birthday?

C Well, last year, I started [MC] dance with some of my friends.

C And I decided [MC] to do [INF] it again this year.

C And I started [MC] last week.

C So far, it's been [MC] really fun.

C And last year, we did [MC] a show at the community center.

C And I liked [MC] it a lot.

C So I'm [MC] pretty excited about that.

E What do you dance, what style?

C I dance [MC] ballet, well, kind of contemporary.

C I do [MC] point on one day, modern on another day, and ballet on another one.

E So you perform all those types of dance per performance?

C Yeah, and we did [MC] the *Tempest* in a kind of dance form.

E Oh really?

E What is the *Tempest*?

C It's [MC] a Shakespeare play about these people who get [REL] shipwrecked on an island.

C And one of the persons on the island who is [REL] already there used [MC] to be [INF] a king.

C And his brother kicked [MC] him out or took [MC] over.

C And then his brother is [MC] the one who gets [REL] shipwrecked on the island.

C And then the first brother does [MC] all this stuff to him to pay [INF] back.

C But in the end, they make [MC] up.

C So it was [MC] all good.

E Do you feel like it was well represented in dance?

C Yeah, I think [MC] so.

C It was [MC] a lot of fun.

C And I can understand [MC] it, which is [REL] a good thing.

C And school just started [MC], eighth grade.

C And it's [MC] kind of weird being [GER] on the top, not having [GER] the other older kids there.

Table 4–4. *continued*

C It's [MC] just strange.

C But I'm kind of getting [MC] used to it.

E Do you like it?

C Yeah, I like [MC] it.

E But it's only one year and then it's back to being a freshman again, next year.

C Yeah, that part isn't [MC] so great.

C And I talked [MC] to some of the people that are [REL] freshmen this year that I knew [REL] last year.

C And they say [MC] it's [NOM] pretty scary.

E Oh no!

C Yeah.

E But you have a lot of friends in your grade?

C Yeah.

E So you'll all go together.

After eliciting a general conversation, the SLP may wish to elicit a conversation about a specific topic of interest, focusing on a favorite hobby or other activity. When conversing about topics of high personal interest, speakers are more likely to use complex syntax compared to when they are talking about topics they find less engaging (Nippold, 2009). For example, the conversational task shown in Table 4–5 was used with speakers who were chess players, and it elicited greater syntactic complexity than did the General Conversation task. The SLP could easily change the topic of conversation from chess to any other hobby, depending on the interests of the child or adolescent (e.g., soccer, golf, tennis, ballet, cheerleading, volleyball), and could make other modifications to customize the interview for a specific activity. However, it is important to remember that eliciting a conversation about such topics is quite different from eliciting an expository sample that focuses on those same topics, and it will yield different results.

Table 4–6 contains an example of a conversation about chess with a 9-year-old boy. It can be seen that many of his responses to the examiner's questions were short and to the point until he began talking about topics of greater personal interest. For example, when the boy talked about playing bughouse, playing chess on a computer, or why he enjoyed chess, the complexity of his language increased, revealing a fairly sophisticated level of syntactic development.

Table 4–5. Chess Conversation Task (Nippold, 2009, p. 860)

Introduction: Now I'd like to ask you about chess:

    A. How long have you played chess?

    B. How old were you when you first started to play?

    C. Who taught you how to play chess?

    D. Do you have a chess rating? (if yes) What is it?

    E. Do you have a chess coach or teacher? (if yes) Tell me about him or her.

    F. Do you belong to a chess club? (if yes) Which one?

    G. How often do you play chess, say, in a typical week?

    H. Who do you play with the most?

    I. Can you name any famous chess players? (if yes) Tell me something about him or her/them.

    J. Do you ever play chess on a computer? Tell me about that.

    K. Now tell me why you enjoy chess.

Table 4–6. Conversation About Chess Between the Examiner and a Boy, Age 9;10 (from the Author's Files). E = examiner; C = child

---

Boy, Age 9;10 Conversing About Chess (TCU = 41; MLCU = 7.32; CD = 1.41)

E How long have you played chess?

C About two years.

E And how old were you when you first started to play?

C Seven.

E And who taught you how to play chess?

C My friend.

C His name was [MC] Michael.

C And I think [MC] he was [NOM] 16 years old.

C Anything more you needed [REL] to ask [INF] me?

E Anything more you can tell me about Michael?

C (He umm started playing) I knew [MC] him when I was [ADV] first born because he was playing [ADV] with my older brother, Frank.

C And that is [MC] all I know [REL].

C And he still lives [MC] with his parents.

E Do you have a chess rating?

C I am [MC] first in club so far.

C I have not been beat [MC] for a while, except by my uncle.

C He is [MC] 19.

C He beat [MC] me just barely.

C And that is [MC] all.

E Do you belong to a chess club?

Table 4–6. *continued*

C Yes.

E Do you have a chess coach or teacher?

C Yeah, I have [MC] a chess teacher.

C But I do not know [MC] his name though because he is [ADV] new.

C Our old teacher had [MC] to move [INF].

C Yeah, I learned [MC] a lot from him.

E Can you tell me any more about him?

C (umm) He is [MC] usually late.

C And (umm) he has taught [MC] me a game.

C It is [MC] bughouse.

C It is [MC] when you are [NOM] on a team.

C And if you take [ADV] somebody's piece, if your partner takes [ADV] somebody else's piece, you get it [MC].

C And if you take [ADV] somebody else's piece, you give [MC] them that piece to them.

C And they get [MC] to set [INF] it up anywhere else.

C They can set [MC] anywhere on the board they want [REL] except it has [ADV] to be [INF] on their side and the pawns cannot be [ADV] on the back.

C Anything else?

E How often do you play chess?

C About every day.

E So, who do you play with the most?

C My brother Timothy.

E Can you name any famous chess players?

C I do not think [MC] so.

E Okay, do you ever play chess on a computer?

C Yes, I got [MC] Chess_master, the 10th edition.

C And it is [MC] pretty challenging.

C And I have [MC] Battle_chess_III.

C And it is [MC] three_D when you have [ADV] actually these real (umm) war pieces that you move [REL].

C And you can actually make [MC] them fight [INF].

C It is [MC] pretty cool.

E How often do you play on the computer?

C About every day.

E So you play a computer every day and you also play a person.

E Now tell me why you enjoy chess.

C It is [MC] a pretty challenging sport.

C And you have [MC] to know [INF] a bunch of strategies to basically know [INF] how to play [INF].

C And it is [MC] really fun to challenge [INF] people because you have [ADV] to use [INF] a bunch of mathematics.

Analysis of Conversational Language Samples

As with preschool children, analysis of conversational language samples elicited from school-age children and adolescents should focus on the use of complex syntax, a foundational language domain. This can be assessed with two standard metrics, mean length of C-unit (MLCU) and CD, as explained in Chapter 12. In examining the use of complex syntax, it is important also to determine if the speaker can use all types of subordinate clauses, including adverbial (ADV), nominal (NOM), relative (REL), gerundive (GER), infinitive (INF), and participial (PRT), which are explained in Chapter 10. Once the conversational language sample has been transcribed, entered into SALT, and segmented into C-units, SALT will automatically calculate MLCU. To determine CD, the SLP could individually code each main clause and each type of subordinate clause in the sample and allow SALT to report the total number of clauses produced. Then, the SLP could divide the total number of clauses by the total number of C-units produced to determine CD. Alternatively, the SLP could simply insert the SI code at the end of each C-unit and allow SALT to automatically calculate and report the SI composite score. To determine if the speaker's performance is within normal limits, the SLP could consult SALT's conversational database as a point of reference for ages 3 to 13 years.

In addition to the SALT reference database, the SLP could refer to normative data collected by Walter Loban (1976) during his longitudinal study of a group of children ($n = 211$) he followed from kindergarten through the 12th grade. Every year, each child participated in a conversational interview with an adult examiner who asked the child to talk about common topics such as games, friends, television shows, books, and, as they got older, parties they had attended and their plans for the future. Each interview was audio-recorded, transcribed verbatim, and segmented into C-units. Table 4–7 contains the average MLCU for grades 1 through 12 (ages 6–18 years) reported by Loban for a subgroup of participants ($n = 35$) who represented "typical" language abilities, the so-called "random group." The data show that MLCU gradually increased as the students grew older.

In addition to examining MLCU and CD, key measures of syntactic development, the student's level of verbal productivity should also be reported. This can easily be accomplished by examining metrics that are automatically reported by SALT. These include the total number of utterances or C-units produced and the total number of words produced, as explained in Chapter 12. Verbal productivity gradually increases during the school-age and adolescent years but is often deficient in students who have language disorders.

Implications for Intervention

School-age children and adolescents with language disorders often struggle to express themselves when talking with their peers, leading to frustra-

Table 4–7. Longitudinal Data Collected by Loban (1976, p. 27) from Conversational Interviews of Students in the "Random Group" ($n = 35$) in Grades 1 Through 12 (Ages 6–18 Years), Reporting Their Average Mean Length of C-unit (MLCU)

Grade	MLCU
1	6.88
2	7.56
3	7.62
4	9.00
5	8.82
6	9.82
7	9.75
8	10.71
9	10.96
10	10.68
11	11.17
12	11.70

tion, embarrassment, and social rejection. These problems may occur when the student is unsure of what to talk about; lacks sufficient knowledge of current events or other popular topics of conversation; uses inaccurate, vague, or overly general words; or speaks in a monotonous, redundant, or fragmentary manner that taxes the listener. For example, consider the following string of simple sentences:

> I went to the coast. There was a storm. The storm tore off some pieces. The pieces were on the cabin. It was loud. I was so scared.

When the same information is expressed more efficiently through the use of subordinate clauses and some well-chosen words, the story suddenly becomes more exciting:

> When I went [ADV] to the coast, there was [MC] a fearsome windstorm that blew [REL] some shingles off the cabin. It caused [MC] a creepy commotion.

When school-age children and adolescents learn to speak in a more engaging manner, their peers may be more inclined to listen to them and to seek them out as conversational partners.

At a basic level, speakers must have the ability to use complex syntax, literate vocabulary, and appropriate grammar. If they are lacking these fundamental skills, language intervention must address their limitations. Then, once students have acquired those skills, they must be prompted to use them in natural communication settings. In order to do so, however, school-age children and adolescents must have information to share that is of interest to others. Thus, it is worthwhile to encourage students to learn about events that are happening at school or in the community. Examples might include the upcoming play, concert, football game, homecoming dance, student election, science fair, or the opening of a new restaurant, movie theater, or skating rink in the local area. Being well informed about a variety of topics, continuously adding to the knowledge base, will help build the cognitive foundation needed to sustain rich conversations. In addition, students working in small groups with the SLP could practice their conversational skills using materials such as Animal Talk (http://www.usgamesinc.com) or Chat Pack Favorites (http://www.TheQuestion Guys.com). Animal Talk, which is more appropriate for younger students, consists of cards that contain information about animals and questions that prompt discussion. For example, one card shows a picture of a Dalmatian accompanied by following paragraph and questions:

> Like people, dogs have competitions and contests. The American Kennel Club establishes the rules and regulations of competitions for dogs in certain categories. A dog earns the title of champion after it receives a certain number of points in AKC contests. What contests have you participated in that had rules and regulations? What did you have to do to earn the right to compete?

The SLP or a student in the group could read the paragraph aloud, followed by the questions to prompt the group to engage in a friendly and lighthearted conversation. For older students, including adolescents, Chat Pack Favorites could be used during intervention by posing a set of questions that could potentially stimulate an engaging conversation—for example:

> What is your favorite thing to do with your friends? Tell me about it.

> What is your favorite snack to buy at a movie theatre? Tell me about it.

> What is the best museum that you've ever visited? Tell me about it.

> What is your favorite thing about America? Tell me about it.

> What is your favorite item from your favorite fast-food restaurant? Tell me about it.

As school-age children and adolescents practice conversing with their peers about topics of mutual interest, they should be encouraged to use complex syntax and appropriate words in order to express themselves in a way that is accurate, clear, and efficient. They should also be encouraged to use positive pragmatic behaviors that promote peer interactions. Examples include listening attentively; allowing others to speak; complimenting; asking questions; expressing feelings calmly and without criticism; using humor; understanding others' values, beliefs, and perspectives; and ignoring unpleasant remarks (Schickedanz, Schickedanz, Forsyth, & Forsyth, 2001). When students with developmental language disorders learn to use good social skills with their peers—such as showing kindness and empathy—it can help increase their opportunities for happiness, personal satisfaction, and success in life (Conti-Ramsden & Durkin, 2016).

Table 4–8 contains a list of behaviors that young people who are proficient conversationalists often display, and Table 4–9 contains a list of behaviors that are sometimes observed in students who have language disorders. When a student's conversational skills are deficient, the

Table 4–8. Conversational Behaviors of Older Children and Adolescents With Typical Language Development

---

Students who are proficient conversationalists do the following (Nippold, 2000, 2007).

As **listeners**, they:

- Allow others to speak without excessive interruptions
- Listen attentively and think about what is being said
- Understand and accept different perspectives and opinions
- Ask relevant and thoughtful questions that draw others out
- Smile, nod, and make normal eye contact
- Exercise discretion with personal information
- Remain optimistic, encouraging, and supportive of others

As **speakers**, they:

- Make relevant comments that extend the topic of conversation
- Talk about topics of general interest to others
- Stay on topic, remain organized, and speak coherently
- Allow others to ask questions, comment, and otherwise contribute
- Make smooth transitions to new or related topics
- Entertain others through humor, drama, and appropriate body language
- Avoid gossiping, swearing, and making hurtful comments

SLP can assist the individual to acquire positive conversational skills by serving as a supportive scaffold. A list of possible intervention goals is contained in Table 4–10, and key features of effective intervention are

Table 4–9. Conversational Behaviors of Some Students Who Have Language Disorders

---

As conversationalists, some older children and adolescents with language disorders may do the following (Brinton, Robinson, & Fujiki, 2004; Paul & Norbury, 2012; Paul et al., 2009):

- Make few topic-relevant comments
- Fail to ask the speaker questions that clarify or extend the topic
- Have little to say of interest to others
- Talk excessively about topics of high personal interest
- Pay little attention to what others are saying (poor listening skills)
- Provide too little or too much information, based on needs of listener
- Show little awareness of listener's background (knowledge, opinions, feelings)
- Respond poorly to listener's verbal and nonverbal cues (e.g., boredom, sadness, interest, empathy)
- Make hurtful, biased, or inaccurate comments about others
- Laugh inappropriately (e.g., at others' misfortunes, foibles)

Table 4–10. Possible Intervention Goals for Older Children and Adolescents With Deficient Conversational Skills

---

During conversations with peers, the student will:

- Identify topics that are of high interest to others, especially to peers
- Learn about a range of topics of general interest to others
- Make appropriate transitions to new or related topics of interest to others
- Listen closely to others in order to ask questions and make topic-relevant comments
- Ask appropriate questions at the right time
- Attend closely to verbal and nonverbal cues indicating others' mental states (e.g., boredom, sadness, interest, empathy)
- Show empathy, understanding, and concern for others in verbal and nonverbal ways, including positive tone of voice, facial expressions, and body language
- Make validating and positive comments (e.g., that compliment, agree, encourage, comfort)
- Share information that is appropriate in terms of the type and amount
- Speak in an organized and coherent fashion that others can follow

---

listed in Table 4–11. In addition, Hoskins (1996) has written an excellent guidebook on how to build conversational skills in school-age children and adolescents, focusing on syntax, the lexicon, and pragmatics. Other helpful sources of information on how to design intervention to support students' conversational skills may be found in Brinton, Robinson, and Fujiki (2004) and Paul and Norbury (2012). During adolescence, it is especially important to address pragmatic skills in the context of conversations. This is because between ages 12 and 18 years, young people spend increasing amounts of time in conversations with peers—in person or on phones—sharing information, building solidarity, and helping each other solve complex problems (Nippold, 2007). The ability to use language to convey subtle and sophisticated thoughts to peers is essential for an adolescent's social development, self-esteem, personal identity, and well-being (Schickedanz et al., 2001).

Table 4–11. Key Features of Effective Intervention for Conversational Skills in Older Children and Adolescents (Adapted from Walker, Schwarz, & Nippold, 1994)

- The SLP directly and systematically teaches the targeted behavior(s) through explanation, modeling, use of video clips, and role-play.

- The student practices the targeted behavior(s) with peers in small group settings.

- The SLP provides clear, specific, and corrective feedback on the student's performance.

- When ready, the student practices the new behavior(s) in settings beyond the treatment room (e.g., cafeteria, gymnasium, classroom, school bus, shopping mall).

- The SLP provides feedback to the student on the targeted behavior(s) in natural communication settings (e.g., through coaching, cueing, and debriefing).

- The SLP provides tangible or social rewards for appropriate conversational behaviors.

CHAPTER 5

Narrative Discourse

Narrative discourse is the use of language to tell stories based on real (factual) or imaginary (fictional) events, or a combination of the two. Factual narration occurs, for example, when a 10-year-old boy tells his parents about an event that happened at school, but fictional narration occurs when he tells his brother a fairy tale (e.g., *Jack and the Beanstalk*). However, when that same boy entertains his classmates with a story based on real and imagined events, he is engaging in creative narration. In all cases, narrative discourse, a monologue, is a more challenging genre than conversational discourse, mainly because the narrative speaker bears the primary responsibility for the production of discourse that is clear, organized, and understood by others. In contrast, the dialogic nature of a conversation offers the speaker greater support from the listener who can interrupt, make comments, ask questions, or request additional information.

Narrative speaking is essential for building relationships with others by sharing thoughts, experiences, and cultural differences. However, it can be especially difficult for preschool children (Frizelle, Thompson, McDonald, & Bishop, 2018), and thus it is often not assessed by speech-language pathologists (SLPs) until children are at least 5 years old and in kindergarten. During the school-age and adolescents years, narrative discourse gradually develops as the stories that are formulated or retold become longer and more detailed, better organized, contain longer and more complex sentences, and include a greater number and variety of literate words (Nippold, 2016). In addition, older children and adolescents evidence better perspective-taking ability and therefore tend to say more about the thoughts, feelings, and attitudes of the characters.

However, many school-age children and adolescents who have language disorders struggle with narrative discourse. For example, during story retelling tasks, these students, compared to their age-matched peers with typical language development, often produce shorter and simpler stories that contain fewer complex sentences and more grammatical errors, and they are less likely to comment on the internal states of the characters in a story such as their thoughts, beliefs, emotions, plans, or perspectives (Fey, Catts, Proctor-Williams, Tomblin, & Zhang, 2004; Gillam & Johnston, 1992; Guo, Eisenberg, Schneider, & Spencer, 2020; Guo & Schneider, 2016; Liles, 1987; McFadden & Gillam, 1996; Merritt & Liles, 1987; Norbury & Bishop, 2003; Strong & Shaver, 1991; Wetherell, Botting, & Conti-Ramsden, 2007).

There are several reasons to address narrative discourse during intervention for children and adolescents who have language disorders. First, the ability to tell engaging stories can contribute to positive interactions with peers, adults, and others, helping build strong relationships through the life span. Second, students in elementary, middle, and high school are often evaluated on their ability to read, retell, and discuss stories from the classroom, such as folk tales, legends, and fables. Third, proficiency with narrative speaking, listening, reading, and writing is a prominent part of the Common Core State Standards (CCSS) beginning in second grade and continuing through high school (National Governors Association Center for Best Practices and Council of Chief State School Officers, 2010). Fourth, intervention for narrative discourse presents the opportunity to address multiple aspects of later language development, including syntax, the literate lexicon, and pragmatics. Samples of narrative discourse, if properly elicited, transcribed, and analyzed, can provide useful information about a student's competence with this genre, thereby offering direction for establishing goals and carrying out intervention.

NARRATIVE LANGUAGE SAMPLING TASKS

Table 5–1 contains a list of tasks that can be used to elicit narrative language samples, indicating the age range for which each task is appropriate. These tasks are described next

SALT's Narrative Story Retell Database

The Systematic Analysis of Language Transcripts' (SALT) Narrative Story Retell Database (Miller, Andriacchi, & Nockerts, 2019) contains stories that are appropriate for children between the ages of 4 and 12 years, or in preschool through sixth grade. They include *Frog, Where Are You?* (FWAY; Mayer, 1969), *Pookins Gets Her Way* (PGHW; Lester, 1987), *A Porcupine*

Table 5–1. Language Sampling Tasks for Narrative Discourse

Language Sampling Task	Age Range
SALT's Narrative Story Retell Database (Miller et al., 2019)	4;4–12;8
Frog, Where Are You? (FWAY; Mayer, 1969)	4;4–7;5
Pookins Gets Her Way (PGHW; Lester, 1987)	7;0–8;11
A Porcupine Named Fluffy (APNF; Lester, 1986)	7;11–9;11
Doctor De Soto (DDS; Steig, 1982)	9;3–12;8
Edmonton Narrative Norms Instrument (ENNI; Schneider et al., 2005)	4;0–9;11
Expression, Reception & Recall of Narrative Instrument (ERRNI; Bishop, 2004)	4;0–15;0+
Fables Task: Mice in Council + Monkey & Dolphin (Nippold, Frantz-Kaspar, et al., 2014)	13;0–24;11
What Happened One Day (Sun & Nippold, 2012)	10;5–17;10

Named Fluffy (APNF; Lester, 1986), and *Doctor De Soto* (DDS; Steig, 1982). Using these materials, the SLP can elicit a spoken narrative sample. The sample should be audio-recorded, transcribed verbatim, and entered into SALT software for analysis. The child's performance can then be compared to that of age-matched or grade-matched typical peers selected from the SALT database, in which norms are available for measures such as mean length of utterance in words (MLU-w), mean length of utterance in morphemes (MLU-m), total number of words, and total number of different words. For some stories, norms for the subordination index (SI) composite are also available. All participants in the normative data collection project spoke English, were living in the United States (California or Wisconsin), and represented a range of socioeconomic backgrounds and ability levels. All had typical language development.

The story FWAY, for ages 4;4 to 7;5, is accompanied by a wordless picture book and a script for the examiner to use. As the child looks at the pictures, the examiner tells the story by following—but not reading—the script. The child is then asked to tell the story back to the examiner, looking at the pictures, one at a time. For PGHW (ages 7;0–8;11), APNF (ages 7;11–9;11), and DDS (ages 9;3–12;8), the procedures are similar. However, for these three stories, there are two versions of each book—one with pictures and printed words and the other with pictures only. To present a story, the examiner uses the book that has both pictures and words, and reads the story to the child while pointing to the pictures. Then, the examiner presents the wordless book to the child and asks him or her to retell the story while looking at the pictures. These materials can be purchased through SALT's website (http://www.saltsoftware.com).

In addition to the narrative retell databases from English-speaking children, SALT also has databases from bilingual Spanish–English-speaking children ages 5 through 7 years (kindergarten through third grade) retelling frog stories. These stories include FWAY (Mayer, 1969) for ages 5;0 to 9;9; *Frog Goes to Dinner* (Mayer, 1974) for ages 5;5 to 8;11, and *Frog on His Own* (Mayer, 1973) for ages 6;0 to 7;9. All bilingual children who participated in the normative data collection project spoke Spanish as their native language, were living in the United States (Texas or California), and represented diverse socioeconomic levels. The reader is referred to Rojas and Iglesias (2019) and Miller et al. (2019, Appendix G) for details on how to use these stories and databases with Spanish–English bilingual children.

Edmonton Narrative Norms Instrument

The Edmonton Narrative Norms Instrument (ENNI; Schneider, Dubé, & Hayward, 2005) is a narrative speaking task for children ages 4 through 9 years that uses a story formulation approach. So rather than retelling a story told by the examiner, as with the SALT story retells, the child views a set of pictures in sequence that depict a story. After studying the pictures carefully, the child tells the story to the examiner while looking at each picture in sequence. The child's story is audio-recorded, transcribed verbatim, and may be entered into SALT for analysis and calculation of factors such as the mean length of C-unit (MLCU), clausal density (CD), the total number of utterances or C-units (TCU) produced, and the total number of words (TWD) produced.

Six stories and a training story are available. The stories range from simple to complex, involve two to four cartoon characters, and depict the interactions between animals such as a giraffe and an elephant, and a rabbit and a dog. For example, in a story called *Airplane*, a giraffe is showing his toy airplane to an elephant, who then grabs it from him and accidentally drops it into a swimming pool, where it begins to sink. Unfortunately, neither character is able to reach the airplane to retrieve it. When another elephant, a lifeguard, attempts to reach the airplane, he too is unsuccessful. However, a third elephant who is swimming in the pool sees the airplane, grabs it before it sinks, and returns it to the giraffe, leading to a happy ending for all.

All materials including the pictures and directions are freely available for download from the ENNI website. In addition, normative data were collected for the ENNI from 377 English-speaking children aged 4;0 to 9;11, living in Edmonton, Canada, and norms are available for metrics such as MLCU, subordination index, and TWD.

Expression, Reception, and Recall of Narrative Instrument

The Expression, Reception, and Recall of Narrative Instrument (ERRNI; Bishop, 2004) is a tool that may be used to elicit spoken narrative language samples from children and adolescents. Normative data for MLU-w in the form of percentiles and standard scores are available for speakers aged 3 to 15 years or older. All participants in Bishop's (2004) normative data collection project spoke British English and were living in England. Data reported by Bishop for MLU-w at various ages are contained in Table 5–2.

Table 5–2. Normative Data from the *Expression, Reception, and Recall of Narrative Instrument* (ERRNI) [Data Adapted from Bishop (2004), Normative Tables, pp. 112–145]

	MLU-w*	
Age Range	**Fish Story**	**Beach Story**
4;0–4;3	4.50–4.74	5.75–5.99
4;4–4;7	5.00–5.24	6.25–6.49
4;8–4;11	5.50–5.74	6.50–6.74
5;0–5;3	6.00–6.24	6.75–6.99
5;4–5;7	6.25–6.49	7.00–7.24
5;8–5;11	6.75–6.99	7.25–7.74
6;0–6;5	7.00–7.24	7.75–7.99
6;6–6;11	7.50–7.74	8.00–8.24
7;0–7;5	7.75–7.99	8.25–8.49
7;6–7;11	8.00–8.24	8.50–8.74
8;0–8;5	8.25–8.49	8.50–8.74
8;6–8;11	8.50–8.74	8.75–8.99
9;0–9;11	8.50–8.74	9.00–9.24
10;0–10;11	8.75–8.99	9.25–9.49
11;0–12;11	8.75–8.99	9.50–9.74
13;0–14;11	9.00–9.24	9.75–9.99
15;0 or older	10.25–10.49	10.25–10.49

*The MLU-w range is at or near the 50th percentile for each age group.

Like the ENNI, the ERRNI uses a story formulation procedure, but the ERRNI was designed for a broader age range than the ENNI. With the ERRNI, two stories are available, *The Beach Story* and *The Fish Story*. For each story, the speaker is shown a series of 15 colorful pictures of children, adults, and animals that depict an unusual event (e.g., a bird steals a girl's wristwatch left lying on the beach). After studying the pictures, the speaker is asked to tell the story to the examiner, focusing on one picture at a time, in sequence. The examiner audio-records the story and later transcribes it verbatim, breaking it into utterances, where each utterance consists of "a main clause together with any dependent clauses" (Bishop, 2004, p. 27), which is essentially a communication unit (C-unit). The speaker's narrative sample can then be interpreted using age-based normative data consisting of percentiles and standard scores provided by the ERRNI. The ERRNI also allows the examiner to score the speaker's story content using a check sheet that lists the essential ideas or propositions expressed in the story. Alternatively, the SLP can enter the transcribed narrative sample into SALT; insert the SI code after each utterance; and allow SALT to calculate MLU-w, the SI composite, total utterances, and other key variables.

There are two parallel forms of the ERRNI, *The Fish Story* and *The Beach Story*, which can be used for pre- and post-intervention purposes. After the initial storytelling has been completed, the ERRNI also provides the option of having the speaker recall the story and retell it from memory, without looking at the pictures. After the story recall activity has been completed, the examiner can ask questions to examine literal (e.g., "What sort of pet does the boy have?") and inferential (e.g., "How did the boy feel when he found the doll in his bag?") comprehension, allowing the speaker to refer to the pictures. Thus, the purpose of the recall activity is to determine how well the speaker remembered the details of the story and understood its meaning. The ERRNI is available for purchase through the publisher (https://www.pearsonclinical.co.uk).

Although normative data are available for children as young as age 3 years, Bishop (2004) reported that children younger than age 5 years often had difficulty formulating a story and instead simply described the pictures. This suggests that language sampling with preschool children should involve story retelling or play-based conversations rather than story formulation tasks. Table 5–3 contains a narrative sample produced by a 10-year-old boy with specific language impairment who was telling *The Beach Story* (Bishop, 2004, pp. 41–42). For demonstration purposes, I entered the boy's sample into SALT; segmented it into C-units; inserted the SI after each C-unit; and examined the results in relation to SALT's Narrative Story Retell database, matched on age and gender. Although the ERRNI uses a story formulation task rather than a retelling task, SALT's Retell database was the closest available set of detailed normative information. The analysis indicated that the boy performed significantly below average on all key variables: MLU-w (5.97), SI composite score (0.97), total

Table 5–3. Narrative Language Sample Elicited from a 10-Year-Old Boy With SLI, Telling the *Beach Story* from the ERRNI (Used with Permission from Bishop, 2004, pp. 41–42)

MLU-w = 5.97
SI composite score = 0.97
Total complete and intelligible utterances = 30
Number of total words = 179
Number of different words = 79

C A lady talking to her brother or the dad [SI-1].
C Her asking her to go to the beach on her own [SI-2].
C Her go in her bedroom [SI-1].
C Get her things she need, a towel, a bag, and her trunks [SI-2].
C Her go on her bike to the beach [SI-1].
C Her near the beach [SI-0].
C He see a friend of hers [SI-1].
C (it s a xxxxx with a dog) [SI-X].
C Him going fishing [SI-1].
C Them at the beach [SI-0].
C Her wave to her another friend [SI-1].
C Here sand [SI-0].
C Her sand in the middle of the bike [SI-0].
C Her put everything down, her towel, bag, hat, bag and watch [SI-1].
C And bird come and nick her watch [SI-2].
C Her friend come [SI-1].
C (Doing xxx do nt know) [SI-X].
C And her come back out the water [SI-1].
C And finding her watch [SI-1].
C She can t see it [SI-1].
C Her packing away [SI-1].
C Her going to the beach again with her friend [SI-1].
C Them friend come up [SI-1].
C Him come at the field [SI-1].
C And we play with the dog [SI-1].
C We ve chased the dog [SI-1].
C Her friend holding the dog [SI-1].
C (her fixing) the man doing a star [SI-1].
C And she find her watch [SI-1].
C Then her finish [SI-1].
C And his friend going back home [SI-1].
C And the other person staying in the field [SI-1].

---

complete and intelligible utterances (30), number of total words (179), and number of different words (79). In addition, informal inspection of his sample indicated numerous morphosyntactic errors in obligatory context, including the substitution of object pronouns (her, them) for subject pronouns (she, they), the substitution of present tense (come, nick, find) for past tense (came, nicked, found) verbs, the omission of auxiliary and copula verbs (is, are), and the omission of the third person present tense marker (go for goes, put for puts). Collectively, these patterns confirm a serious deficit in expressive language development and indicate that intervention should address both morphosyntax and the production of complex sentences.

Fables Task

To evaluate narrative speaking in adolescents, Nippold, Frantz-Kaspar, et al. (2014) created the Fables Task, which involved the retelling of two fables, *The Mice in Council* and *The Monkey and the Dolphin*. Each fable was accompanied by a colorful illustration. The protocol used to present the stories and to elicit the retelling of each is shown in Table 5–4. Fables were used to elicit narrative samples in adolescents because these stories, although superficially simple, deal with complex themes (e.g., pride, collaboration, honesty, pretense) that might be of interest to adolescents, given their cognitive, social, and emotional development. It was predicted that the abstract nature of the stories would prompt complex thought and hence the use of complex syntax as the adolescents retold the fables, and that syntactic complexity during the narrative task would be greater than when those same adolescents were engaged in a formal conversational task with the examiner. The conversational task used in this study involved a structured interview in which the speaker was asked to talk about family, friends, work, travel, or hobbies.

To examine those predictions, Nippold, Frantz-Kaspar, et al. (2014) individually interviewed 40 adolescents (20 boys and 20 girls) with a mean age of 14 years. All participants had typical language development and were native speakers of American English. Each conversational and narrative sample was transcribed verbatim, coded for the use of main and subordinate clauses, and examined for MLCU and CD. Results showed that the narrative task prompted greater syntactic complexity compared with the conversational task.

In a subsequent study, Nippold, Frantz-Kaspar, and Vigeland (2017) administered the same tasks—conversational speaking and fable retelling —to 40 young adults with a mean age of 22 years who were native speakers of American English and believed to have typical language development. Results indicated that syntactic complexity was greater during the narrative task than during the conversational task, measured in terms of

Table 5–4. Narrative Speaking Task Using Fables (Nippold, Frantz-Kaspar, et al., 2014, p. 884)

(Interviewer reads the following slowly and clearly . . .)

"This is a storytelling activity that involves fables. Fables are imaginary stories about animals that act like people. I am going to read you two different fables. Please listen to each one carefully. Be ready to tell each story back to me, in your own words. Try to remember as much as you can so that you can tell the whole story back to me. After you finish, I will ask you some questions about the story. There are no penalties for incorrect answers. I just want to know what you think about the stories. Are you ready? . . . Here's the first one."

SHOW FABLE CARD TO PARTICIPANT . . .

The Mice in Council

The mice lived in constant terror of the cat, whose greatest pleasure was toying with them and eating them up. The mice called a meeting to try to solve their problems. Many plans were discussed but none seemed right. What to do about the great cat?

At last a small mouse leaped up. He drew himself up to his full height. "I propose," he said, "that a bell be hung around the cat's neck so that whenever he approaches, we will hear the bell tinkle and we shall be able to escape." All the mice applauded, and the young mouse took a few bows and then sat down.

After the motion was seconded and passed, a wise old mouse slowly rose to his feet. "My friends, fellow mice, our young friend has proposed a brilliant solution to end our constant fear and jeopardy from the cat. Only a mouse of great genius could have conceived such a simple solution, for indeed with the bell around his neck, we shall all most certainly hear Mr. Cat's no longer stealthy approach. But one question occurs to this old head. Who, may I ask, shall bell the cat?"

Moral: Some things are easier said than done (Lawrence, 1997, p. 19).

Interviewer asks participant to retell the story. . . . (Turn on audio recorder)

TURN OVER CARD TO SHOW NEXT FABLE

"Here's the next story, the last one. Listen carefully and be ready to tell it back to me."

The Monkey and the Dolphin

It was an old custom among sailors to take with them on their voyages monkeys and other pets to amuse them while they were at sea. So it happened that on a certain voyage a sailor took with him a monkey as a companion on board ship.

Off the coast of Sunium, the famous promontory of Attica, the ship was caught in a violent storm and was wrecked. All on board were thrown into the water and had to swim for land as best they could. And among them was the monkey.

A dolphin saw him struggling in the waves, and taking him for a man, went to his assistance. As they were nearing the shore just opposite Piraeus, the harbor of Athens, the dolphin spoke. "Are you an Athenian?" he asked.

"Yes, indeed," replied the monkey, as he spat out a mouthful of sea water. "I belong to one of the first families of the city."

"Then, of course, you know Piraeus," said the dolphin.

"Oh yes," said the monkey, who thought Piraeus must be the name of some distinguished citizen, "he is one of my very dearest friends."

Disgusted by so obvious a falsehood, the dolphin dived to the bottom of the sea and left the monkey to his fate.

Moral: Those who pretend to be what they are not, sooner or later, find themselves in deep water (Grosset & Dunlap, 1947, pp. 198–199).

Interviewer asks participant to retell the story. . . . (Turn on audio recorder)

MLCU and CD. In addition, upon comparing the adults to the adolescents in Nippold, Frantz-Kaspar, et al. (2014), results indicated that the groups did not differ in terms of syntactic complexity on the narrative task; however, the adults outperformed the adolescents on the conversational task on both measures of syntactic complexity, with the results reported in Table 5–5. Although these two studies did not contain enough participants to justify calling the results reported in Table 5–5 "normative data," the means for MLCU and CD may be useful as general points of reference if SLPs choose to administer the fables retelling task to adolescents and would like to interpret a student's performance informally.

It is also interesting to compare the means for MLCU in narrative speaking reported in Table 5–5 to the means for MLU reported in Table 5–2 for MLU on the ERRNI (Bishop, 2004) for the two oldest groups of participants (ages 13–14 and 15+ years). Participants in the Nippold studies spoke American English, and those in the Bishop study spoke British English; the samples were not otherwise matched, but similar procedures were used across studies for segmenting utterances and calculating MLU/MLCU. Inspection of Table 5–5 indicates that the means are higher for the Fables Task than *The Fish Story* or *The Beach Story*. Before drawing any conclusions, however, research is necessary to formally compare the two tasks with the same groups of participants to determine if the tasks differ in their capacity to elicit complex syntax.

Table 5–6 contains an example of an adolescent girl's retelling of both fables used in the Nippold, Frantz-Kaspar, et al. (2014) study. She produces

Table 5–5. Measures of Syntactic Complexity on Conversational and Narrative Speaking (Fables Task) for Adolescents and Adults (Adapted from Nippold, Frantz-Kaspar, et al., 2017, p. 1343)

	Conversational Speaking		Narrative Speaking (Fables)	
	Adolescents	Adults	Adolescents	Adults
Mean length of C-unit				
Mean	7.84	9.58	13.27	13.29
SD	1.18	1.61	2.86	2.11
Range	5.22–10.00	5.64–13.44	7.75–23.11	9.35–18.38
Clausal density				
Mean	1.36	1.68	2.46	2.49
SD	0.20	0.26	0.55	0.39
Range	0.79–1.70	1.05–2.25	1.35–4.00	1.84–3.29

Table 5–6. Adolescent Girl's Retelling of Two Fables (from the Author's Files)

Note: Each retelling has been coded for clause types. TCU = total communication units; MLCU = mean length of C-unit; CD = clausal density; MC = main clause; NOM = nominal clause; ADV = adverbial clause; REL = relative clause; INF = infinitive clause; PRT = participial clause; GER = gerundive clause.

Girl, Age 14;2

Retelling The Mice in Council (TCU = 12; MLCU = 11.92; CD = 2.17)

E Can you retell that story?

C Yeah, so the story is [MC] about a council of mice.

C And they're trying [MC] to figure [INF] out what they can do [NOM] about their problem.

C And their problem is [MC] that there's [NOM] a cat who takes [REL] advantage of them and plays [REL] with them and eats [REL] them.

C And that's [MC] obviously not good for the mice.

C So they're trying [MC] to think [INF] of a solution.

C And this little teeny mouse (he says) well he stands [MC] up.

C And he says [MC] let [NOM]'s put [INF] a bell around the cat's neck.

C And everybody's [MC] like, wow that's [NOM] amazing.

C (And the) and then (um they) they vote [MC] on it.

C And then (the) it passes [MC].

C So they're [MC] in agreement.

C And then one of the elder mice, who's obviously thought [REL] the solution out more than everybody else, (he says) he says [MC] this is [NOM] a great proposal but who is going [NOM] to put [INF] the bell on the cat?

E Nice.

E Thank you.

Retelling The Monkey and the Dolphin (TCU = 20; MLCU = 10.75; CD = 1.85)

E Can you retell the story?

C Kay, so there were [MC] (uh) sailors.

C And they were [MC] out on their ship with their pets.

C And (there) there was [MC] a storm.

C And (they got) they were stranded [MC] (I guess) in the middle of the sea.

C And (uh) they were all trying [MC] to swim [INF] back to shore.

C And some of them were probably drowning [MC] and stuff.

C And it was [MC] horrible.

C (And) and a dolphin came [MC] up to one of the pets and (uh) asked [MC] if he was [NOM] a citizen of Athens (I guess).

C And (the) the monkey decided [MC] to play [INF] up to the dolphin cause he (I guess he uh) thought [ADV] (that) that (would make) the dolphin would obviously take [NOM] him to land and he'd be [NOM] safe.

continues

81

Table 5–6. *continued*

C He'd (um) benefit [MC] from playing [GER] up the dolphin.

C And (uh) so the dolphin was asking [MC] him stuff.

C And (he was being) he was kind of boasting [MC] about it.

C And he was [MC] like oh yeah I'm [NOM] rich and famous.

C And then the dolphin asked [MC] him a pretty simple question.

C And he took [MC] it the wrong way.

C And it was [MC] obviously a lie because that's [ADV] not what it was [REL] (that's and um and).

C And the dolphin decided [MC] that he was [NOM] n't worth it because he was lied [ADV] to.

C (Um) (he wasn't) he wasn't [MC] truthful about himself (so).

E Nice.

C Do you want [MC] the moral?

E You can tell the moral, too.

C The moral was [MC] that if you pretend [ADV] to be [INF] something other than yourself, you might just find [NOM] yourself in deeper water than you were [ADV] before.

E Nice.

E Yeah, I really like the way you said that.

---

a number of long and complex utterances that contain multiple levels of clausal embedding, as in the following example from *The Mice in Council*:

> And then one of the elder mice, who's obviously thought [REL] the solution out more than everybody else, (he says) he says [MC] this is [NOM] a great proposal but who is going [NOM] to put [INF] the bell on the cat?

A similar level of syntactic complexity occurs when she states the moral of *The Monkey and the Dolphin*:

> The moral was [MC] that if you pretend [ADV] to be [INF] something other than yourself, you might just find [NOM] yourself in deeper water than you were [ADV] before.

In summary, the results of the Nippold, Frantz-Kaspar, et al. (2014) study indicate that fables can elicit the use of complex syntax in the narrative speaking of young adolescents. Future studies are needed to examine narrative speaking in adolescents with language impairments, using fables.

"What Happened One Day"

To learn about the development of written narrative production in older students, Sun and Nippold (2012) conducted a study in which 11-year-old children, 14-year-old adolescents, and 17-year-old adolescents (n = 40 per group) wrote essays at school in their classrooms. All students spoke Standard American English as their primary language and had typical language development. Titled "What Happened One Day," the essay asked them to write a story—real or imaginary—about something funny, sad, or scary that happened to them and a friend. The students were given an outline that prompted them to address a set of story grammar elements. They were also given booklets of lined paper in which to write their stories, and they were allowed 20 minutes to complete it. The task, as presented to the students, is shown in Table 5–7.

Table 5–7. Narrative Writing Task, "What Happened One Day" (Sun & Nippold, 2012, p. 12)

At this time, I would like you to write a story. Please write a story about something funny, sad, or scary that happened to you and a friend. You get to decide what to write about. It can be anything that was funny, sad, or scary. If you can't think of something that really happened, you can make it up. It doesn't have to be a true story. You can use your imagination, if you want. It's up to you.

The following outline will help you organize your thoughts and write a good story. In your story, be sure to do the following:

1. Tell where the events took place (the setting).
2. Tell who the main people are (characters).
3. Tell everything that happened in the story (plot).
4. Tell about the problems that came up (problems).
5. Explain what the characters tried to do (attempts).
6. Explain how things turned out (outcome).
7. Tell how everyone felt during the events (thoughts).

Keep this list of points in front of you as you write your story. As you address each point, try to write a full paragraph of your own ideas. You will have 20 minutes to complete your work. I have given you a booklet of lined paper to use in writing your story. Please put your name, age, and grade level on the booklet.

As you do this work, please use your best writing style with complete sentences and correct grammar, spelling, and punctuation. If you aren't sure how to spell a word, make your best guess. Try to write neatly, using a pen or pencil. If you make a mistake, just cross it out or use an eraser. Keep going until I ask you to stop writing.

Do you have any questions?

The title of your story is "What Happened One Day."

The results of the study, reported in Table 5–8, indicated that the 17-year-olds outperformed the 14- and 11-year-olds on total T-units (i.e., sentences), a measure of language productivity, and that both the 17- and 14-year-olds outperformed the 11-year-olds on mean length of T-unit (MLTU), a measure of syntactic complexity. In addition, the 14-year-olds outperformed the 11-year-olds on CD, another measure of syntactic complexity. It was also found that the oldest group used a greater number of abstract nouns (e.g., apathy, accomplishment, imagination) and metacognitive verbs (e.g., assume, reflect, ignore) than did the youngest group. Importantly, all groups appeared to enjoy the narrative activity, with many

Table 5–8. Results of Sun and Nippold (2012; Adapted from p. 6)

	Age 11	Age 14	Age 17
Total T-units (age 17 > age 14, age 11)			
Mean	19.10	23.80	30.70
SD	8.86	9.93	7.99
Range	8–46	4–44	15–46
Mean length of T-unit (age 17, age 14 > age 11)			
Mean	9.14	11.19	11.27
SD	2.22	3.93	2.07
Range	6.23–16.70	6.11–30.75	8.00–17.07
Clausal density (age 14 > age 11)			
Mean	1.50	1.71	1.63
SD	0.26	0.34	0.27
Range	1.00–2.26	1.17–2.75	1.20–2.73
Abstract nouns* (age 17 > age 11)			
Mean	8.65	14.52	19.94
SD	13.67	19.42	12.26
Range	0–84.62	0–100.00	0–46.67
Metacognitive verbs* (age 17, age 14 > age 11)			
Mean	8.29	16.42	18.99
SD	8.24	17.69	8.29
Range	0–35.00	0–91.67	7.89–36.36

*Reported as the percentage of T-units containing at least one occurrence.

of them requesting to continue writing their stories, even after the time limit had been called. This pattern suggested that the task was appropriate for students of these ages.

Table 5–9 contains examples of two narrative essays produced by participants in the Sun and Nippold (2012) study—an 11-year-old boy (Writer #1) and a 13-year-old boy (Writer #2). For each writer, MLTU and CD are reported. In addition to finite clauses (MC, REL, NOM, ADV), all nonfinite clauses are coded in these examples and included as part of the CD calculation. Nonfinite clauses include infinitives (INF), gerundives (GER), and participials (PRT). Although the two boys performed similarly in terms of MLTU, the older boy produced a higher level of CD than did the younger one, reflecting a greater amount of subordination in his essay. This can be seen by comparing each writer's longest sentence:

Writer #1: Then we had [MC] to walk [INF] way down and around the whole outside of the whole huge mall. (17 words)

Writer #2: When she went [ADV] inside to tell [INF] his dad about it, he didn't believe [MC] it either until he came [ADV] outside and saw [ADV] the broken tent and deer prints. (28 words)

Writer #1's sentence of 17 words contains only one subordinate clause, with an infinitive clause modifying the main clause. In contrast, Writer #2's sentence of 28 words contains four subordinate clauses modifying the main clause that add detailed information. Because the greater use of subordination is characteristic of more advanced syntactic development, both sentence length (MLTU) and the amount of CD in an essay should be examined.

IMPLICATIONS FOR INTERVENTION

Intervention for narrative discourse with children and adolescents who have language disorders presents an opportunity to address numerous aspects of later language development. These include organization, coherence, social perspective-taking, verbal productivity, morphosyntax, and the use of complex syntax and literate vocabulary including mental state terms such as metacognitive verbs (e.g., know, think, feel, believe). When designing intervention, macro- and microstructural elements of narrative discourse should be considered.

The macrostructure is the larger framework that includes the reasons for telling a story; the individuals who will be listening to it or reading it; and key story grammar elements that include the setting, characters,

Table 5-9. Narrative Essays Written by Two Boys With Typical Language Development (from the Author's Files)

Each essay has been coded for clause types. Note: TTU = total T-units; MLTU = mean length of T-unit; CD = clausal density; MC = main clause; NOM = nominal clause; ADV = adverbial clause; REL = relative clause; INF = infinitive clause; PRT = participial clause; GER = gerundive clause.

Writer #1: Boy, Age 11;7 (TTU = 11; MLTU = 12.18; CD = 1.73)

One day at the mall, me and my friend went [MC] to the Home Town Buffet.

I towered [MC] three to four plates of food, one dessert plate, and two sundaes.

On the other hand, my friend had [MC] very little.

Little did I know [MC] that we had [NOM] to walk [INF] all over in the mall.

So every time I saw [ADV] a bench, I would lay [MC] down for as long as I could [ADV].

Then we went [MC] to Harry Ritchie's, Game Crazy, Radio Shack, Target, and to another video game store.

My stomach was aching [MC] the whole time.

Me and my friend both agreed [MC] I ate [NOM] way too much.

Then we had [MC] to walk [INF] way down and around the whole outside of the whole huge mall.

Then we went [MC] to the other mall and walked [MC] around.

I learned [MC] never to eat [INF] that much again.

Writer #2: Boy, Age 13;8 (TTU = 12; MLTU = 12.58; CD = 2.42)

It all started [MC] when I went [ADV] to my friend's house to spend [INF] the night.

We set [MC] up a tent to sleep [INF] in.

Jim and I were playing [MC] games when we heard [ADV] something.

And the next thing we know [REL], a deer fell [MC] on his tent in the backyard.

It was [MC] pretty freaky.

We tried [MC] to kick [INF] him off the tent.

But it just kept [MC] moving [GER] around.

In the end, it got [MC] up and ran [MC] off back into the woods.

When we went [ADV] inside to tell [INF] his mom about it, she did not believe [MC] it at first because it was [ADV] pretty unbelievable.

But when she came [ADV] outside and saw [ADV] the broken tent and deer prints, she believed [MC] us.

When she went [ADV] inside to tell [INF] his dad about it, he didn't believe [MC] it either until he came [ADV] outside and saw [ADV] the broken tent and deer prints.

All in all, it was [MC] one weird night.

problems, attempts, outcomes, reactions, and ending. By talking with students about this framework and providing them with a written outline that lists the story grammar elements, the SLP can assist students to tell a well-organized, coherent story that is engaging to others. For students who do not read well, icons or pictographs can be placed next to each story grammar element so that they too can benefit from this structure. Moreover, it is important to remember that before students can tell a good story, they must have something to say. Therefore, if students are being asked to formulate a story, they must be able to make sense of the events or stimuli they will talk about, such as pictures, videos, or situations they have experienced. Similarly, if they are expected to retell a story, they must be able to comprehend and recall the main events and details and draw inferences from that information. Once these conditions are in place, students can write quick notes next to each story grammar element or icon on the outline to support the telling of a good story, which requires them to access the appropriate spoken language skills. Hence, the microstructure of a story focuses on the use of complex syntax and literate vocabulary—aspects of language that will allow students to express themselves with accuracy, clarity, and efficiency. The use of complex syntax and literate vocabulary can be addressed during storytelling or retelling activities in which sentences that contain subordinate clauses and precise and/or imaginative words are modeled by the SLP, followed by activities that are supported by evidence-based research such as sentence-combining activities (Eisenberg, 2006; Graham & Perin, 2007; Saddler & Graham, 2005; Scott & Nelson, 2009). Table 5–10 presents an overview of intervention for narrative discourse.

An example of how to carry out narrative intervention with school-age children is now offered, using a story that was drawn from a second-grade classroom, *The Drum: A Folktale from India* (Cleveland, 2006). Folk tales are often discussed in elementary school classrooms in an attempt to familiarize students with aspects of cultural diversity. As it turns out, however, folk tales often convey universal messages that speak to people from all cultures. For example, *The Drum* is a folk tale that illustrates how an attitude of kindness, generosity, and caring is like a boomerang—it comes back to the individual, bringing unexpected joy. Cleveland's version of the story is accompanied by colorful drawings of the setting, characters, objects, and events, providing contextual support for each episode and illustrating the emotions of the characters.

The Drum is a story about a young boy growing up in India with his mother. Although the boy and his mother are poor and have few possessions, the mother asks him what he would like from the market. The boy replies that he would like a drum. The mother is sad because she cannot afford to buy him a drum. However, she meets a stranger along the road who gives her a magic stick, which she gives to her son. The boy

Table 5–10. Overview of an Intervention Approach for Narrative Discourse

- The SLP works with students in small groups that meet frequently.
- Students are encouraged to support each other and to use appropriate pragmatics.
- Stories are chosen from the regular education curriculum (e.g., folk tales, legends, fables).
- The understanding of stories is promoted to support their retelling.
- Written language is used to support spoken language.
- A graphic organizer is used for each story, highlighting key story grammar elements:
  - Setting
  - Characters
  - Problems
  - Solutions/attempts
  - Outcomes
  - Reactions
  - Ending/resolution
- Students fill in the graphic organizer before attempting to retell the story.
- As a student retells a story, it is entered into a laptop computer.
- The document is saved, and changes are made as the students make progress.
- Sentence-combining activities are used to encourage complex syntax.
- Students discuss the meanings of difficult words and complex concepts contained in the story.
- Students are encouraged to think about the meaning of the story in relation to their own lives.

accepts the stick graciously, and one day when he is out walking with it, he encounters a woman who needs wood in order to light a fire to cook bread. The boy gives the stick to the woman, who lights the fire and cooks her bread. In return, she gives the boy a piece of bread. The boy then gives the bread to a hungry child, whose mother thanks the boy by giving him a large pot, which he then gives to a washer man. Through a series of similar exchanges, the boy eventually receives a drum and is thrilled beyond belief.

The Drum is a rather long story, consisting of an introduction, six episodes, and a conclusion (total of 30 pages). For this reason, when using this folk tale to work on narrative discourse with school-age children who have language disorders, the SLP may wish to break it into manageable sections and to spend one or more sessions on each part of the story, allowing time for practice and review to ensure that the children understand the story and can retell it with confidence. To illustrate how to accomplish this, let us consider a hypothetical scenario.

The SLP is working with a group of three 9-year-old boys, each having a diagnosis of specific language impairment. The group meets with the SLP at school two times per week for 30-minute sessions. Although the focus of intervention is on narrative discourse, pragmatic skills are also targeted through modeling and positive reinforcement during each session. So, based on teacher report and informal observation, it was determined that each boy needed to improve his peer interaction skills in terms of (1) listening attentively when someone else is speaking, (2) not interrupting, (3) taking turns speaking and listening, (4) making eye contact, and (5) being supportive by showing kindness and not teasing or laughing at others' mistakes or struggles.

During formal assessment, a narrative language sample using the story retelling task, *A Porcupine Named Fluffy* (Lester, 1986), was elicited from each boy. It was then transcribed and analyzed using SALT software, and the following long-term goals were established:

Goal #1: The student will understand stories drawn from the classroom.

Goal #2: The student will retell stories drawn from the classroom by:
   A. Using a greater number of subordinate clauses
   B. Using a greater number of precise words (including meta-cognitive verbs)
   C. Increasing the total number of words produced
   D. Increasing the total number of utterances produced by:
      1. Including a greater number of story grammar elements
      2. Including more references to the thoughts and feelings of the characters

For the first session, each student holds a copy of *The Drum* and follows along as the SLP reads the introduction aloud, clearly and slowly, while pointing to the illustrations. Then, each student is offered the opportunity to read the introduction, taking turns reading one sentence at a time. The SLP reads the introduction again while the students listen. The SLP then begins to ask the students some questions regarding the facts of the story to ensure that they understand it, such as "Where do the boy and his mother live?" and "What did the boy want as a gift from his mother?" Questions that require inferencing are also posed, such as "Why did the boy tell his mother, 'I know you cannot get me a drum'?" and "How did his mother feel about being unable to get a drum?" Once these questions are answered successfully, the students are ready to begin retelling the story in their own words. In doing so, they can refer to the illustrations on each page while the text is covered. Their responses could be entered into a laptop computer by the SLP or an assistant, who displays the screen for the students to see. The students can then take turns reading their sentences aloud. Next, the SLP can encourage the students to combine the simple sentences they see on the screen into one or more complex sentences through modeling, sentence imitation, sentence combining, and sentence completion activities. For example, assume that the three students produced the following simple sentences in retelling part of the introduction:

A boy lived in India.

He lived with his mother.

They did not have very much money.

Through modeling and prompting, the SLP could help the boys combine the simple sentences into one complex sentence that contains a relative clause, rewriting it as follows:

A boy and his mother *who lived in India* [REL] did not have very much money.

Following these same steps, the remainder of the introduction could be read, interpreted, and retold as the students add to the story before moving on to each of the six episodes and finally to the conclusion. During these activities, the use of subordinate clauses and precise vocabulary (e.g., magic, shivering, replied) can be prompted through the production of sentences such as the following:

The boy's mother felt [MC] sad because she could not buy [ADV] her son a drum.

Walking [PRT] along the road, she met [MC] an old man who gave [REL] her a stick.

The man told [MC] the mother that the stick might have [NOM] some magic in it.

One day, the boy met [MC] another man who was [REL] all wet and shivering [REL].

When the boy asked [ADV] the man what had happened [NOM], he replied [MC] that a robber had stolen [NOM] his clothes and had pushed [NOM] him into the river.

To encourage social perspective-taking, the students could be taught to use metacognitive verbs such as felt, feared, or worried, as they talk about the characters' thoughts in the following way:

> The boy *felt* [MC] happy when the hungry child ate [ADV] the bread.

> The washer man *feared* [MC] he would have [NOM] no pot for washing [GER] clothes.

> The father *worried* [MC] that his son's marriage would have [NOM] bad luck.

The students should practice reading these complex sentences frequently because repeated oral reading helps build fluency and reading comprehension (Reutzel, 2009; Robertson, 2009).

Eventually, the students could be prompted to retell the entire folk tale in their own words while looking at the illustrations but not reading the story or the sentences on the screen of the laptop computer. To assist with organization and content, they could refer to the story grammar outline with its highlighted words or icons as they retell the introduction, episodes, and conclusion.

Each student's progress could be monitored on a daily basis by using a check sheet that allows the SLP to record such things as how often a student used a metacognitive verb, newly learned adjective, or nominal, relative, or adverbial clause, or how often a student combined two simple sentences into one complex sentence. Following several months of intervention, another narrative language sample could be elicited, transcribed, and analyzed, again using *A Porcupine Named Fluffy* (Lester, 1986), and progress could be measured on factors such as MLCU, CD, TWD, and TCU.

It is acknowledged that assessment using language samples and intervention for narrative discourse as just described requires patience, practice, and persistence, and there is a strong need for evidence-based intervention studies in this area. Nevertheless, most SLPs have the knowledge, skill, and expertise to carry this out successfully. Our clients are counting on us.

CHAPTER 6

Expository Discourse

Expository discourse is the use of language to convey information. When working with school-age children and adolescents, it is essential that the speech-language pathologist (SLP) evaluate students' ability to express themselves using expository discourse. The reason is that expository discourse is often called upon in academic and social situations as when students give oral reports in classes such as language arts, history, and social studies or describe to their teachers and classmates how to conduct a chemistry or physics experiment. Beyond the classroom, expository discourse is called upon when children and adolescents must explain complex matters, such as how to repair a broken clock, play a new video game, or care for an injured pet. Information on the development of expository discourse is available in Nippold (2016), which emphasizes the role of epistemology as a key factor that underlies growth.

Unlike the dialogic nature of conversation, expository discourse is a monologue in which the speaker bears the primary responsibility for successful communication. It is also heavily knowledge driven (Nippold, 2010a, 2016), and for this reason, language sampling for expository discourse often focuses on academic topics, making it relevant to classroom success. Although classroom teachers are responsible for ensuring that students acquire knowledge of a particular subject, such as science, history, or mathematics, the SLP can work closely with teachers in those classes, helping build the knowledge base required to support expository discourse. This can be accomplished by targeting meaningful classroom assignments such as upcoming speeches or reports in which it is necessary to use complex syntax, literate vocabulary, and appropriate pragmatics in spoken or written language. Language samples elicited under those conditions can provide a wealth of information about the ability of school-age children and adolescents to express themselves with accuracy, clarity, and efficiency. Activities that can be implemented to build students' expository discourse skills are discussed later in this chapter.

EXPOSITORY LANGUAGE SAMPLING TASKS

In addition to collecting expository language samples in classroom settings, a number of formal tasks, drawn from the research literature, can be used. These include the Favorite Game or Sport (FGS) task (Nippold, Hesketh, Duthie, & Mansfield, 2005) and the Peer Conflict Resolution (PCR) task (Nippold, Mansfield, & Billow, 2007). Compared with conversational and narrative speaking tasks, expository tasks such as the FGS or PCR will often elicit longer and syntactically more complex utterances as the speaker calls upon specialized knowledge to explain complicated matters (Nippold, 2009, 2016). Designed by Nippold for a study of children, adolescents, and adults (Nippold, Hesketh, et al., 2005), the original FGS task (shown in Table 6–1), or a variation of it, has been used in studies with school-age children and adolescents having typical language development (TLD), specific language impairment (SLI), nonspecific language impairment (NLI), autism spectrum disorders (ASD), and traumatic brain injury (TBI) (e.g., Heilmann & Malone, 2014; Moran & Gillon, 2010; Nippold & Hesketh, 2009; Nippold, Hesketh, et al, 2005; Nippold, Mansfield, Billow, & Tomblin, 2008; Nippold, Moran, Mansfield, & Gillon, 2005; Westerveld & Moran, 2011, 2013). In addition, Systematic Analysis of Language Transcripts (SALT; Miller, Andriacchi, & Nockerts, 2019) has a large expository database using the FGS task for American English-speaking students

Table 6–1. The Favorite Game or Sport (FGS) Task (Nippold, Hesketh, et al., 2005, p. 1052)

Interviewer: I am hoping to learn what people of different ages know about certain topics. There are no penalties for incorrect answers.

1. What is your favorite game or sport?

2. Why is [e.g., chess] your favorite game?

3. I'm not too familiar with the game of [chess], so I would like you to tell me all about it. For example, tell me what the goals are, and how many people may play a game. Also, tell me about the rules that players need to follow. Tell me everything you can think of about the game of [chess] so that someone who has never played before would know how to play.

4. Now I would like you to tell me what a player should do in order to win the game of [chess]. In other words, what are some key strategies that every good player should know?

(n = 354) with TLD, ages 10 through 18 years. One unique feature of SALT's version of the FGS task is that the speaker is given a graphic organizer, or planning sheet, that lists the different questions and is encouraged to think about those questions and to write brief notes before beginning to speak. This procedure is thought to more closely resemble common academic tasks in which written language is used to support spoken language.

Favorite Game or Sport Task

With the original FGS task, the child or adolescent is asked to name a preferred game or sport and to talk about it by explaining a number of key features, including the rules, goals, and strategies needed to win the competitive activity. Because the speaker chooses the game or sport, it is assumed that he or she has some knowledge or familiarity with it. In some studies (Nippold & Hesketh, 2009; Nippold, Hesketh, et al., 2005; Nippold et al., 2008), students' performance on the FGS task was compared with their performance on a task similar to the General Conversation task shown in Table 4–3. The findings showed that both tasks were sensitive to development in the production of complex syntax during childhood and adolescence (Nippold, Hesketh, et al., 2005). However, it also was found that the FGS task elicited longer utterances with greater amounts of subordination than did the General Conversation task for students with TLD, SLI, and NLI (Nippold et al., 2008). Although the conversational task did not reveal any differences between groups, the FGS task indicated that adolescents with TLD outperformed those with SLI and NLI and that those with SLI outperformed those with NLI on standard measures of syntactic development, including mean length of C-unit (MLCU) and clausal density (CD). This suggests that the FGS expository task could be administered to gain insight into the use of complex syntax in children and adolescents with diagnosed or suspected developmental language disorders.

Table 6–2 contains excerpts from the samples of two 13-year-old boys during the FGS task. Both boys were explaining how to play football. The first speaker has SLI, and the second one has TLD. Both excerpts were entered into SALT and coded for main and subordinate clauses, including finite and nonfinite clauses. Although both excerpts are relatively short, there are some interesting points to consider. Speaker #1 produced about half as many C-units as Speaker #2, suggesting that his knowledge of football was less extensive. In addition, Speaker #1 produced shorter C-units, on average, used a smaller number and variety of subordinate clauses, and was less likely to embed subordinate clauses compared with Speaker #2, who produced C-units such as the following:

And if it's [ADV] fourth down, and you don't think [ADV] you're going [NOM] to make [INF] it, then you can punt [MC] and put [MC] the other team further in their territory.

Table 6–2. Excerpts from the Samples of Two 13-Year-Old Boys Explaining How to Play Football During the FGS Task (from the Author's Files)

Speaker #1 has SLI, and Speaker #2 has TLD. Each sample has been coded for clause types. All mazes are enclosed in parentheses. Note: TCU= total C-units; MLCU= mean length of C-unit; CD = clausal density; MC = main clause; ADV = adverbial clause; NOM = nominal clause; REL = relative clause; INF = infinitive clause; PRT = participial clause; GER = gerundive clause.

Speaker #1 (SLI): TCU = 11; MLCU = 11.00; CD = 1.73

C (OK) All you have [REL] is [MC] 11 people (on) for offense at a time.

C You only have [MC] 11 on the field at a time for your team on offense or defense.

C (um) The goal is [MC] to (run the ball) get [INF] the ball down on the other side of the field where the end zone is [REL].

C And you score [MC] six points.

C If you make [ADV] a field goal, you get [MC] one point.

C And if you go [ADV] (for two for an extra poi) for a two point conversion, you get [MC] two points.

C You kick [MC] the ball.

C If you score [ADV], you kick [MC] the ball off to the other team.

C And they run [MC] it.

C (and then you get a chance to like) There's [MC] four downs.

C And if you only get [ADV] the four downs for the first ten yards, (and) you got [MC] to (like) give [INF] the ball to the other team.

Speaker #2 (TLD): TCU = 21; MLCU = 12.10; CD = 2.29

C (OK) There are [MC] 11 people on each team (that can) that's [REL] on the field at a time.

C So there's [MC] 22 total.

C (um) Positions are [MC] quarterback who throws [REL] the ball for people to catch [INF].

C And then there's [MC] the receivers who try [REL] to catch [INF] passes.

C (um) There's [MC] a running back.

C There's [MC] actually three running backs.

C There's [MC] a running back, a tailback, and a fullback (um) who all get [REL] hand offs and try [REL] to run [INF] up field.

C And then the rest are [MC] linemen who protect [REL] the quarterback and make [REL] holes for the running backs.

C And the whole object of the game is [MC] for your offense to take [INF] the ball down the field and score [INF] a touchdown which is [REL] worth six points.

C And then after that, you kick [MC] an extra point.

C So a touchdown, if you get [ADV] the extra point, is [MC] worth seven.

C On defense, the object is [MC] to stop [INF] the other team's offense from scoring [GER].

Table 6–2. *continued*

C You get [MC] (four tries) four downs.

C And in those four downs, you have [MC] to get [INF] ten yards.

C And you get [MC] to keep [INF] the ball.

C And so (if you don't get four downs or) if you don't make [ADV] ten yards on four downs, then you lose [MC] the ball.

C And it's [MC] the other team's ball.

C And if it's [ADV] fourth down, and you don't think [ADV] you're going [NOM] to make [INF] it, then you can punt [MC] and put [MC] the other team further in their territory.

C And some of the rules are [MC] you have [NOM] to stay [INF] on your side of the line of scrimmage until the ball's hiked [ADV].

C (um) You can't block [MC] someone from behind.

C And there's [MC] no late hits or anything like that.

Peer Conflict Resolution Task

The PCR task, shown in Table 6–3, like the FGS task, has been used in research with adolescents having TLD, SLI, NLI, and ASD (Nippold & Hesketh, 2009; Nippold et al., 2007; Nippold, Mansfield, Billow, & Tomblin, 2009). However, unlike the FGS task, which can also be used with younger school-age children, the PCR task is most appropriate for students who are at least 10 years old. Adapted from Selman, Beardslee, Schultz, Krupa, and Podorefsky (1986), the PCR task requires the student to listen to a set of conflicts between young people and to retell each one to the examiner. After retelling a conflict, the student is asked a set of questions that prompt him or her to reflect on the underlying issues, suggest ways they might be resolved, explain why those solutions might be successful, and speculate on how the characters then might feel as a result of using the suggested strategies. In answering those questions, the student engages in expository discourse.

The PCR task is most appropriate for adolescents because they are in a developmental stage in which peer interaction is of primary importance as they learn about appropriate social behavior. Peers also are a major source of emotional support for many adolescents. Because interpersonal conflicts can be challenging to resolve and may be approached from multiple perspectives, the PCR task may stimulate complex thought and sophisticated reasoning as the issues are considered. Hence, the task may prompt adolescents to access and employ the complex syntax (i.e., subordinate clauses) that they do possess as they articulate their views.

Table 6–3. Peer Conflict Resolution Task (Nippold et al., 2007, p. 187)

Interviewer: People are always running into problems with others at school, at work, and at home. Everyone has to work out ways to solve these problems. I am going to read you two different stories that illustrate these types of problems. I would like you to listen carefully and be ready to tell each story back to me, in your own words. Then I will ask you some questions about the story. There are no penalties for incorrect answers. I just want to know what you think about the issues and how they should be handled.

(In presenting the task, the interviewer should use male names with male students, and female names with female students. This pattern may increase the likelihood that students would be able to relate to the characters' actions, challenges, and emotions.)

Story A: "The Science Fair"

John's (Debbie's) teacher assigned him (her) to work with three other boys (girls) on a project for the science fair. The boys (girls) decided to build a model airplane that could actually fly. All of the boys (girls) except one, a boy (girl) named Bob (Melanie), worked hard on the project. Bob (Melanie) refused to do anything and just let the others do all the work. This bothered John (Debbie) very much.

Now I'd like you to tell the story back to me, in your own words. Try to tell me everything you can remember about the story . . .

Now I'd like to ask you some questions about the story:

1. What is the main problem here?
2. Why is that a problem?
3. What is a good way for John (Debbie) to deal with Bob (Melanie)?
4. Why is that a good way for John (Debbie) to deal with Bob (Melanie)?
5. What do you think will happen if John (Debbie) does that?
6. How do you think they both will feel if John (Debbie) does that?

Story B: "The Fast-Food Restaurant"

Mike and Peter (Jane and Kathy) work at a fast-food restaurant together. It is Mike's (Jane's) turn to work on the grill, which he (she) really likes to do, and it is Peter's (Kathy's) turn to do the garbage. Peter (Kathy) says his (her) arm is sore and asks Mike (Jane) to switch jobs with him (her), but Mike (Jane) doesn't want to lose his (her) chance on the grill.

Now I'd like you to tell the story back to me, in your own words. Try to tell me everything you can remember about the story . . .

Now I'd like to ask you some questions about the story:

1. What is the main problem here?
2. Why is that a problem?
3. What is a good way for Mike (Jane) to deal with Peter (Kathy)?
4. Why is that a good way for Mike (Jane) to deal with Peter (Kathy)?
5. What do you think will happen if Mike (Jane) does that?
6. How do you think they both will feel if Mike (Jane) does that?

As with the FGS task, the PCR task was sensitive to developmental growth in syntax in terms of MLCU, CD, and the use of nominal and relative clauses (Nippold et al., 2007). In addition, findings revealed that adolescents with TLD outperformed their peers with SLI and NLI on measures of syntactic development, which included MLCU, CD, and nominal clause production (Nippold et al., 2009). As with the FGS task, performance on the PCR task in students with ASD yielded mixed findings (see Chapter 8), with some of them requiring significant amounts of scaffolding to perform the task.

Table 6–4 contains excerpts from the samples of two 15-year-old boys during the PCR task. Speaker #1 has SLI, and Speaker #2 has TLD. In terms of the quantitative measures, Speaker #2 outperformed Speaker #1 on all key variables: TCU, MLCU, and CD. Qualitatively, it is interesting to examine the content of their responses to the examiner's questions, with Speaker #2 showing slightly more insight into the complexity of the issues than Speaker #1, who tended to respond in a simplistic fashion. For example, in response to the question, "How do you think they both will feel if John does that?" Speaker #2 suggested that John would have mixed emotions (feeling fine but also disappointed), whereas Speaker #1 suggested that John would be happy. Speaker #2 also used more sophisticated vocabulary (e.g., *confronts, decides, refuses, disappoint, displeased*) than Speaker #1 (e.g., *tell, like, happy, angry, mad*) in his responses.

Table 6–4. Excerpts from the Spoken Language Samples of Two 15-Year-Old Boys During the PCR Task (from the Author's Files)

Speaker #1 has SLI, and Speaker #2 has TLD. Each sample has been coded for clause types. All mazes are enclosed in parentheses. Note: TCU= total C-units; MLCU= mean length of C-unit; CD = clausal density; MC = main clause; ADV = adverbial clause; NOM = nominal clause; REL = relative clause; INF = infinitive clause; PRT = participial clause; GER = gerundive clause.

Speaker #1 (SLI): TCU = 10; MLCU = 10.44; CD = 2.20

E What is the main problem here?

C John didn't like [MC] what Bob was doing [NOM].

E Why is that a problem?

C Because John doesn't like [MC] when people don't help [NOM] on projects that they're assigned [REL] to.

E What is a good way for John to deal with Bob?

C Go [MC] to the teacher and tell [MC] the teacher Bob wasn't doing [NOM] it.

C And have [MC] Bob removed [PRT] from the group.

E What do you think will happen if John does that?

continues

Table 6–4. *continued*

C Either Bob will get [MC] mad (and help) and tell [MC] the teacher that he'll help [NOM] more.

C (or he'll just take ou get out get taken out of the) Or he'll respect [MC] the teacher (and not get) and get taken [MC] out of that and put [MC] in a different group.

E How do you think they both will feel if John does that?

C (angry)

C (he) He'll be [MC] happy.

C John will be [MC] happy, more satisfied.

C and Bob will be [MC] angry because he's gonna [ADV] get [INF] a failed grade for not helping [GER].

Speaker #2 (TLD): TCU = 13; MLCU = 13.00; CD = 2.77

E What is the main problem here?

C Bob will not work [MC].

E Why is that a problem?

C (uh) When you have [ADV] one person unwilling [PRT] to do [INF] any work, that means [MC] your other people in the group have [NOM] to work [INF] harder and pick [INF] up the slack for him.

E What is a good way for John to deal with Bob?

C (uh) He can confront [MC] Bob and ask [MC] him to work [INF].

C And if Bob still refuses [ADV], he can go [MC] to the teacher and ask [MC] that Bob be switched [NOM] or removed [NOM].

E What do you think will happen if John does that?

C Well, if he confronts [ADV] Bob, and Bob decides [ADV] "(fine) I'll work" [NOM], Bob will work [MC], not very well, and very disgruntily.

C If he confronts [ADV] the teacher about it, the teacher will ask [MC] the other members of the group.

C And if they all (give) give [ADV] the same answer, Bob will be removed [MC] from group.

C He will either be replaced [MC].

C Or they will end [MC] up working [PRT] by themselves still.

E How do you think they both will feel if John does that?

C John will be [MC] (uh) fine with it because now he won't have [ADV] to make [INF] up for someone else's slack.

C But it will also disappoint [MC] him because he'd still have [ADV] to do [INF] more work.

C Bob will be [MC] displeased.

C He'll have [MC] to do [INF] his own project.

Written Language

The Nature of Friendship Task

To examine the development of expository discourse in written language, Nippold and Sun (2010) conducted a study in which 11-year-old children (fifth grade) and 14-year-old adolescents (eighth grade; $n = 40$ per group) were asked to write an expository essay in their classrooms at school. The expository essay, titled "The Nature of Friendship," asked the students to discuss friendship and its importance, activities that friends enjoy, and factors that can build or damage friendships. The students were given an outline or graphic organizer that contained a list of points they should address as they wrote their essays. They also were given a booklet of lined paper in which to write their essays and were allowed 20 minutes to complete their work. The task and the graphic organizer are shown in Table 6–5.

Table 6–5. Expository Writing Task, "The Nature of Friendship" (Nippold & Sun, 2010, p. 102)

At this time, I would like you to write an essay. Please write an essay on the topic of friendship. Friendship is very important to people of all ages—children, adolescents, and adults. Most people say they enjoy spending time with their friends. They like to talk with their friends in person or on the phone and spend time together.

The following outline will help you organize your thoughts and write a strong essay. In your essay, be sure to explain the following:

1. What is friendship?
2. Why is it important to people?
3. How can friendship make life more enjoyable?
4. What kinds of things do friends like to do together?
5. How can people become good friends?
6. What kinds of actions can damage friendships?
7. How can people remain good friends over time?

Keep this list of questions in front of you as you write your essay. As you answer each question, try to write a full paragraph of your own ideas. You will have 20 minutes to complete your work. I have given you a booklet of lined paper to use in writing your essay. Please put your name, age, and grade level on the booklet.

As you do this work, use your best writing style with complete sentences and correct grammar, spelling, and punctuation. If you aren't sure how to spell a word, make your best guess. Try to write neatly, using a pen or pencil. If you make a mistake, just cross it out or use an eraser. Keep going until I ask you to stop writing.

Do you have any questions?

The title of your essay is "The Nature of Friendship."

Nippold and Sun (2010) found that the eighth graders outperformed the fifth graders on total words and sentences produced and on mean length of T-unit (MLTU). Table 6–6 contains examples of expository essays written by two students who participated in the study, an 11-year-old girl (Writer #1) and a 13-year-old girl (Writer #2). Both MLTU and CD are

Table 6–6. Excerpts of Expository Essays Written by Two Girls with Typical Language Development (from the Author's Files)

Each essay has been coded for clause types. Note: TTU = total T-units; MLTU = mean length of T-unit; CD = clausal density; MC = main clause; NOM = nominal clause; ADV = adverbial clause; REL = relative clause; INF = infinitive clause; PRT = participial clause; GER = gerundive clause.

Writer #1: Girl, Age 11;0 (TTU = 22; MLTU = 12.05; CD = 2.64)

Do you know [MC] what friendship is [NOM]?

I do [MC].

So let [MC] me tell [INF] you.

Friendship is [MC] something you have [REL] between someone, someone you can trust [REL] and rely [REL] on.

They should be [MC] nice and thoughtful.

Also, they should never do [MC] mean or bad things to you or others.

It is [MC] important to people because you have [ADV] someone you can let [REL] something out to.

Plus they feel [MC] they have [NOM] someone always there for them.

Maybe also because then if they get [ADV] picked on, they have [MC] someone to have [INF] to help [INF] them out.

And it is [MC] fun to have [INF] friendship.

Friendship can make [MC] your life more enjoyable because you have [ADV] someone to laugh [INF] with and play [INF] with.

You can have [MC] at least someone to talk [INF] to and listen [INF] to.

When you have [ADV] a friend, you can do [MC] a lot of things like go [NOM] to the mall in addition play [NOM] board games.

They also like [MC] to just hang [INF] out with each other.

You can become [MC] a good friend by not yelling [GER] at people and using [GER] bad words because that makes [ADV] people think [NOM] you are [NOM] a bad person.

People will find [MC] out that you are [NOM] like that.

Table 6-6. *continued*

And nobody will want [MC] to be [INF] your friend.

Also you never want [MC] to lie [INF].

Or people won't trust [MC] you.

A lot of things can ruin [MC] your friendship like telling [GER] people their private things like family history, who they like [NOM], what they don't like [NOM] about people, and telling [GER] about embarrassing moments.

Also if someone moves [ADV] or leaves [ADV] for awhile, get [MC] their email address or phone number.

I hope [MC] your friendship lasts [NOM] a long time.

Writer #2: Girl, Age 13;10 (TTU = 15; MLTU = 16.47, CD = 3.87)

Friendship is [MC] a strong bond between two or more people.

It is [MC] important to people because it is [ADV] someone they can talk [REL] to, hang [REL] out with, or share [REL] secrets.

Friendship is [MC] an important part of life.

It makes [MC] life more enjoyable because you are [ADV] not depressed all the time and sad and lonely.

They make [MC] life more fun.

Best friends usually hang [MC] out together, sometimes go [MC] to the mall, watch [MC] a movie, stay [MC] the night at each other's house, share [MC] their problems, and give [MC] advice.

They pretty much do [MC] everything together.

Becoming [GER] someone's best friend includes [MC] earning [GER] trust, honesty, being [GER] nice.

Most friends have [MC] a lot in common or share [MC] the same interests.

The type of actions that can damage [REL] friendships are [MC] like backstabbing [GER] most of the time, lying [GER], or being [GER] rude, fighting [GER] in most girls' friendships, fighting [GER] over boys and who likes [NOM] who.

Stealing [GER] your friend's stuff could ruin [MC] a friendship.

Keeping [GER] a friendship and making [GER] it last a lifetime means [MC] being [GER] trustworthy, being [GER] honest, sharing [GER] your problems, trying [GER] not to fight [INF] with them or make [INF] them mad at you.

If you think [ADV] you two have [NOM] a problem and no one is trying [NOM] to work [INF] it out, just ignoring [GER] it, then try [MC] to talk [INF] to them about it and be [MC] open, help [MC] them with their problems, and help [MC] them through life, helping [PRT] make [INF] important decisions.

Just always be [MC] there for them all the time by their side all day every day.

That is [MC] what friendship is [NOM] all about, right?

substantially higher in the older girl's essay. The longest sentence in each girl's essay is shown here:

Writer #1: A lot of things can ruin [MC] your friendship like telling [GER] people their private things like family history, who they like [NOM], what they don't like [NOM] about people, and telling [GER] about embarrassing moments.

Writer #2: If you think [ADV] you two have [NOM] a problem and no one is trying [NOM] to work [INF] it out, just ignoring [GER] it, then try [MC] to talk [INF] to them about it and be [MC] open, help [MC] them with their problems, and help [MC] them through life, helping [PRT] make [INF] important decisions.

The sentence produced by Writer #1 contains four subordinate clauses, and each modifies the main clause; no subordinate clauses in this sentence are embedded within other subordinate clauses. Hence, there is only one level of hierarchical complexity. In contrast, the sentence produced by Writer #2 contains four coordinated main clauses, eight subordinate clauses, and three levels of hierarchical complexity where subordinate clauses that modify main clauses are themselves modified by other subordinate clauses.

Enhancing Expository Discourse in Young School-Age Children

Intervention for expository discourse is an opportunity to promote the use of complex sentences in young school-age children with language disorders. With kindergarten and first-grade children, this can be accomplished during cognitively stimulating activities such as science experiments tied to the curriculum. For example, the SLP can encourage children, working in small groups, to talk about the results of a science experiment while providing frequent exposure to sentences that contain subordinate clauses (Curran & Owen Van Horne, 2019). For example, complex sentences that contain *adverbial* clauses can be elicited through questions, recasts, and modeling, as in this hypothetical exchange between the SLP and a group of kindergarten children during a science lesson on how different colors are formed:

SLP: Why did the blue paint turn green?

Child: Cause I add yellow paint.

SLP: Yes, the blue paint **turned** green because you **added** yellow paint!

SLP: Now you tell me all about it.

Child: Blue paint turn green 'cause I add yellow!

SLP: Yes, the blue paint **turned** green because you **added** yellow! (speaking slowly)

Similarly, *relative* clauses can be elicited during science lessons when, for example, children are learning about different types of foods and are prompted to talk about them, as in this example:

SLP: Who can find a fruit that is very large, green on the outside, and red on the inside?

Child: I can! I can! It a watermelon!

SLP: Yes, a watermelon is a fruit that is very large.

SLP: Now you tell me all about a watermelon.

Child: It a fruit. It large!

SLP: Yes, it is a fruit **that** is very large and green on the outside. (speaking slowly)

Nominal clauses can be taught by focusing on early metacognitive verbs, such as "know," "think," and "believe," and asking children what they have learned, as in this example:

SLP: Who knows what is inside the watermelon?

Child: I know! I know! Juice and seeds!

SLP: Yes, you know what is inside the watermelon.

SLP: Tell me all about it. What do you know?

Child: I know what inside the watermelon—juice and seeds!

SLP: Yes, you know that juice and seeds are inside a watermelon! (speaking slowly)

Of course, before children with language disorders can produce such sentences on their own, they will require a great deal of modeling and other scaffolding techniques where they are frequently asked to imitate main clauses, subordinate clauses, and full sentences; to complete those sentences when provided with just a prompt (e.g., "I know that watermelons . . . "); and to combine simple sentences (e.g., "I know something about watermelons. They have juice and seeds inside"; "They are green on the outside. They are red on the inside.") into longer, complex sentences (e.g., "I know that watermelons have juice and seeds inside"; "Although watermelons are green on the outside, they are red on the inside."). In these contexts, the SLP will also need to spend time addressing common errors in the use of grammatical morphemes (e.g., past tense -*ed*, copula verb *is*). However, this type of intervention for complex syntax can and should proceed before children have fully mastered these and other grammatical morphemes, because the ability to use complex syntax will enable them to express their own thoughts and ideas more efficiently than if they were limited to producing a string of fragments or simple sentences.

Enhancing Expository Discourse in Older Children and Adolescents

An example of how to carry out intervention for expository discourse with older children and adolescents is now described, using a hypothetical but realistic scenario. The highlights of this approach are listed in Table 6–7. The scenario is that three 15-year-old boys with SLI have been assigned by their biology teacher to work as a group to make an oral report in class. The report will take place in approximately 4 weeks. Together, the boys choose the topic, "Life in the Grasslands." Table 6–8 presents a passage from their textbook, which will serve as a major source of information for their report. Note, however, that the passage contains many literate words that have been highlighted. In Table 6–9, the same passage is shown with

Table 6–7. Highlights of an Intervention Approach for Expository Discourse

---

- Target meaningful assignments from the classroom, e.g., oral reports.
- Work with classroom teacher to build the knowledge base in a specific domain (e.g., biology) as a foundation for strong expository discourse.
- Assign students to work cooperatively in pairs or in small groups.
- Support students as they produce an expository document.
- Use laptop computers to create a running record of the document.
- Save and continuously modify the document.
- Use sentence-combining and sentence completion activities.
- Combine the literate lexicon with complex syntax:
  o Subordinate conjunctions with adverbial clauses
  o Metacognitive/metalinguistic verbs with nominal clauses
  o Aristotelian definitions and relative clauses
- Use repeated oral reading of complex sentences.
- Encourage summarization of content.
- Provide many practice sessions of oral report to build confidence.

Table 6–8. Reading Material for Oral Report, with Literate Words Highlighted in **Bold** (Adapted from Biggs et al., 2002, p. 83)

> Textbook Passage: "Life in the Grasslands"
> Literate Vocabulary: **Nouns, Verbs, Adjectives**

Grasslands are large **communities** covered with grasses and **similar** small plants. They occur in **climates** that **experience** a dry **season**, where **insufficient** water **exists** to **support** forests. Called **prairies** in Australia, Canada, and the United States, **grasslands** contain fewer than ten to 15 trees per **hectares**, though larger numbers of trees are found near streams and other water **sources**. This **biome occupies** more area than any other **terrestrial biome**, and it has a higher **biological diversity** than deserts, often with more than 100 **species** per acre. Because they are **ideal** for growing cereal grains such as oats, rye, and wheat, which are different **species** of grasses, **grasslands** have become known as the **breadbaskets of the world**.

Source: Biggs, A., Gregg, K., Hagins, W. C., Kapicka, C., Lundgren, L., Rillero, P., & National Geographic Society, *Biology: The Dynamics of Life*, page 83, Copyright 2002, The McGraw-Hill Companies, Inc.

Table 6–9. Reading Material for Oral Report With Subordinate Clauses Highlighted in **Bold** (Adapted from Biggs et al., 2002, p. 83)

> Textbook Passage: "Life in the Grasslands"
> Subordinate Clauses: **Adverbial, Participial, Relative**

Grasslands are large communities **covered with grasses and similar small plants**. They occur in climates that **experience a dry season**, where **insufficient water exists to support forests. Called prairies** in Australia, Canada, and the United States, grasslands contain fewer than ten to 15 trees per hectares, **though larger numbers of trees are found near streams and other water sources**. This biome occupies more area than any other terrestrial biome, and it has a higher biological diversity than deserts, often with more than 100 species per acre. **Because they are ideal** for **growing cereal grains** such as oats, rye, and wheat, **which are different species of grasses**, grasslands have become known as the breadbaskets of the world.

Source: Biggs, A., Gregg, K., Hagins, W. C., Kapicka, C., Lundgren, L., Rillero, P., & National Geographic Society, *Biology: The Dynamics of Life*, page 83, Copyright 2002, The McGraw-Hill Companies, Inc.

the subordinate clauses highlighted. An examination of this passage suggests that it will be challenging to the boys because it places high demands on their language skills. For example, given their documented deficits in lexical and syntactic development, they can be expected to have difficulty comprehending the passage as it is read aloud to them and when they attempt to read it to themselves. The passage also assumes some background knowledge of related topics (e.g., geography, climatology, edible plants). Despite these challenges, much can be done to help the boys succeed with their oral report, particularly when the SLP establishes reasonable goals, has a systematic plan for helping them achieve those goals, is able to work with them frequently, and maintains a positive attitude. Hence, the SLP at this school has established the following goals for each group member:

Goal #1: The student will understand passages from the biology text.

Goal #2: The student will explain the content of the passages as follows:

    A. Using a greater number of complex sentences, including

        1. Adverbial clauses

        2. Relative clauses

        3. Nominal clauses

    B. Using a greater number of words and utterances

    C. Using domain-specific technical vocabulary

To begin, it is helpful if the boys have access to a laptop computer, know how to use it, and have reasonably accurate keyboarding skills. This will allow them to create a running record of their oral report, which will be written in the expository genre. If necessary, a scribe or speech assistant may be called upon to write down what the students would like to say. This document will then be saved and modified over time as the boys make improvements to it, adding new information and using complex sentences and literate words with each intervention session.

For this group of boys, the SLP has chosen to read short excerpts of the biology passage to them because they often become frustrated with independent reading assignments. As the SLP reads the passage aloud, the boys follow along with their own printed copies of it. Then the boys are asked individually to retell as much of the excerpt as they can remember, in their own words. The exact words and sentences that they use are entered into the computer as they watch the screen. Here is what the boys have said:

Grasslands are large pieces of land.

They are covered with grasses and small plants.

Trees do not grow well in grasslands.

But sometimes trees can grow near streams or rivers.

Although this is a good start, the SLP notes that the students have produced all simple sentences. To increase their use of complex syntax, and hence the efficiency of their communication, the SLP decides to engage the boys in some sentence-combining activities, knowing that this technique is supported by research (e.g., Eisenberg, 2006; Graham & Perin, 2007; Saddler & Graham, 2005; Scott & Nelson, 2009). The SLP begins by modeling an example of this. This is what the SLP says:

Trees grow well. It rains often.

Trees grow well when . . . it rains often.

After presenting several more examples, the SLP asks the boys to combine two of the simple sentences that they have written into one complex sentence. They begin with the following sentences, which appear on the screen of the laptop computer:

Grasslands are large pieces of land.

They are covered with grasses and small plants.

To assist the boys, the SLP reads the first sentence aloud, pauses, and then prompts them to complete it with the second sentence by providing an appropriate relative pronoun:

Grasslands are large pieces of land *that* . . .

This leads the boys to produce a complex sentence that contains a relative clause:

Grasslands are large pieces of land *that are covered with grasses and small plants.*

This revised sentence is then entered into the computer, and the two simple sentences are deleted. It is noteworthy that the complex sentence the boys have just produced is actually an Aristotelian definition, which follows the formula, "An *X* is a *Y* that *Z*." Aristotelian definitions constitute a clear and efficient way to express meaning, and for this reason, they frequently occur in formal communication (Nippold, Hegel, Sohlberg, & Schwarz, 1999), including textbooks used at school (Nippold, 2016). Moreover, the ability to produce these definitions is associated closely with academic achievement in adolescents (Nippold, 1999). Table 6–10 contains an Aristotelian definition that occurred in a science textbook. It shows how multiple levels of embedding can be organized to express a large amount of information efficiently.

Table 6–10. Example of an Aristotelian Definition Contained in a Science Textbook (Biggs et al., 2002, p. 83)

| Aristotelian definitions commonly occur in expository passages: |

Other important prairie animals include prairie dogs, which are [REL] seed-eating rodents that build [REL] underground "towns" known [PRT] to stretch across mile after mile of grassland, and the foxes and ferrets that prey [REL] on them.

Source: Biggs, A., Gregg, K., Hagins, W. C., Kapicka, C., Lundgren, L., Rillero, P., & National Geographic Society, *Biology: The Dynamics of Life*, page 83, Copyright 2002, The McGraw-Hill Companies, Inc.

Next, the SLP moves to the second set of simple sentences, which appear on the computer screen:

Trees do not grow well in grasslands.

But sometimes trees can grow near streams or rivers.

Once again, the SLP reads the first sentence aloud and then pauses. This time, however, the SLP prompts the students to complete it by providing an appropriate subordinate conjunction:

Trees do not grow well in grasslands *unless* . . .

But sometimes trees can grow near streams or rivers.

This leads them to produce a complex sentence with an adverbial clause:

Trees do not grow well in grasslands *unless they are near streams or rivers*.

As before, the new sentence is entered into the laptop, and the old sentences are deleted.

Thus far, the intervention activities have prompted the boys to produce complex sentences that contain relative and adverbial clauses. To prompt the use of nominal clauses, the SLP decides to focus on some metacognitive (e.g., *assume*) and metalinguistic (e.g., *claim*) verbs that occur in other passages of the biology book.

The goal will be for the boys to produce complex sentences such as the following:

Biologists assume *that thousands of buffalo once roamed [NOM] the grasslands*.

Botanists claim *that some wildflowers grow [NOM] well in grasslands*.

These types of sentences might be elicited by asking specific questions, which require knowledge of the subject matter, and then offering a sentence to be completed:

Q: What do biologists assume?

A: They assume that . . .

Q: What do botanists claim?

A: They claim that . . .

As the boys make progress with this type of exercise, they can be encouraged to produce sentences that contain embedded subordinate clauses, for example:

Q: Why do botanists make that claim?

A: They make that claim *because they know [ADV] that certain flowers, such as blazing stars, are [NOM] drought-resistant.*

At each intervention session with the SLP, the boys will add several complex sentences to the document they are writing concerning life in the grasslands, using these types of activities. As each new sentence is added, each boy will be requested to read and reread the entire document aloud, a technique called *repeated oral reading* that helps build reading fluency and comprehension (Reutzel, 2009; Robertson, 2009). It also provides an opportunity for the boys to practice using complex sentences in oral language. Then, after repeatedly reading the document aloud, they will each be asked to summarize, in their own words, what they have written. Over time, these oral summaries should contain greater amounts of relevant information, conveyed through an increased use of complex sentences and literate words.

After spending time on these intervention activities, the boys will need to practice delivering their oral report in order to refine their speaking abilities and build their confidence. During these practice sessions, they will be allowed to refer to note cards. However, they will be expected to present their report by speaking primarily from their knowledge base, because it is their understanding of the topic that will support their use of complex syntax and literate words during expository discourse. As they practice, the SLP will provide feedback on additional factors that will impact their delivery, such as speech rate, articulation, vocal intensity, facial expressions, and eye contact. The SLP will also need to address any grammatical errors that occur, such as the failure to use past irregular verb forms correctly. This can occur in the context of carrying out intervention for complex syntax by providing numerous examples of past tense irregular verbs, drawing students' conscious attention to those words, and having them use those words in meaningful contexts.

In summary, activities that encourage students to combine literate vocabulary (e.g., abstract nouns, subordinate conjunctions, metacognitive verbs) with complex syntax (e.g., relative clauses, adverbial clauses, nominal clauses) as they discuss the material they are learning in the classroom provide needed practice in using expository discourse in formal speaking contexts. A long-term goal is that they will be able to express themselves with greater accuracy, clarity, and efficiency when speaking in the expository genre about many different topics. Given the SLP's knowledge and understanding of the complex nature of spoken and written communication, it is clear that this professional can make a unique contribution to the academic success of school-age children and adolescents with developmental language disorders.

CHAPTER 7

Persuasive Discourse

With persuasive or argumentative discourse, a speaker or writer takes a position on a controversial topic and tries to convince others to agree with his or her point of view (Gage, 1991). According to British philosopher Stephen Toulmin (1958), to be effective, the persuasive speaker or writer must support claims with evidence, acknowledge and rebut the opposing point of view, and draw logical conclusions based on the information presented.

During childhood, adolescence, and into adulthood, performance on spoken and written persuasive or argumentative tasks gradually improves, with measurable growth occurring in the ability to consider both sides of an issue, to appeal to others' values and beliefs, to present multiple reasons for a particular claim, and to use complex syntax and literate vocabulary to communicate clearly and efficiently (Nippold, 2007; Nippold & Ward-Lonergan, 2010; Nippold, Ward-Lonergan, & Fanning, 2005). However, children and adolescents with language disorders often struggle to produce spoken and written persuasive discourse that is well-organized, rich in content, addresses diverse points of view (Wong, Butler, Ficzere, & Kuperis, 1996), and employs complex sentences and literate vocabulary. Moreover, the ability to generate counterarguments is especially challenging, as it is even for students who have typical language development.

Given the cognitive and linguistic demands required by persuasive discourse, language sampling in this genre presents an opportunity to "stress the system" (Lahey, 1990) of the speaker or writer, potentially revealing the individual's strengths and weaknesses in complex syntax, vocabulary, perspective-taking, reasoning, and critical thinking. Assessing persuasive discourse is particularly relevant for adolescents in middle school and high school. For example, Table 7–1 presents the Common Core State Standards in English/Language Arts for Grade 8 in speaking, listening,

Table 7–1. Common Core State Standards in English/Language Arts for Grade 8 Related to Persuasive Discourse (National Governor's Association Center for Best Practices and Council of Chief State School Officers, 2010)

Speaking and Listening:

Comprehension and Collaboration:

- Engage effectively in a range of collaborative discussions (one-on-one, in groups, and teacher-led) with diverse partners on grade 8 topics, texts, and issues, building on others' ideas and expressing their own clearly. CCSS.ELA-LITERACY.SL.8.1

- Analyze the purpose of information presented in diverse media and formats (e.g., visually, quantitatively, orally) and evaluate the motives (e.g., social, commercial, political) behind its presentation. CCSS.ELA-LITERACY.SL.8.2

- Delineate a speaker's argument and specific claims, evaluating the soundness of the reasoning and relevance and sufficiency of the evidence and identifying when irrelevant evidence is introduced. CCSS.ELA-LITERACY.SL.8.3

Writing:

Write argument to support claims with clear reasons and relevant evidence. CCSS.ELA-LITERACY.W.8.1

- Introduce claim(s), acknowledge and distinguish the claim(s) from alternate or opposing claims, and organize the reasons and evidence logically.

- Support claim(s) with logical reasoning and relevant evidence, using accurate, credible sources and demonstrating an understanding of the topic or text.

- Use words, phrases, and clauses to create cohesion and clarify relationships among claim(s), counterclaims, reasons, and evidence.

- Establish and maintain a formal style.

- Provide a concluding statement or section that follows from and supports the argument.

and writing (National Governors Association Center for Best Practices and Council of Chief State School Officers, 2010), underscoring the complexity of this genre.

LANGUAGE SAMPLING TASKS

In a developmental study, Nippold, Ward-Lonergan, et al. (2005) examined the ability of children, adolescents, and adults to write a persuasive essay on the controversial topic of training animals to perform in circuses. Mean ages of the three groups, respectively, were 11, 17, and 24 years ($n = 60$ per group). The task employed in their study is shown in Table 7–2.

Each participant was allowed 20 minutes to complete the essay. Each handwritten essay was subsequently typed and entered into Systematic Analysis of Language Transcripts (SALT; Miller, Andriacchi, & Nockerts, 2019) and coded for selected aspects of syntactic, semantic, and pragmatic development.

The results of the Nippold, Ward-Lonergan, et al. (2005) study indicated age-related improvements in language productivity (essay length); syntactic development (mean length of T-unit and relative clause production); and lexical development as measured by the use of adverbial conjuncts (e.g., however, finally, in conclusion), abstract nouns (e.g., realization, essence, kindness), and metacognitive verbs (e.g., realize, assess, determine). In terms of pragmatics, an age-related increase occurred in the participants' ability to consider multiple points of view in their essays. Whereas children were more likely to view the conflict from only one perspective, either favoring or rejecting the circus, adolescents and adults were more likely to consider multiple perspectives. Examples of essays written by three participants in this study—a child, an adolescent, and an adult—are presented in Table 7–3. In each essay, the use of three types of literate words has been highlighted: adverbial conjuncts, metacognitive verbs, and abstract nouns.

Table 7–2. Persuasive Writing Task, "The Circus Controversy" (Nippold, Ward-Lonergan, & Fanning, 2005, p. 129)

People have different views on animals performing in circuses. For example, some people think it is a **great idea** because it provides lots of entertainment for the public. Also, it gives parents and children something to do together, and the people who train the animals can make some money. However, other people think having animals in circuses is a **bad idea** because the animals are often locked in small cages and are not fed well. They also believe it is cruel to force a dog, tiger, or elephant to perform certain tricks that might be dangerous.

I am interested in learning what **you** think about this controversy and whether or not **you** think circuses with trained animals should be allowed to perform for the public. I would like you to spend the next 20 minutes writing an essay. Tell me exactly what you think about the controversy. Give me lots of good reasons for your opinion.

Please do your own work and don't share ideas with your neighbors. Be sure to double space your essay. Also, please use your best writing style, with correct grammar and spelling, and good handwriting. If you aren't sure how to spell a word, just take a guess. Do you have any questions?

Table 7–3. Persuasive Essays Produced by Participants in the Study by Nippold, Ward-Lonergan, and Fanning (2005)

These examples (from the author's files) were analyzed by Fanning (2004), who coded instances of three types of literate words: adverbial conjuncts [AC], metacognitive verbs [MCV], and abstract nouns [ABN]. The code follows each word (in bold). Consistent with SALT conventions for coding words, the word code was placed immediately next to the word, with no space, as shown below.

Boy, Age 11 Years

I **think**[MCV] it is a bad **idea**[ABN] to have animals in the circus because animals should be free to do what they **want**[MCV].

They're stuck in small cages.

So[AC] there is barely enough room to get their adequate exercise. People don't **like**[MCV] to be imprisoned.

So[AC] we should let them go.

Then[AC] they won't be forced to do tricks.

I **think**[MCV] it is cruel to train animals to do a trick because if they don't do it right, the trainers will hit them.

These are the **reasons**[ABN] why I **think**[MCV] circuses should not be allowed. For the animals' **sake**[ABN].

Boy, Age 17 Years

A common **controversy**[ABN] is often whether or not circuses are good or bad for the **community**[ABN].

I **like**[MCV] the clowns because often times they are also animal trainers.

However[AC], there is a **downside**[ABN] to all these beneficial **factors**[ABN].

Frequently[AC], the animals are underfed and are kept in small cages.

This alone **infuriates**[MCV] animal enthusiasts everywhere.

Circuses can be cruel to animals.

Therefore[AC], they should be closed down.

If animals **feel**[MCV] threatened, they could be dangerous when they fight back.

What I **believe**[MCV] is that a circus could hire more people and have them go to clown school.

Everybody **likes**[MCV] clowns, right?

The hardest **part**[ABN] of this would be training all those clowns.

Still[AC], with a little **creativity**[ABN] and some **ingenuity**[ABN] I **think**[MCV] a clown school could be possible.

Overall[AC], I **think**[MCV] animals should not be in circuses.

Table 7–3. *continued*

Man, Age 24 Years

A trip to the circus can be an exciting **event**[ABN] for both children and adults. The circus is a place where kids can see and almost touch their favorite wild and exotic animals.

Otherwise[AC] kids may only see the animals in books or on television.

I am not entirely against animals performing in a circus.

In addition[AC], I **believe**[MCV] there should be strict **regulations**[ABN] about proper humane **care**[ABN] for animals.

Adults tend to **perceive**[MCV] the circus through more critical eyes, **analyzing**[MCV] every trick, **assessing**[MCV] the **status**[ABN] of animals, or the **behavior**[ABN] of clowns.

Obviously[AC], there is a **dispute**[ABN] about animal **cruelty**[ABN] in **terms**[ABN] of the traveling caravan thus bringing the circus from the **heights**[ABN] of magical **essence**[ABN] to the **pits**[ABN] of **criticism**[ABN].

Sadly[AC], this **issue**[ABN] may continue for a long time to come.

In the study by Nippold, Ward-Lonergan, et al. (2005), writers of all ages showed interest in the task, and many of them were passionate in expressing their views about the ethical treatment of circus animals. This pattern, coupled with the finding that the task was sensitive to developmental gains in syntax, semantics, and pragmatics, suggests that it is a useful tool for examining the ability of middle school and high school students to write persuasive essays. After a student has completed an essay, the speech-language pathologist (SLP) may wish to analyze it syntactically, semantically, and pragmatically, as described in this investigation.

In addition to the Circus Controversy task (Nippold, Ward-Lonergan, et al., 2005), Table 7–4 contains a list of topics potentially of interest to students in middle school and high school. To assess persuasive discourse in adolescents, the SLP could encourage students to choose one of those topics and work to prepare a speech or essay in which they take a position and argue their point of view effectively. It is helpful if students are allowed to plan their speech or essay in advance, using a graphic organizer or outline, such as the one in Table 7–5. In addition, SALT (Miller et al., 2019) has a similar list of topics thought to be of interest to adolescents (p. 279). SALT also has a large referential database of American and Australian adolescents ($n = 179$) ages 12 through 18 years, speaking in the persuasive genre. Details on the manner in which the SALT persuasive language samples were collected and analyzed are available in Heilmann, Malone, and Westerveld (2020). As with the SALT expository database, described

Table 7–4. Topics for Persuasive Speaking and Writing, Potentially of Interest to Adolescents (Adapted from Kelly, 2020a, 2020b)

- Should physical education classes be required of all high school students?
- Should all high school students be required to perform community service?
- Should school uniforms be required in middle school and high school?
- Should smokers be required pay an extra health tax?
- Should junk food be banned from schools?
- Should people be required to attend parenting classes before having children?
- Should all students be required to learn a foreign language in middle school?
- Should all students be required to take a cooking class in middle school?
- Should all students be required to take a shop or practical arts class?
- Should all students be required to take a performing arts class?
- Should all students be required to learn computer programming?
- Should all students be required to attend school year round?
- Should all students be required to study history?
- Should citizens who do not vote be fined?
- Should the legal voting/driving/drinking age be lowered or raised?
- Should teachers be replaced by computers?
- Is it ever appropriate for the government to restrict freedom of speech?
- Is democracy the best form of government?
- Is the right to bear arms a necessary constitutional amendment today?

in Chapter 6 and reported in Heilmann and Malone (2014), adolescents in the Heilmann et al. (2020) study were provided with a planning sheet that listed the key features of a good persuasive speech and were encouraged to write quick notes next to each point before beginning to talk.

IMPLICATIONS FOR INTERVENTION

Intervention designed to build students' persuasive speaking and writing skills presents an opportunity for the SLP to work collaboratively with classroom teachers to help students succeed academically. In middle schools and high schools today, it is common practice in classes such as science, history, health, and literature for students to be asked to engage

Table 7–5. Graphic Organizer for Planning a
Persuasive Speech or Essay

What is the controversial topic?

What do I believe? Why?

    I believe X

    My reasons are as follows:

        First,

        Next,

        Also,

What do other people believe? Why?

    On the other hand, some people believe . . .

    Their reasons are as follows:

        First,

        Next,

        Also,

Which view is stronger? Why?

    After considering both sides,

    Nevertheless,

    To sum up,

    In conclusion,

in debates with their classmates, to give speeches, and to write persuasive essays, either alone or with peers, in which they must take a position and defend it with solid arguments. However, to be successful at persuasive speaking or writing tasks, students must know something about the topic, be motivated to discuss it, and believe that their efforts will make a difference.

It is important, therefore, that students be allowed to select the topic they will address and that they be encouraged to learn more about that topic by reading books, magazines, and informative articles available through the Internet. It is helpful also if they can work together in small groups in which different points of view can be expressed and discussed. Two hypothetical but realistic examples of how this type of intervention might be carried out are presented next (also see Nippold & Ward-Lonergan, 2010). Table 7–6 lists the highlights of the approach, and Table 7–7 lists some key features to examine when monitoring progress in persuasive discourse over time.

Table 7–6. Highlights of an Intervention Approach for Persuasive Discourse

- SLP works collaboratively with classroom teacher (e.g., history, science, health).
- Students work together in small groups with SLP.
- Students in consultation with SLP and teacher select topic to debate.
- Students are encouraged to learn more about the topic.
- Brainstorming activities occur to stimulate discussion about the topic.
- Subgroups defend own point of view and consider other side of issue.
- Reasons are offered, based on documented information.
- Points on both sides of the issue are typed into the laptop computer.
- The document is saved and modified as more information is added.
- Students are encouraged to use literate vocabulary and complex syntax.
- Students use full sentences with correct grammar and spelling.
- Students use words that are precise, accurate, and engaging.
- Students use graphic organizer to write persuasive essay:
  - State topic and explain why it is controversial.
  - State own opinion clearly (in my opinion . . .).
  - Give different reasons for own opinion (first of all, second, third, finally).
  - State what others believe (on the other hand, some people believe . . .).
  - Explain why they believe that way (they believe this because . . .).
  - Summarize own opinion and conclude the essay (nevertheless, I still believe . . . I believe this because . . . In conclusion . . .).

Table 7–7. Monitoring Progress During Intervention for Persuasive Discourse

Compare samples of persuasive discourse (spoken or written) over time.

Look for measurable growth in:

    Mean length of C-unit

    Clausal density

    Literate vocabulary (e.g., metacognitive verbs, abstract nouns, adverbial conjuncts)

    Sequencing, organization, coherence

    Perspective-taking

    Use of counterarguments

    Number of C-units or T-units (amount of language)

Intervention Scenario: Leisure-Time Activities

In an eighth-grade health class, a group of six students [two of whom have developmental language disorders (DLDs)] decide to debate the issue of leisure-time activities. Three of the students strongly believe that young people their age should participate in physical activities after school, such as playing basketball, tennis, and baseball, or hiking, running, and swimming. However, the other three students strongly believe that after a full day of school, it is more beneficial to engage in less active pastimes such as watching television, playing video games, reading, texting, e-mailing, or talking on the phone with friends.

For the two students with DLDs, the SLP has established the following goals:

Goal #1: The student will write an essay that considers both sides of an issue.

Goal #2: The student will write an essay that is well-organized.

Goal #3: The student will write an essay that includes complex language:

  A. Literate vocabulary

    1. Adverbial conjuncts (e.g., consequently, therefore, however)

    2. Metacognitive verbs (e.g., expect, assume, infer)

    3. Abstract nouns (e.g., accomplishment, satisfaction, affection)

  B. Complex sentences that contain major types of subordinate clauses

    1. Adverbial (e.g., *When people exercise*, they lose weight.)

    2. Relative (e.g., People *who exercise* are healthier.)

    3. Nominal (e.g., I believe *it is better to relax at home.*)

Before the students begin writing their essays in which they argue their own point of view and attempt to convince others to agree with them, the SLP engages the entire group in a series of brainstorming sessions, with each session lasting approximately 30 minutes. During the first session, a fundamental question is posed: "How should adolescents in the eighth grade spend their afterschool leisure hours?" The two opposing points of view quickly surface. A student representative from each subgroup is asked to come to the white board and make two columns, marked "Reasons For" and "Reasons Against" their point of view. Thus, each subgroup is expected not only to argue in favor of its own point of view but also to consider the opposite point of view. Next, the representative will ask each member of the subgroup to contribute at least one reason under each column, which then is written on the whiteboard. During this process, another student in the subgroup, the recorder, will be asked to copy the information from the white board into a document to be stored on a laptop computer. The document will then be saved and later modified when the subgroup meets again. During subsequent brainstorming sessions, the students in each subgroup will be expected to add to the list of items under the two columns and to do so by collecting facts from authoritative sources. For example, one subgroup may locate scientific evidence that indicates how physical activity can increase the body's strength and flexibility, build endurance, control weight, maintain blood pressure, and improve sleep. In contrast, the subgroup favoring more sedentary activities may locate scientific evidence indicating that laughter that occurs when talking on the phone with friends can increase endorphins in the brain, leading to feelings of well-being and relaxation. This subgroup also reports a study indicating that time spent talking with others can increase one's social network, providing the opportunity to gain emotional support, collaborate on homework assignments, plan recreational outings, and build solidarity with peers. During the process of reading topic-related articles, an additional benefit is that students are likely to encounter literate vocabulary (e.g., *contentment, coordination, encouragement, metabolism*) that they can then incorporate into their lists and later into their persuasive essays.

After each subgroup has completed its list of items both for and against their point of view, they edit their document, ensuring that all points are written in full sentences that are grammatically correct and free of spelling errors. This presents an opportunity for the students with DLDs to focus on the production of complex sentences containing literate vocabulary. For example, with guidance from the SLP, the following three sentences could be combined into the fourth more efficient sentence, which contains an embedded subordinate clause and a technical term (*hypertension*):

1. Walking home from school every day is good exercise.

2. Walking helps you lose weight.

3. Losing weight can prevent hypertension.

4. Walking [GER] home from school every day is [MC] good exercise because it helps [ADV] you lose [INF] weight, which can prevent [ADV] hypertension.

Next, they are asked to share their information with the entire group by having different members of the subgroup take turns reading each point aloud from the printed document. After each group has had its turn, an open discussion will occur in which all students are encouraged to make comments, ask questions, and express their opinions respectfully.

Following these brainstorming and discussion sessions, students will be asked to write their essays, using a graphic organizer that provides an outline of the essential features of a strong persuasive argument. The following is an example of such a tool:

1. State the topic and explain why it is controversial.

2. State your own opinion clearly.

3. Give at least three different reasons for your opinion.

4. State what other people believe (the other side of the controversy).

5. Try to explain why other people believe that way.

6. Summarize your opinion and conclude the essay.

In addition, students will be reminded to attend to the following points:

■ Use full sentences with correct grammar and spelling.

■ Use words that are precise, accurate, and engaging.

It is expected that students will need time to write, edit, and revise their essays before the final product is ready to be read by their teacher and classmates. Because good writing requires patience and persistence, students should be encouraged to approach the task systematically and to remember that the goal is to produce an essay that will influence others. It also can be expected that students may change their minds as they work on their essays, tempering their views after they have considered the evidence on both sides of the controversy. This should be encouraged because it means the students are grappling with the complexities of the topic and are realizing that few issues are as simple or as "black or white" as they first may appear. Indeed, when students move from an extreme position to a more balanced and flexible one, it shows they have benefited from the experience of debating an issue and attempting to persuade others.

Intervention Scenario: Letters to the Editor

In this scenario, the SLP collaborates with a classroom teacher of English, language arts, or journalism at a middle school or high school, and students are assigned to write letters that could potentially be published in the local newspaper in the "Letters to the Editor" section. Students could work independently or in small groups. If working in groups, they would have the opportunity to adjust to the different personalities and communication skills of their classmates, discuss a variety of ideas, and edit each other's work in the context of building their own spoken and written language skills in relevant social and academic contexts.

Because a letter to the editor must convince the readership of a particular point of view, it has the quality of authenticity and can be expected to motivate students to use their best spoken and written language skills. Goals for this persuasive writing assignment would be to address students' ability to use complex syntax and literate vocabulary while attempting to convince other people to accept certain beliefs or to perform specific actions. Students who are assigned to this activity could produce a letter on a controversial topic that is of strong interest to them. Topics might include if students should be allowed to use cell phones in class, if students should be required to wear school uniforms, or if teachers should contact parents when students perform poorly on examinations or projects. During the process of writing these letters and evaluating their own progress, students could use the following list of questions to guide their self-assessment:

Does the letter . . .

1. State the topic and explain why it is controversial?

2. State the author's opinion clearly?

3. Give at least three different reasons for the author's opinion?

4. State what other people believe (the other side of the controversy)?

5. Attempt to explain *why* other people believe that way?

6. Summarize the author's opinion?

7. Use full sentences with correct grammar and spelling?

8. Use words that are precise, accurate, and engaging?

To teach students this process of assessment, the SLP might ask them to evaluate the following letter, written by an eighth-grade girl, Willow, and her classmates and published in a local newspaper ("Teachers Need to Be Healthy," 2009). The letter concerns a ban on the consumption of junk food at a school, and the controversy centers on whether or not the ban, directed at students, should also include teachers. Willow and her classmates wrote as follows:

> We think that the ban of junk foods in schools should include teachers. Sodas and other junk foods are just as unhealthy for teachers as they are for students. The teachers need to set a good example for the students. If students see that the ban on junk food includes teachers as well as themselves, they might be more willing to go along with the ban. To have a mind and body that functions the best they can, you need to eat the proper amount of nutrients.

You do not get these nutrients from junk foods and soda. Because of this, you do not function as well as you could. We think it is important for teachers to have healthy bodies and minds, so that they will teach the students better than otherwise. If teachers eat or drink junk food or soda, they will not teach as well. If the teachers really cannot live without the junk food, they can very easily just eat it at their homes. It should not be that hard for them to wait the seven or eight hours that their jobs take up to eat junk food if they need it that badly. After all, students can.

In reviewing a persuasive letter such as this, students with DLDs may benefit by focusing their attention on the last two points (#7 and #8), determining whether sentences are well constructed and whether appropriate words are used. With the SLP acting as a scaffold, they could be encouraged to rewrite any sentences that are incomplete or that contain grammatical errors or misspelled words and to substitute more appropriate words, with the goal of improving the clarity of the letter. They also could be encouraged to identify sentences that contain different types of clauses and to discuss with the SLP how those clauses improve the sentence by adding specific pieces of information. For example, the following sentence from Willow's letter contains four subordinate clauses:

If students see [ADV] that the ban on junk food includes [NOM] teachers as well as themselves, they might be [MC] more willing [PRT] to go [INF] along with the ban.

After discussing how the adverbial clause in this sentence communicates a certain condition, they might discuss how the metacognitive verb *see* introduces the nominal clause and how both of those subordinate clauses support and modify the main clause. By examining the main clause in isolation (i.e., "they might be more willing to go along with the ban") and comparing it with the full sentence, students might be assisted to understand the role of subordinate clauses in providing essential information in a clear, precise, and efficient manner.

CHAPTER 8

Autism Spectrum Disorders

In this chapter, language sampling is discussed in relation to children and adolescents who have been diagnosed with autism spectrum disorders (ASD). This is a condition that refers to a set of developmental disabilities characterized by severe and pervasive deficits in communication and social interaction, accompanied by restricted, repetitive, and ritualistic behaviors (Nelson, 2010). In 2020, the Centers for Disease Control and Prevention's Autism and Developmental Disabilities Monitoring Network reported that ASD affects approximately 1 in 54 children from all racial, ethnic, and socioeconomic backgrounds and that boys are four times more likely to be diagnosed with ASD than girls (https://www.cdc.gov/ncbddd/autism/data.html; accessed June 14, 2020). In schools today, speech-language pathologists (SLPs) play a central role in the diagnosis, assessment, and treatment of communication disorders in students with ASD, whose numbers continue to increase. Because ASD is a lifelong condition, SLPs are expected to address the communication needs of students with ASD at all educational levels. Nevertheless, given the behavioral challenges of these students, it can be difficult to evaluate their language skills and to obtain useful information during formal testing sessions, especially when attempting to administer norm-referenced standardized language tests. For this reason, it is strongly recommended that SLPs elicit language samples from students with ASD in order to obtain information that can be used to evaluate their ability to communicate in real-world settings. However, this is not necessarily an easy process. Hence, this chapter discusses some of the challenges that arise when working with children and adolescents who have ASD. It also describes a study that employed language samples to evaluate four students with ASD.

127

LANGUAGE DEVELOPMENT IN STUDENTS WITH ASD

Children and adolescents with ASD are heterogeneous in their language and cognitive development (Howlin, 2005; Loveland & Tunali-Kotoski, 2005; Sigman & McGovern, 2005; Tager-Flusberg, 2004). Although many students with ASD are delayed in these areas, others perform above average, and still others fall somewhere in between (Baron-Cohen et al., 2005). Despite this variability, it is common for students with ASD to have deficits in language development (Tager-Flusberg, 2004). For example, they often have difficulty comprehending directions, explanations, and nonliteral forms of language such as sarcasm, jokes, idioms, and metaphors (Paul, 2007). Problems in verbal expression may include articulation errors, stereotypic phrases, echolalia, neologisms, unusual intonational and prosodic patterns, and the failure to employ certain types of words such as mental state verbs (e.g., *know, think, believe*; Shea & Mesibov, 2005; Tager-Flusberg, Paul, & Lord, 2005). Difficulties with narrative discourse also occur, especially in their ability to understand and explain the emotions and mental states of characters in a story (Loveland & Tunali-Kotoski, 2005).

Although children and adolescents with ASD often improve in their receptive and expressive language abilities as they develop, the majority experience lifelong deficits in communication (Howlin, 2005; Tager-Flusberg et al., 2005). Indeed, a hallmark of ASD is the existence of serious deficits in pragmatics, the social use of language (Geurts & Embrechts, 2008; Paul, Orlovski, Marcinko, & Volkmar, 2009; Volden, Coolican, Garon, White, & Bryson, 2009). For example, for some students with ASD who engage in conversations, social communication deficits may be evidenced in their failure to follow conventional rules of politeness, such as taking turns, making topic-relevant comments, shifting topics gracefully, sharing the conversational floor (Tager-Flusberg et al., 2005), and responding to others with appropriate amounts of information (Paul et al., 2009). During conversations, they also may show an obsessive focus on a narrow range of topics (e.g., city bus routes, baseball statistics), the use of inappropriate comments or questions (Loveland & Tunali-Kotoski, 2005), and unusual vocal patterns in speaking (Paul et al., 2009).

Some students with ASD also experience deficits in specific domains of language such as syntax, the structural foundation of sentences (Bennett et al., 2008; Landa & Goldberg, 2005; Lewis, Murdoch, & Woodyatt, 2007). Although norm-referenced standardized language tests often are used to identify syntactic deficits in children and adolescents with ASD, those tests do not necessarily indicate how a speaker uses syntax to communicate in natural speaking situations. To obtain this type of functional and clinically useful information, it is necessary to elicit language samples.

A STUDY OF SYNTACTIC DEVELOPMENT

To learn more about syntactic development in speakers with ASD, we conducted a small, exploratory study (Nippold & Hesketh, 2009) in which we elicited conversational and expository language samples from children and adolescents who had received an educational diagnosis of ASD from their school district (n = 4; mean age = 12;3; age range = 10;0–14;3). Based on the report of a school-based SLP, degrees of autism included mild (n = 2), mild–moderate (n = 1), and moderate–severe (n = 1). Each student with ASD was matched individually to a student with typical language development (TLD) (n = 4; mean age = 12;7; age range = 10;11–14;1) on the basis of chronological age and gender. According to their teachers, all students in the TLD group were free of any known disorders of language, learning, or cognition and were making acceptable progress in school. There were two boys and two girls in each group. All students in the study spoke Standard American English as their primary language and were attending schools in western Oregon (United States). Before any testing took place, the parents of each student had signed a consent form, giving formal permission for their son or daughter to participate in the study. In addition, each child or adolescent involved in the study had signed an individual assent form, indicating his or her own agreement to perform the tasks.

Tasks

Each participant was interviewed by a trained graduate student at school or at the University of Oregon Speech-Language-Hearing Center. Each interview began with a general conversation (CON) about common topics such as family, pets, and school, using procedures similar to those described in Chapter 4 (General Conversation task). Following the conversation, two expository tasks were administered, the Favorite Game or Sport (FGS) task and the Peer Conflict Resolution (PCR) task, both of which were described in Chapter 6. When the PCR task was presented to children and adolescents with ASD, pictures of the main characters accompanied each story. It was decided that pictures might increase their attention to the task, given their autistic behaviors. However, when the task was presented to students with TLD, the pictures were not used as they did not appear to be necessary to maintain their attention.

Transcription, Coding, and Analysis

Each language sample (CON, FGS, and PCR) was transcribed into its own Systematic Analysis of Language Transcripts file (Miller & Chapman, 2003), segmented into communication units (C-units), and coded for main and subordinate clauses. A C-unit consists of a main clause and optionally may contain one or more subordinate clauses. The sentence, "Mike enjoys flipping burgers even though it gets hot in the kitchen," is a 12-word C-unit that consists of a main clause ("Mike enjoys flipping burgers") and one adverbial clause ("even though it gets hot in the kitchen") that is linked to the main clause. Any utterances that were less than a C-unit in that they did not contain a subject or a predicate (i.e., fragments) were placed within parentheses and excluded from analyses. All mazes (e.g., false starts, repetitions) were also parenthesized and ignored for purposes of this study. All C-units were examined for the presence of three types of subordinate clauses: relative, adverbial, and nominal. Only clauses that contained finite verbs were coded, a procedure that had been employed in past studies using the same tasks (Nippold, Hesketh, Duthie, & Mansfield, 2005; Nippold, Mansfield, Billow, & Tomblin, 2008, 2009). After each sample had been coded for main and subordinate clauses, clausal density was determined by summing the total number of main and subordinate clauses and dividing this sum by the total number of C-units produced. The total number of C-units served as a measure of language productivity, while mean length of C-unit (MLCU) and clausal density (CD) served as measures of syntactic complexity. All samples were coded for main and subordinate clauses by one investigator (MN) and rechecked by the other investigator (LH). The initial agreement level for clause coding was 99%. All disagreements were resolved, resulting in 100% agreement.

Results

The performance of each speaker with ASD (A) and the matched peer with TLD (T) is reported in Tables 8–1, 8–2, and 8–3, respectively, for the CON, FGS, and PCR tasks. Thus, in each table, there are four pairs of speakers: A1–T1, A2–T2, A3–T3, and A4–T4. Variables of interest include total C-units, a measure of language productivity; and MLCU, CD, and relative, adverbial, and nominal clause use—measures of syntactic development in school-age children and adolescents (Nippold, Hesketh, et al., 2005; Nippold, Mansfield, & Billow, 2007).

Individual Differences

Because of the small number of participants in the study, the data were analyzed informally rather than with traditional statistical tests. In the following sections, the performance of each speaker with ASD is compared with the performance of the matched peer with TLD in terms of syntactic complexity and language productivity. These comparisons allow for a

Table 8–1. Performance of Individual Speakers in the ASD (A) and TLD (T) Groups on the General Conversation Task

	A1	T1	A2	T2	A3	T3	A4	T4
Total C-units	020	033	042	042	047	066	047	027
Mean length of C-unit	05.75	06.73	08.19	06.29	08.60	05.85	06.98	07.67
Clausal density	01.10	01.12	01.21	01.19	01.36	01.09	01.23	01.44
Relative clause use*	00.00	00.09	00.10	00.07	00.15	00.00	00.00	00.11
Adverbial clause use*	00.05	00.00	00.05	00.05	00.00	00.00	00.09	00.26
Nominal clause use*	00.05	00.03	00.07	00.07	00.21	00.09	00.15	00.07

*Reported as percent of C-units per sample.

Table 8–2. Performance of Individual Speakers in the ASD (A) and TLD (T) Groups on the Favorite Game or Sport Task

	A1	T1	A2	T2	A3	T3	A4	T4
Total C-units	023	031	108	085	078	073	032	037
Mean Length of C-unit	04.83	09.74	12.21	09.76	07.21	09.60	10.16	11.00
Clausal Density	01.00	01.55	01.77	01.49	01.23	01.55	01.34	01.76
Relative Clause Use*	00.00	00.10	00.17	00.04	00.05	00.07	00.00	00.11
Adverbial Clause Use*	00.00	00.29	00.40	00.33	00.04	00.25	00.16	00.38
Nominal Clause Use*	00.00	00.16	00.20	00.13	00.14	00.23	00.19	00.27

*Reported as percent of C-units per sample.

detailed analysis of each speaker, providing naturalistic information about language development. They also provide information about the effectiveness of the language sampling tasks and how, in some cases, they needed to be modified for the individual student. In addition, the analyses offer

Table 8–3. Performance of Individual Speakers in the ASD (A) and TLD (T) Groups on the Peer Conflict Resolution Task

	A1	T1	A2	T2	A3	T3	A4	T4
Total C-units	028	031	048	049	069	022	053	051
Mean Length of C-unit	05.39	10.45	11.27	11.92	07.10	11.00	11.68	10.02
Clausal Density	01.07	01.61	01.56	02.02	01.14	01.45	01.43	01.53
Relative Clause Use*	00.00	00.19	00.02	00.08	00.03	00.05	00.06	00.04
Adverbial Clause Use*	00.04	00.26	00.25	00.33	00.07	00.23	00.13	00.18
Nominal Clause Use*	04	00.16	00.29	00.61	00.04	00.18	00.25	00.31

*Reported as percent of C-units per sample.

some clinical implications. Thus, for each speaker with ASD, areas that might be targeted during intervention are listed.

Pair #1

A1, a 14-year-old boy with moderate to severe autism, willingly participated in the activities, evidenced by his efforts to comply with the examiner's requests throughout the interview. However, his utterances frequently consisted of fragments that did not meet the criteria for complete C-units. Of his total utterances, 67% were fragments in the CON task, 66% were fragments in the FGS task, and 64% were fragments in the PCR task. Hence, his total number of C-units, a measure of language productivity, was lower than that of T1, his matched peer, particularly on the CON and FGS tasks. In addition, many of his utterances contained grammatical errors (e.g., "Batgirl never to talk," "A lots of bugs," "Wearing the glasses black one"), and his MLCU for all three tasks (5.75, 4.83, and 5.39, respectively) was shorter than would be expected for his age (Nippold et al., 2007; Nippold, Hesketh, et al., 2005). Throughout the tasks, A1 produced no relative clauses and few adverbial or nominal clauses, and the restricted use of subordination resulted in low clausal density scores (CON = 1.10; FGS = 1.00; PCR = 1.07). Unfortunately, he did not increase the complexity of his utterances as he moved from conversational to expository discourse, which is in marked contrast to the expected pattern for a speaker his age (Nippold, Hesketh, et al., 2005). These behaviors in a 14-year-old boy indicate a significant delay in syntactic development (Nippold et al., 2007; Nippold, Hesketh, et al., 2005) and are consistent with research linking syntactic deficits with more severe autism (Bennett et al., 2008).

Regarding the content of his discourse, many of his responses suggested that he did not understand the examiner's prompts or was unable to formulate appropriate replies. For example, during the FGS task, when asked to explain some strategies needed to win a Batman game, the activity he indicated was his favorite, he replied as follows:

> I win. A lot of fun. I win. I beat Mister Freeze. I looked at Victor.
> Got scared first. . . . My chase after the Poison Ivy with Weiner
> car. I shoot it. The Great Monster. Insider the hide. I came to see
> Poison Ivy. What do you know?

During the PCR task, A1 was unable to retell either of the stories, so the examiner modified the task by pointing to the pictures, rephrasing parts of the stories, and asking simpler questions. This spontaneous scaffolding resulted in the production of utterances that bore at least some relevance to the situation. For example, during the Fast Food scenario, when asked to explain the problem between Mike and Peter, A1 replied,

> Mike can't get to work there. Mike did not work the grill. Mike
> is leaving again. Ouch! That feels bad. He breaks it. French fries.
> That does taste good.

Then, when asked how Mike might help solve the problem with Peter's arm, he replied,

> Mike cannot help his arm. It cannot be fixed. He looks so scared.
> He must not help him. I can't help his arm. Mike's arm is broken
> again. He must go.

In summary, this boy required a great deal of patience, flexibility, support, and positive reinforcement from the examiner in order to perform the tasks at a basic level. Had the examiner been unwilling to deviate from the scripted activity, A1's ability to achieve at least some degree of success with the three tasks would not have been revealed.

The contrast with A1's matched typical peer, T1, also a 14-year-old boy, was striking. As reported in Tables 8–1, 8–2, and 8–3, T1's MLCU was consistently greater than A1's on all three tasks (CON = 6.73; FGS = 9.74; PCR = 10.45), as were his CD scores (CON = 1.42; FGS = 2.03; PCR = 2.35), reflecting the use of relative, adverbial, and nominal clauses. The tables also indicate that his syntactic complexity increased as he moved from conversational to expository discourse, with MLCU and CD scores higher on FGS and PCR than on CON, a pattern that is found in typically developing speakers his age. He also produced more C-units than A1, particularly on the CON and FGS tasks. Consistent with this pattern, T1 readily replied to the examiner's questions and prompts, supplying topic-relevant comments that were grammatically correct, complete, and to the point. For example, when asked to explain how to win a basketball game, T1 replied as follows:

> Usually I don't let them pass me. I try and stay on their butt so that they either go around me or stay where they're at. So I just pretty much stay put there and keep them from getting the ball. Offense is when you have the ball.

Behaviors to Target with A1

Inspection of T1's performance on the three speaking tasks offers guidance concerning the level of functional communication that can be expected of a 14-year-old boy. By comparison, A1's performance on the tasks indicated a severe deficit in syntactic development, marked by fragments, grammatical errors, and little use of subordination. A1 also showed difficulty answering questions with topic-relevant comments. The information obtained from A1's conversational and expository samples suggests that it would be useful to target the following behaviors during language intervention:

1. Increase the production of complete and grammatically correct sentences during natural speaking situations of conversational and expository discourse.

2. Increase the production of complex sentences in spoken language through the use of relative, adverbial, and nominal subordinate clauses.

3. Increase the production of topic-relevant comments in response to questions concerning favorite activities and stories that involve peer conflicts.

Pair #2

Standing in marked contrast with A1, A2, a 13-year-old boy with mild autism, was one of the most talkative participants in the study, particularly during the FGS task, in which he produced 108 C-units while explaining the game of Pokémon. Although his language productivity on this task exceeded that of his matched peer, his productivity on the other two tasks, CON and PCR, was nearly identical to that of his peer. It was also found that A2's syntactic development was appropriate for his age on all three tasks (see Tables 8–1, 8–2, and 8–3) in terms of MLCU, CD, and the use of different types of subordinate clauses. He also employed greater syntactic complexity in expository discourse than in conversational, reflecting a pattern found in typically developing speakers of all ages (Nippold, Hesketh, et al., 2005). For example, his ability to produce complex sentences containing multiple adverbial clauses was displayed in the following utterance during the FGS:

> Like your status, if you have really bad status or your status
> is very low or if your defense is very low but your attack is
> very high, I would recommend getting a high physical attack
> or something to raise your defense or protect you from really
> powerful attacks.

Regarding the content of his discourse, he generally responded to the examiner's prompts with topic-relevant comments. Nevertheless, he tended to provide an excessive amount of detail, particularly during the FGS task, and he often used terminology that was specific to the game (e.g., "You either choose a grass, a fire, or a water depending on which one you want best") without defining those terms. Although it was often difficult to follow his explanations because of this pattern, he proceeded as if the listener understood his comments and shared his background knowledge, suggesting a deficit in perspective taking. For example, when asked to explain some key strategies about Pokémon that every good player should know, he replied as follows:

> A key strategy someone should know is the rule of elements,
> accuracy, and power moves, what each move does and how it
> may affect one player and another. Some of the moves affect
> three players. Some only affect two. It varies. There's a thing
> called a double battle. It's where you and an ally versus two
> other players. And you don't want to hurt your ally because who
> knows how much life points it has. Because you need to use
> something if they're both grass and you're a fire type. I would
> suggest finding a move that takes two of them out at once, like a
> move called heat wave.

As with A1, the interview with A2 required patience, flexibility, and a positive attitude from the examiner. But unlike A1, A2 was a loquacious speaker who needed little prompting to produce long and complex explanations of a topic he knew well. However, he did not appear to focus on the needs of the listener when his message was unclear.

Regarding the PCR task, A2 retold both scenarios appropriately and provided relevant responses when asked to explain the nature of the problem in each situation and how it might be resolved. It is possible that the greater structure offered by the PCR task, with its brief scenarios and focused questions, assisted A2 to organize his thoughts and to speak more coherently than during the FGS task. However, there was a tendency for him to focus on the perspective of only one of the characters in each story. For example, regarding the Science Fair scenario, he explained that the main problem was that Bob was going to "get in trouble," "miss out on the assignment," or "have to do it again," without commenting on the implications of the conflict for the other members of the group.

A2's matched typical peer, T2, also a 13-year-old boy, produced levels of syntactic complexity that were slightly lower than A2's scores for MLCU and CD on the CON and FGS tasks (see Tables 8–1 and 8–2). However, his performance equaled or slightly exceeded A2's on the PCR task (see Table 8–3). One salient difference between these two speakers was that T2 replied to the examiner's prompts with the appropriate amounts of information, addressing the main issues in a coherent fashion, and consistently defining key terms, as when he was asked to explain the term *turnover*:

> A turnover could be like if you're dribbling down the court and somebody hits the ball away and steals it. Or if you're going up for a shot and they reject you that means they hit the ball away. That could be a turnover. A turnover could be also if you accidentally go out of bounds, the ball does, if you miss a pass or something. A turnover is a mistake that your team makes.

Another difference between these speakers was that, during the PCR task, T2 appeared to view the conflicts from multiple perspectives, expressing concern for larger issues such as the success of the project and the boys' friendship, reflecting a more mature developmental level (Selman, Beardslee, Schultz, Krupa, & Podorefsky, 1986). For example, with the Science Fair scenario, he explained as follows:

> The main problem I think is Bob won't work. And they need him to work to help make the project go along faster. And he won't. And it makes the other people mad which makes their group not so good. . . . And it's a problem because it probably makes them not friends anymore.

Areas to Target with A2

Inspection of A2's performance on the tasks indicated that he possessed many strengths as a communicator, which included high levels of syntactic complexity and language productivity. However, in comparison with T2, he demonstrated some weaknesses that may be socially penalizing. For example, the content of his discourse was sometimes difficult to follow, particularly when he used terms that were unfamiliar to the listener, and he often appeared to be unaware of the listener's confusions during the interview. To improve the clarity of A2's discourse, while building on his strengths, it would be useful to target the following behaviors during intervention:

1. Increase his attention to the needs of the listener by training him to watch for nonverbal signs of comprehension (e.g., nodding) and confusion (e.g., frowns).

2. Increase his sensitivity to the knowledge base of others by training him to ask if his message has been understood, while using his skill with complex syntax (e.g., "Are you familiar with a strategy that is called a heat wave?").

3. Increase his ability to define key terms when discussing a topic of high personal interest by calling upon his proficiency in using relative clauses (e.g., "In the game of *Pokémon*, a heat wave is a move *that takes out two players at once*").

Pair #3

A3, an 11-year-old girl with mild to moderate autism, frequently spoke in simple utterances during each of the three tasks. Because many of her utterances were less than a complete C-unit (e.g., "everything," "brain," "too many questions"), they could not be included in the calculation of her MLCU and CD scores (see Tables 8–1, 8–2, and 8–3). Of her total utterances, 27% were fragments in the CON task, 14% were fragments in the FGS task, and 14% were fragments in the PCR task. Hence, on the CON task, she produced fewer C-units than her matched peer, T3. On the other two tasks, FGS and PCR, A3 produced a greater number of C-units than did T3. However, as explained later, those scores must be interpreted cautiously because the examiner deviated from the scripted interview in an attempt to respond flexibly to some challenging behaviors that A3 exhibited.

Similar to the behavior of A1, A3 did not increase the complexity of her utterances as she moved from conversational to expository discourse. Although her MLCU exceeded that of her matched peer during the CON task, she lagged behind her peer on the two expository tasks. However, during the expository tasks, she occasionally produced long, grammatically correct sentences that contained subordinate clauses, indicating that her syntax was developmentally appropriate. At one point, she stated as follows:

I know what a lot of people my age don't. The cell is the smallest unit that has all the characteristics of life. Now if you want to know what general people my age know about games and sports, you shouldn't have picked me because I can bring a lot that I and only I know.

It was also noteworthy that although A3 claimed to be knowledgeable of games and sports, she exhibited difficulty explaining how to play her favorite game, which she reported was Truth or Dare. Despite the examiner's suggestion that she choose another game to discuss, A3 protested that she did not like any games, that they were boring, and that the examiner was asking too many questions. Once the examiner agreed to stop asking questions, A3 began to talk about her interest in natural modes of transportation. At that point, with A3 in control of the interview, she produced a continuous string of 11 C-units on this topic, quite coherently, and with appropriate subordination:

> I also have a bike. But I want to expand my modes of transportation. And to go with my horse, I want a covered wagon. And plus I always ride my bike everywhere I go. And Mama drives the horrible, smelly, stinky car. But I'm natural. And I go a different way. In fact, it's not just modes of transportation. It's not just going places where I want to be natural. I never want to see a nonnatural thing in my house. Next I might want to get a Pterodactyl.

During the PCR task, A3 listened attentively to the stories and retold each one successfully. However, when the examiner began to ask her to explain the nature of the conflict and how it could be resolved, A3 protested that she did not know ("I don't know." "I have no idea." "Does this look like I know anything?" [shrugs shoulders, turns palms upward]). Despite the examiner's efforts to simplify the questions, A3 attempted to control the interaction by repeatedly telling the examiner to stop asking questions ("No more questions") and requesting that they talk about something different. For example, during the Fast Food scenario, she stated as follows:

> I want to have another story. Only can they not be people because I don't like people. And you know what? Are all the stories with girls? Are they all with people? Any other creatures? What about in any other stories? Other creatures, I said, and no people.

In summary, when asked to explain the rules of a game or to discuss interpersonal issues, A3 expressed frustration, criticized the tasks, and attempted to change the subject. However, when she was allowed to direct the interaction and talk about topics of high personal interest, her affect improved markedly, as did her communication skills.

A3's matched peer, T3, also an 11-year-old girl, used simpler syntax on the CON task than did A3 in terms of MLCU, CD, and subordinate clauses (see Table 8–1). However, she used higher syntactic complexity on the two expository tasks than did A3 (see Tables 8–2 and 8–3). For example, T3's MLCU was 2.39 words higher than A3's on the FGS task and 3.9 words higher than A3's on the PCR task. Although T3's syntactic complexity was lower than A3's on the CON task, her syntactic complexity increased as she moved from the conversational to the expository tasks, reflecting the expected, typical pattern in spoken discourse. Moreover, during both expository tasks, T3 readily responded to each of the examiner's prompts with detailed explanations that were organized, coherent, and relevant. For example, when asked to explain how to play the game of Monopoly, she began as follows:

> Well, first you have to choose your pieces and then find out who's going to be banker. But if you're the banker, you have to choose, are you going to play the game too and be the banker, or are you going to be the banker and not play? And then the banker has to give you two five hundreds, two fifties, two one hundreds, six ones, six tens, six fives, and six twenties. And then you roll to see who goes first. And then you can't buy anything until you go around once.

Similarly, during the PCR task, T3 provided reasonable explanations that reflected concern for everyone involved, suggesting that both conflicts could be resolved by having the characters talk to each other to find out what the other was thinking. During the Science Fair scenario, when asked to explain why that was a good strategy, T3 replied that through talking, "you can let the other person know that you really do care." Thus, her comments evidenced a developmentally mature approach to resolving conflicts (Selman et al., 1986).

Areas to Target with A3

The interview with A3 indicated that she was able to use age-appropriate syntax. However, she did so only when she could direct the conversation and select the topic. Unfortunately, her communication skills quickly broke down when she was asked to discuss a topic about which she was less knowledgeable or one that she disliked. By collaborating with A3's teacher, the SLP could generate a list of topics that would be relevant to A3's school success (e.g., science) and potentially of interest to her (e.g., alternative methods of home heating, organic farming techniques, how recycled plastic bottles can be used to build fences and decks). The SLP and teacher could work together to promote A3's knowledge of those and other meaningful topics, which would support her ability to talk about them. Then, in this way, language intervention could target the following behaviors:

1. Increase the number and range of topics that A3 can discuss in a positive manner, using complete sentences with complex syntax.

2. Increase the frequency of answering topic-specific questions with positive, informative replies, using complete sentences with complex syntax.

3. Increase A3's willingness to engage in conversations about topics that are new or less familiar to her but of high interest to others (including her peers).

Pair #4

A4, a 10-year-old girl with mild autism, began the conversational task hesitantly, speaking slowly and producing utterances that were less than a C-unit (e.g., "or both, oh yeah, all right, good yeah"). Gradually, she began to produce longer utterances (e.g., "Oh and also I really like to draw pictures. And now I can draw horses cantering") as the examiner remained patient and supportive. For the FGS task, A4 chose dog training as her topic. Speaking guardedly, she required multiple prompts and the rephrasing of questions by the examiner in order to continue the interaction. In addition, because dog training is not a game or a sport, it was necessary to modify the questions to suit the topic (e.g., Examiner: "What are the goals of dog training? What are you trying to get your dog to do?"). Even with these modifications, A4 tended to produce only one utterance at a time rather than a string of topic-relevant utterances, responding directly to each prompt, with little spontaneous elaboration. Thus, with frequent scaffolding from the examiner, the FGS task became a conversation rather than an expository monologue. Because the tasks were modified in this way, A4's scores for language productivity must be interpreted cautiously. Had the examiner not responded in this flexible manner, it is likely that A4 would have produced far fewer total C-units on the CON and FGS tasks.

Nevertheless, A4's performance improved markedly during the PCR task, which she appeared to find more interesting than the FGS task. For this task, she retold each scenario accurately and completely, and did so without additional prompting from the examiner, and the suggestions she offered for resolving the conflicts were creative and sophisticated. For example, for the Science Fair scenario, she indicated that it was important for the group members to try to talk with each other as a first step and that, if that did not succeed, to bring in a facilitator to avoid making people mad or hurting their feelings. It was noteworthy also that she offered a number of spontaneous comments about the stories. During the Fast Food scenario, she pointed out that if the characters "needed to be in a rush to get someone's order down," then they "wouldn't have time to talk this out slowly like at school." She also discussed the importance of "sharing responsibility," explaining insightfully how "it does take a lot of work to own a restaurant."

A4's syntactic complexity increased as she moved from conversational to expository discourse, reflecting the expected pattern. Note also that her syntactic complexity was higher during the PCR task than the FGS task, evidenced by her MLCU and CD scores (see Table 8–3). Thus, it appears that the PCR task, which seemed to engage her interests more fully, helped reveal her ability to use language in a more complex, creative, and sophisticated manner. Her performance on this task indicated that her syntactic development was appropriate, as her scores were similar to those of T4, the 10-year-old girl who served as her matched peer.

However, despite their similar scores on the PCR task, T4's overall performance differed markedly from that of A4. During the conversation, T4 spoke freely about preferred activities, producing multiple utterances on the same topic (e.g., "I am kind of good at tetherball. But there's only a couple of people that I can beat. And I like playing with someone that's the same as me"). Then, for the FGS task, with little prompting, T4 chose the game of Sorry and proceeded to explain the details of this favorite activity in a clear, efficient, and organized fashion. For example, in one uninterrupted string of 19 C-units, she described how to set up the board, how to determine which player starts, how to use the playing pieces and cards, how to disadvantage an opponent, and how to win. Then, when asked about key strategies, she explained that "you have to be smart," "think about the other players," and trade only with those who are "closest to your home."

Similarly, during the PCR task, T4 showed a clear understanding of what was being asked of her and a mature understanding of interpersonal issues. After retelling the scenarios, she explained the nature of each conflict and offered solutions that involved compromising, making the activities more enjoyable, not making other group members angry, and not requiring authority figures to intervene. These observations suggested that she was an insightful young lady who took responsibility for resolving interpersonal conflicts.

Goals for A4

Similar to A3, A4 demonstrated the ability to use age-appropriate syntax when she spoke about topics that interested her and about which she was knowledgeable (working in a restaurant, resolving interpersonal conflicts). However, her communication skills broke down when she was asked to talk about less familiar topics. This suggests that it would be worthwhile to expand the range of topics about which A4 can converse comfortably and fluently. As with A3, this might be accomplished by consulting with her teacher and generating a list of topics that would be interesting to her and relevant to school success (e.g., the solar system, how glaciers were formed, the life cycle of an oak tree). Language intervention then could assist her to talk about those topics in a confident and informed manner. Thus, the following behaviors could be targeted for A4:

1. Increase the range of topics she can discuss confidently, using complete sentences with complex syntax.

2. Increase the frequency of answering topic-specific questions by having A4 elaborate on her replies with multiple utterances that contain complex syntax.

3. Increase her willingness to engage in conversations about topics that are new or less familiar to her but of high interest to others (including her peers).

Discussion

In this exploratory study, syntactic development was examined in school-age children and adolescents with ASD, using language sampling tasks to elicit conversational and expository discourse. Prior to this study, little was known about the ability of students with ASD to employ complex syntax in natural speaking tasks, particularly during expository discourse.

The findings of the study were interpreted informally because of the small number of participants, coupled with the high degree of variability that occurred, particularly in the ASD group. Under these conditions, three of the four speakers with ASD demonstrated age-appropriate syntactic development and one speaker with ASD evidenced a severe syntactic deficit. In addition, three speakers with ASD had difficulty with the tasks, requiring the examiner to spontaneously adapt the activities by modifying the questions and providing additional prompts and supports. Nevertheless, even under these modified conditions, the tasks revealed helpful information about the strengths and weaknesses of each speaker with ASD.

For example, A1, a boy with moderate to severe autism, produced a large number of fragments, and many of his utterances contained grammatical errors. Those factors, combined with a short MLCU and low CD scores, indicated the presence of a syntactic deficit. In addition, he did not show the expected pattern of increasing the complexity of his utterances as he moved from the conversational to the expository tasks, which suggested a restricted ability to use subordination. Similarly, A3 found the expository tasks challenging, requiring the examiner to adapt the activities in a flexible manner. Indeed, A3 was able to continue the interaction only when she could talk about topics of her own choosing, primarily in the conversational genre. Thus, her MLCU and CD scores did not increase as she moved through the tasks. Nevertheless, under those modified conditions, she produced developmentally appropriate, complex sentences. By remaining calm and flexible with these two speakers, the examiner obtained clinically useful information, identifying a syntactic deficit in one speaker and ruling out such a deficit in the other. The two remaining speakers with ASD, A2 and A4, also demonstrated age-appropriate syntactic development. However, qualitative analyses of their performance indicated other unique challenges. For example, during the FGS task, A2 tended to provide excessive detail when talking about his favorite game, Pokémon, and he did not attend closely to the listener's needs when his explanations lacked clarity, suggesting a problem with perspective taking. Similarly, during the PCR task, he tended to focus on the needs of only one of the characters, ignoring all others in the story. Those sorts of observations of A2, revealed by the expository tasks, could be helpful in designing intervention to build his awareness of other people's perspectives in situations in which he uses expository discourse, such as at school when talking with teachers and classmates about science, math, or history.

With A4, it was useful to observe the contrast in her behavior during the two expository tasks, with greater syntactic complexity and a more fluent speaking style exhibited during the PCR task. Moreover, she appeared to enjoy the PCR task more than the FGS task, which allowed her to demonstrate her knowledge of how to resolve peer conflicts, a topic she had learned about in school. Had only the FGS task been presented, her ability to speak in this more sophisticated manner would not have been revealed.

CONCLUSIONS

This small pilot study examined syntactic development in children and adolescents with ASD by eliciting samples of conversational and expository discourse. We found that the speaker who exhibited the most severe autism also exhibited the poorest syntactic development. The three other speakers, who had milder autism, exhibited weaknesses in organization, clarity, and perspective taking during the tasks despite having adequate syntactic development. Although the number of participants was too small to draw generalizations, the results are consistent with a pattern in which more severe autism is linked to syntactic deficits (Bennett et al., 2008). Despite the preliminary nature of the study, the findings also suggest that efforts to examine syntactic development in speakers with ASD using natural speaking tasks can be a fruitful clinical activity. However, it is emphasized that the language sampling tasks employed in this study needed to be modified for three of the four speakers with ASD, requiring patience and flexibility from the examiner. Had the examiner been unwilling to make adjustments, it is likely that the levels of language productivity would have been quite low for those speakers. Thus, the tasks were not administered to those speakers in the way in which they had been designed, or in the way in which they had been administered to the typical peers. Nevertheless, even under modified conditions, the tasks yielded useful information about each speaker with ASD, offering practical implications for intervention.

PART II

Grammar Review
and Exercises

Words and

Traditional parts of speech, or "word classes," are nouns, pronouns, adjectives, verbs, adverbs, prepositions, particles, conjunctions, articles, and interjections (Crews, 1977; Quirk & Greenbaum, 1973; Quirk, Greenbaum, Leech, & Svartvik, 1985). This is an ancient but useful method of classifying words that was introduced by the Greek philosopher Aristotle (384–322 BC). Aristotle sought to understand how different words function to express different meanings (*Grammar: Parts of Speech* [2009] http://eslus.com/LESSONS/GRAMMAR/POS/pos1.htm).

PARTS OF SPEECH

Nouns

A noun is often described as a "person, place, or thing" (e.g., *dog, cat, house, tree, car*). Nouns can be pluralized (e.g., *dogs, cats, houses, trees, cars*). They also can be preceded by an article (e.g., *a, an, the, some*). A proper noun is the name of a specific person, place, or thing (e.g., John Smith, Chicago, Tugman Park). Another unique aspect of nouns is that they can be concrete (e.g., *door, siren, fur, apple, flower*) or abstract (e.g., *compassion, empathy, freedom, respect, truth*). Whereas concrete nouns refer to physical objects that one can see, hear, feel, taste, or smell, abstract nouns refer to mental constructs or concepts that lack tangible, physical referents.

Pronouns

A pronoun represents or "stands in for" a noun. There are many types of pronouns, such as personal, possessive, demonstrative, reflexive, relative, indefinite, and interrogative.

1. Personal pronoun: Refers to people or animals and can substitute for specific names of those things (e.g., *I, you, me, he, she, we, they*).

2. Possessive pronoun: Used in place of a noun and implies ownership (e.g., *his* house, *her* mother, *their* books).

3. Demonstrative pronoun: Refers to people, animals, or objects and singles out what they refer to (e.g., *this, these, those, that*; *this* baby is cute; *that* cat is Puff; *those* are Mary's books; *these* shoes are mine).

4. Reflexive pronoun: Refers back to the subject of the sentence (e.g., *himself, herself, themselves, itself, ourselves, yourself*). For example, Mary helped *herself*; Jim and Joe taught *themselves*.

5. Relative pronoun: Introduces a relative clause, which tells about a subject or an object. For example, the boy *who* is late is my brother; the donut *that* you ate was chocolate; you bought the cake *that* was orange; my sister is the one *who* is happy.

6. Indefinite pronoun: Does not refer to a specific person, animal, or thing, but refers to something more general (e.g., *anybody, anyone, one, each, any, everything, everyone, some, all, something, somebody, someone*). Other indefinite pronouns include *what, which, who*, and *whose* (when they are not introducing a relative clause). For example, she knows *what* to do; I know *who* will win; I know *which* cat is mine.

7. Interrogative pronoun: Initiates a question (e.g., *who, what, why, when, how, whom, whose, which*). For example, *What* time is it? *How* are you? *Whose* dog is this?

Adjectives

An adjective describes or modifies a noun (e.g., *old, red, big, happy*). Adjectives can be made comparative and superlative (e.g., the *bigger* cake, the *highest* mountain). Other types of words cannot be made comparative or superlative.

Verbs

A verb expresses action (e.g., *run, jump, fall*) or state of being (e.g., *think, feel, know, believe*). Verbs tell you about the subject of the sentence and can express **simple** present, past, or future tense, as in the following examples, in which "John" is the subject:

John runs three miles every day. (simple present tense)

John ran three miles yesterday. (simple past tense)

John will run three miles tomorrow. (simple future tense)

In addition to the simple present, past, or future tense of the verb, as in the previous examples, there is the **progressive** form of the verb, as in the following examples in which Bob is the subject:

Bob is driving the van today. (present progressive tense)

Bob was driving the van yesterday. (past progressive tense)

Bob will be driving the van tomorrow. (future progressive tense)

Finally, in addition to the simple and progressive verb forms, there is the **perfect** form, which involves the notion of verb **aspect**. Aspect indicates "the point of time from which an action is seen to take place" (Jarvie, 2007, p. 37). This can involve the present, past, or future aspect, as in the following examples, in which Tom is the subject:

Tom has lived in Chicago for 20 years. (present perfect tense)

Tom had lived in Chicago for 20 years. (past perfect tense)

Tom will have lived in Chicago for 20 years next Christmas. (future perfect tense)

Verb Types

There are many types of verbs.

1. Main verb: A sentence must have a main verb. The main verb is most directly related to the subject of the sentence (e.g., Jill *wants* an apple; Bob *runs* fast). Main verbs can express different tenses —past, present, and future. Two types of past tense verbs are past regular and past irregular. Past regular verbs add -*ed* (e.g., yesterday, the boy *walked*; the boy *talked*; the boy *jumped*). Past irregular verbs take an unpredictable form and do not add -*ed* (e.g., *ran*, *wrote*, *drove*, *fell*, *ate*).

2. Copula verb: This is the verb *to be* in its various forms (*is*, *are*, *am*, *was*, *were*, *will be*). For example, the ball *is* red; Bill *was* a cowboy; they *are* spooky; we *were* children. The copula is a finite verb that links or joins the subject of the sentence to the predicate.

It is the main verb of the clause. It is marked for person (first, second, third), tense (present, past, future), and number (singular, plural; see Table 9–1).

3. Auxiliary verb: These are helping verbs that combine with other verbs and work with the main verb (e.g., I *am* driving; he *is* swimming; they *are* running; we *had been* eating). The auxiliary verb (*am, is, are*) expresses person (first, second, third), tense (past, present, future), and number (singular, plural). For example, he *was* swimming; they *were* running. Other auxiliary verbs include *can, will,* and *do.* For example, I *can* read this; she *will* be late; *don't* forget to vote (see Table 9–1).

4. Modal verb: This is a special type of auxiliary verb. Modal verbs help express the mood or attitude of the speaker, or special conditions (e.g., *might, could, should, may, need, will, ought to, used to, would, shall, must*). For example, you *might* like the new book; he *should* do his work; we *may* go shopping tomorrow. Modals can

Table 9–1. How Copula and Auxiliary Verbs Are Marked for Person (1st, 2nd, 3rd), Tense (Present, Past, Future), and Number (Singular, Plural)

Number	Person	Tense		
		Present	**Past**	**Future**
		Copula Verb		
Singular	1st	I am happy.	I was happy.	I will be happy.
	2nd	You are happy.	You were happy.	You will be happy.
	3rd	She/he is happy.	She/he was happy.	She/he will be happy.
Plural	1st	We are happy.	We were happy.	We will be happy.
	2nd	You are happy.	You were happy.	You will be happy.
	3rd	They are happy.	They were happy.	They will be happy.
		Auxiliary Verb		
Singular	1st	I am going.	I was going.	I will be going.
	2nd	You are going.	You were going.	You will be going.
	3rd	She/he is going.	She/he was going.	She/he will be going.
Plural	1st	We are going.	We were going.	We will be going.
	2nd	You are going.	You were going.	You will be going.
	3rd	They are going.	They were going.	They will be going.

express a mood of uncertainty (e.g., you *might* like the movie) or of certainty (e.g., you *must* see the movie).

5. Finite verb: A verb that is marked for person (first, second, third), tense (past, present, future), and number (singular, plural):

I *walked* to the store yesterday.

She *walked* to the store yesterday.

He *will walk* to the store tomorrow.

They *are walking* to the store right now.

He/she/it *walks*; I walk; they *walk* every day.

Mary has *walked* 16 miles today.

6. Nonfinite verb: A verb that is unmarked for person, tense, and number. They include infinitives, gerunds, and participles.

a. Infinitive: This is a verb in its unmarked form, as one would find it in the dictionary. It is often preceded by "to" (e.g., *to go, to run, to dance, to play*). For example, I wanted *to go* home; the teenagers planned *to dance* all night. Sometimes *to* is omitted (e.g., I saw the lion *eat* the meat).

b. Gerund: This verb ends with *-ing* and acts like a noun (e.g., *swimming* is good exercise; *smoking* is bad for you; they enjoy *knitting*; her hobbies are *fishing* and *embroidering*).

c. Participle: This verb ends in *-ing*, *-ed*, or *-en* and acts like an adjective (e.g., the *swimming* boy got to shore; the *crooked* fence fell down; the *broken* cup was on the floor).

Adverbs

An adverb modifies or describes a verb (e.g., he drove *slowly*; the rain fell *quietly*; she ran *quickly*). Adverbs often end in the suffix *-ly* (e.g., *nicely, quickly, hastily, slowly*) but not always (e.g., I will work *now*). There are many types of adverbs—for example:

1. Adverb of time: This answers the question "when." For example, when did she run? She ran *early*. Other examples include *later, tonight, yesterday, before, after, now*.

2. Adverb of place: This answers the question "where." For example, where did she run? She ran *everywhere*. Other examples include *anywhere, here, somewhere, there*.

3. Adverb of manner: This answers the question "how?" For example, how did she drive? She drove *cautiously*. Other examples include *carefully, jokingly, kindly, slowly*.

4. Adverb of magnitude: This expresses the degree of size, amount, or intensity (e.g., *slightly, somewhat, rather, quite, decidedly, extremely, unusually*).

5. Adverb of likelihood: This expresses the degree of probability (e.g., *absolutely, certainly, definitely, maybe, perhaps, positively, possibly, probably*).

Adverbs can modify other types of words besides verbs. For example, they can modify adjectives (e.g., the *very* pretty coat) and other adverbs (e.g., *early* yesterday morning; she ran *very* quickly). In fact, any modifier that is not an adjective or an article is probably an adverb.

Prepositions

A preposition is a small word such as *to, in, under, over, into, on,* or *above*. These words introduce a prepositional phrase (e.g., I went *to the store*; I put it *on the shelf*; the ball rolled *under the bed*). A prepositional phrase consists of a preposition and its object.

Particles

A particle looks like a preposition but does not act like one. Particles are small words such as *up, down, off, in,* and *out* that co-occur with specific verbs as in *look up, roll down, turn off, let in, throw out, cut up,* and *wear out*. Particles, unlike prepositions, can sometimes shift their position to the right of the object. For example, he looked *up* the number/he looked the number *up*; she rolled *down* the window/she rolled the window *down*; he turned *off* the TV/he turned the TV *off*; she let *in* the cat/she let the cat *in*; he threw *out* the trash/he threw the trash *out*.

Conjunctions

A conjunction is a small word that connects other words (within a clause) or connects clauses (within a sentence). They are also called *connectives* (e.g., *and, but, or, for, so, yet, although*). For example, he likes ham *and* eggs; I'll take blue *or* red; he doesn't like jam *but* she does. There are three major types of conjunctions: coordinate, subordinate, and correlative.

1. Coordinate (e.g., *and, but, for, or, so, yet*): These conjunctions introduce an independent (main) clause (e.g., I like strawberry *but* Bill likes chocolate). Coordinate conjunctions often signal a main

clause, one that could stand by itself and make sense (e.g., I went shopping, *and* Mary stayed home).

2. Subordinate (e.g., *after, although, unless*): These conjunctions introduce a dependent (subordinate) clause (e.g., *although* it was raining, we went for a walk). Subordinate conjunctions signal a dependent (subordinate) clause, a clause that usually cannot stand alone and make sense (e.g., *after* the rain stopped, we went outside). Other examples of subordinate conjunctions include the following: *as, as if, as long as, as soon as, as though, because, before, how, if, in order that, provided that, since, though, till, until, when, whenever, where, wherever, while, so that*. Some of these conjunctions also may introduce a phrase rather than a clause (e.g., *Because of his teacher's encouragement*, he applied for a scholarship).

3. Correlative (e.g., *both . . . and; either . . . or; neither . . . nor; not only . . . but also*): Correlative conjunctions occur as groups of words within the same clause. For example, I want *both* coffee *and* pie; George wants *not only* chocolate *but also* vanilla; I'll take *either* pizza *or* spaghetti; he likes *neither* pie *nor* cake.

Adverbial Conjuncts

This is a special type of conjunction that introduces a main clause. For example, *meanwhile, hence, consequently, accordingly, similarly, conversely, contrastively*. These words are frequently found in literate contexts and serve to link ideas in a logical manner. For example, Tim likes Bach; *consequently*, he bought a ticket to the concert.

Articles

An article is a small word that immediately precedes a noun or adjective. The article identifies (or points out) the noun; it doesn't describe it (e.g., *a, the, an*). For example, *the* dog was old; I want *a* big cookie. Articles are either definite (*the*) or indefinite (*a, an*). A definite article identifies a particular object (e.g., *the* dog, *the* girl). An indefinite article doesn't specify any particular object (e.g., I'll take *an* orange; I'd like *a* book).

Interjections

This is an informal expression of emotion (e.g., Ah! Ahah! Good grief! Gosh! Hey! Hurrah! Oh! OK! Ouch! Right! Shh! Ugh! Whew!).

PHRASES

A *phrase* is a small group of words that functions as if it were a specific part of speech (e.g., noun, verb, preposition). A phrase is a larger unit than a word but a smaller unit than a clause because it lacks a subject–predicate relationship (Crews, 1977; Dumond, 1993; Jarvie, 2007).

The main types of phrases are defined next, followed by examples.

Noun Phrase

Definition: A group of words that contains a noun; it may also contain an article (e.g., *a, an, the*) and possibly some modifiers.

Examples:

The snowy mountain range (noun = *range*)

A glorious golden field (noun = *field*)

An acrobatic ski jump (noun = *jump*)

Age zero main sequence (noun = *sequence*)

Verb Phrase

Definition: A group of words that contains a verb and possibly some auxiliaries such as modal verbs (e.g., *could, should, must*).

Examples:

Had been sleeping (main verb = *sleeping*)

Could have been watching (main verb = *watching*)

May have written (main verb = *written*)

Was building (main verb = *building*)

Prepositional Phrase

Definition: A group of words that contains a preposition followed by a noun phrase.

Examples:

Under the rock (preposition = *under*)

Along the winding river (preposition = *along*)

In a colorful clown suit (preposition = *in*)

Over the slippery slope (preposition = *over*)

Prepositional phrases can also post-modify noun phrases:

The sports car *with the silver hub caps* (preposition = *with*)

The very old house *beyond the apple tree* (preposition = *beyond*)

Adjective Phrase

Definition: A group of words that contains an adjective and modifies a noun or noun phrase. The adjective phrase can come either before or after the noun phrase.

Examples:

A *complex and scary* poem (adjectives = *complex, scary*)

An *honest and forthright* mechanic (adjectives = *honest, forthright*)

The dog was *extremely well-behaved* (adjective = *well-behaved*)

The house was *old and dilapidated* (adjectives = *old, dilapidated*)

Adverb Phrase

Definition A: A group of words that contains an adverb that modifies another adverb; as a unit, those words work together to modify a verb in the sentence.

Examples:

She ran *rather quickly* down the street (the adverb *rather* modifies the adverb *quickly*; as a unit, the adverb phrase modifies the verb *ran*)

She counted the money *quite carefully* (the adverb *quite* modifies the adverb *carefully*; as a unit, the adverb phrase modifies the verb *counted*)

He greeted the diners *most cheerfully* (the adverb *most* modifies the adverb *cheerfully*; as a unit, the adverb phrase modifies the verb *greeted*)

He opened the door *somewhat cautiously* (the adverb *somewhat* modifies the adverb *cautiously*; as a unit, the adverb phrase modifies the verb *opened*)

Definition B: An adverb phrase can also begin with a subordinate conjunction and modify a verb. Unlike an adverbial clause (see Chapter 10), an adverb phrase does not contain a verb.

Examples:

He ordered coffee *after midnight* (the adverb phrase tells **when** he ordered coffee)

She will sleep *until the dawn* (the adverb phrase tells **how long** she will sleep)

Because of the rain, they stayed home (the adverb phrase tells **why** they stayed home)

He ate lunch *before noon* (the adverb phrase tells **when** he ate)

They have lived in California *since the earthquake of 1971*.

EXERCISES: WORDS AND PHRASES

Exercise 9–1. Identifying Words in Passages

In passages 1 through 6, circle all of the *nouns* including *gerunds* and *proper nouns* (but not pronouns):

1. Computers can do lots of things. They can add millions of numbers in the twinkling of an eye. They can outwit chess grandmasters. They can guide weapons to their targets. They can book you onto a plane between a guitar-strumming nun and a nonsmoking physics professor. Some can even play the bongos. That's quite a variety! So if we're going to talk about computers, we'd better decide right now which of them we're going to look at, and how (Feynman, 1996, p. 1).

2. Most of the luxuries, and many of the so-called comforts of life, are not only not indispensable, but positive hindrances to the elevation of mankind. With respect to luxuries and comforts, the wisest have ever lived a more simple and meager life than the poor. The ancient philosophers, Chinese, Hindoo, Persian, and Greek, were a class than which none has been poorer in outward riches, none so rich in inward (Thoreau, 2004, p. 14).

3. For a French parent, education is everything. The child must have as many and as important certificates of academic attainment as possible. In American and British business life, experience counts. In French life, the right education and the right certificates count. This is why some experienced American and British teachers wishing to work in France are horrified to find their experience downgraded because they do not have the equivalent degree certificate to the French one (Tomalin, 2003, p. 93).

4. There are two kinds of knowledge. One is the everyday kind of knowledge we have of the world, which we get through our senses (usually called "empirical" knowledge). Plato thought that this kind

of knowledge was useful enough for ordinary people to go about their everyday lives. But it wasn't the real thing. Like Heraclitus, Pythagoras, and maybe Socrates, Plato thought that the empirical world was a kind of illusion, a veil that hid the real truth from us (Robinson & Groves, 2005, p. 62).

5. Plato was probably the greatest philosopher of all time, and the first to collect all sorts of different ideas and arguments into books that everyone can read. He wanted to know about everything and constantly pestered his fellow philosophers for answers to his disturbing questions. He also had resolute ideas of his own, some of which seem sensible enough, and some of which now seem extremely odd. But, from the start, he knew that "doing philosophy" was a very special activity (Robinson & Groves, 2005, p. 3).

6. I propose that educationalists should no longer conceive of children as passive, empty jam jars who need to be stuffed with information, but as independently minded problem solvers who need to be continually challenged. (John Dewey; Robinson & Groves, 2004, p. 111)

In passages 7 through 12, circle all of the *adjectives* including the *participles*:

7. The legacy of Scotland's tumultuous and often violent history can be found in its extraordinary array of prehistoric sites, religious ruins, and other historic attractions. Today these relics offer visitors intriguing insights into some of the defining battles, heroes, and forgotten worlds of the country's rich and turbulent past (Wilson & Murphy, 2008, p. 274).

8. Once Oregon was thought to be immune to earthquakes. Today we know that we have them in three different flavors—devastating subduction earthquakes like the 1700 catastrophe, deep intraplate earthquakes like the Puget Sound temblors of 1949 and 2001, and sharp local jolts like the Spring Break Quake of 1993 (Sullivan, 2008, p. 67).

9. Some artists are finite draftsmen with meticulous drawing skills. Other artists are storytellers. A few invent a new lens of perception. But Sarkis Antikajian is a painter. His work is a bodacious celebration of brush dipped in paint and spread across canvas. While some painters claim they paint light, Sarkis Antikajian paints energy. He leaves his viewer breathless by the onslaught on his transcription. His masterful use of intense chroma ravishes the visual cortex in a heady embrace. Sarkis wields color with the same bravado employed by the trumpeter Maynard Ferguson when he plays C above high C (Moffet, 2006, pp. 18–19).

10. The ancient Greeks made extensive use of honey in salves and potions, in prepared dishes, to make perfume, as libations for the dead, and to appease the gods. Bee-keepers numbered among their ranks the philosopher Aristotle; for Hippocrates, the father of medicine, honey was a favorite remedy. The followers of Pythagoras lived on a diet of bread and honey—and seemed to far outlive any of their contemporaries (Style, 1993, p. 14).

11. French culture once dominated Western civilization. From about 1650 to about 1920, the upper classes in several countries preferred French to their own native languages. French was the official language for diplomatic negotiations and much government business. The achievements of French writers, artists, architects, and composers were widely admired and imitated. Since then, other cultures have moved to the forefront. English has overtaken French as the most widely spoken language (Harris, 1989, p. 167).

12. Mister Fox was just about famished and thirsty too, when he stole into a vineyard where the sun-ripened grapes were hanging upon a trellis in a tempting show, but too high for him to reach. He took a run and a jump, snapping at the nearest bunch, but missed. Again and again he jumped, only to miss the luscious prize. At last, worn out with his efforts, he retreated, muttering, "Well, I never really wanted those

grapes anyway. I am sure they are sour and perhaps wormy in the bargain." ("The Fox and the Grapes," Grosset & Dunlap, 1947, p. 14)

In passages 13 through 17, circle all of the *finite verbs*:

13. Trieste, set on a gulf with rolling hills as a backdrop, is the most important seaport on the northern Adriatic. Because of its geographic position and its history, the cooking of Trieste is eclectic. *Gnocchetti di fegato*, liver dumplings, are a reminder of Austrian ties. Venezia's influence is apparent in its many risotto, including its own version of *risi e bisi*. It also has its own variation of *brodetto*, the fish stew so popular along the entire Italian coastline. Made with local fish, the sauce contains vinegar, wine, and sometimes tomatoes, and is always served with grilled polenta. There are many rich desserts. Typical are *strucoli*, similar to strudel, which like *preniz*, an Easter specialty, are made with a variety of ingredients (Luciano et al., 1991, p. 87).

14. When first I took up my abode in the woods, that is, began to spend my nights as well as days there, which, by accident, was on Independence Day, or the fourth of July, 1845, my house was not finished for winter, but was merely a defense against the rain, without plastering or chimney, the walls being of rough weather-stained boards, with wide chinks, which made it cool at night (Thoreau, 2004, p. 81).

15. The only house I had been the owner of before, if I except a boat, was a tent, which I used occasionally when making excursions in the summer, and this is still rolled up in my garret; but the boat, after passing from hand to hand, has gone down the stream of time. With this more substantial shelter about me, I had made some progress toward settling in the world (Thoreau, 2004, p. 82).

16. Sonja Kovalevsky (1850–1891), earlier known as Sophia Korvin-Krukovsky, was a gifted mathematician. She was born in Moscow to Russian nobility. She left Russia in 1868 because universities were

closed to women. She went to Germany because she wished to study
with Karl Weierstrass in Berlin. It was said that her early interest
in mathematics was due in part to an odd wallpaper that covered
her room in a summer house. Fascinated, she spent hours trying to
make sense of it. The paper turned out to be lecture notes on higher
mathematics purchased by her father during his student days (K.
Smith, 1995, p. 479).

17. In his famous laboratory school at the University of Chicago,
    children were (and still are) encouraged to solve problems by
    inventing hypotheses and testing them. Dewey thought that art
    should be encouraged because it stimulates imaginative "solutions"
    to its own unique "problems" (Robinson & Groves, 2004, p. 111).

In passages 18 through 22, circle all of the *adverbs*:

18. Western Iran extends from the border with Armenia and Azerbaijan in
    the north to the industrial city of Ahvaz near the Gulf. Culturally, it is
    the most diverse part of Iran, with Azaris, Armenians, Loris, Bakhtiaris,
    and Kurds among the distinct ethnic groups you'll encounter.
    Despite this and a wealth of historical, religious, and cultural sights,
    stunning mountain scenery, and great trekking possibilities, few
    travelers see more than Tabriz. Pity them, then take advantage of the
    unspoilt expanses and go yourself (Ham et al., 2006, p. 199).

19. The Middle East is home to some of the world's most significant
    cities—Jerusalem, Cairo, Damascus, Baghdad, and Istanbul. The
    ruins of the once similarly epic cities of history—Petra, Persepolis,
    Ephesus, Palmyra, Baalbek, Leptis Magna, and the bounty of ancient
    Egypt—also mark the passage of centuries in a region where the
    ancient world lives and breathes. The landscapes of the region
    are equally spellbinding, from the unrivalled seas of sand dunes
    and palm-fringed lakes in Libya's Sahara desert to the stunning
    mountains of the north, and the underwater world of the Red Sea
    (Ham et al., 2006, p. 4).

20. Mt. Fuji is the highest mountain in Japan, and by far the most splendid, but during July and August (the open season) it is not a dauntingly hard climb. An athlete, it is said, could leave home in Tokyo in the morning, reach the peak, and be home in time for dinner. Most people prefer to take it at a more leisurely pace, spending a night at the top and greeting the morning sun with a cry of "*Banzai!*" (Popham, 1992, p. 159).

21. I left the woods for as good a reason as I went there. Perhaps it seemed to me that I had several more lives to live, and could not spare any more time for that one. It is remarkable how easily and insensibly we fall into a particular route, and make a beaten track for ourselves. I had not lived there a week before my feet wore a path from my door to the pond-side; and though it is five or six years since I trod it, it is still quite distinct. It is true, I fear that others may have fallen into it, and so helped to keep it open (Thoreau, 2004, p. 313).

22. John Dewey (1859–1952) was a systematic pragmatist or "instrumentalist" who believed that being "philosophical" really meant being critically intelligent and maintaining a "scientific" approach to human problems. Pragmatists like Dewey were great enthusiasts for the successes of science and its methods of inquiry. Dewey was convinced that philosophy could also play a key role in a creative American democracy by contributing to all kinds of knowledge in ethics, art, education, and the newly emerging social sciences. Like Pierce, Dewey was a theoretical "fallibilist," but still firmly a believer in the real possibility of practical progress in human affairs. Society can only progress if its members are educated to be intelligent and flexible (Robinson & Groves, 2004, p. 111).

In passage 23, circle all of the *prepositions*:

23. The year 1877 was an important one in the study of the planet Mars. The Red Planet came unusually close to Earth, affording astronomers

an especially good view. Of particular note was the discovery by
U.S. Naval Observatory astronomer Asaph Hall, of the two moons
circling Mars. But most exciting was the report of the Italian
astronomer Giovanni Schiaparelli on his observations of a network
of linear markings that he termed *canali*. In Italian, the word
usually means "grooves" or "channels," but it can also mean "canals"
(Chaisson & McMillan, 2005, p. 140).

In passages 24 and 25, circle all of the *pronouns*:

24. This country, with its institutions, belongs to the people who inhabit
    it. Whenever they shall grow weary of the existing government,
    they can exercise their *constitutional* right of amending it, or their
    revolutionary right to dismember, or overthrow it. I cannot be
    ignorant of the fact that many worthy and patriotic citizens are
    desirous of having the constitution amended (Emerson, 1841/2009,
    Self-Reliance, p. 41).

25. All the barnyard knew that the hen was indisposed. So one day, the
    cat decided to pay her a visit of condolence. Creeping up to her nest,
    the cat in his most sympathetic voice said, "How are you, my dear
    friend? I was so sorry to hear of your illness. Isn't there something
    that I can bring you to cheer you up and to help you feel like
    yourself again?" "Thank you," said the hen. "Please be good enough
    to leave me in peace, and I have no fear but I shall soon be well."
    Moral: Uninvited guests are often most welcome when they are
    gone. ("The Cat and the Hen," Grosset & Dunlap, 1947, p. 133).

In passage 26, circle all of the *articles*:

26. Starting in the 1870s, another upheaval in the arts resulted from the
    development of a new approach to painting called Impressionism.
    Young artists rejected the long-accepted, conventional ways of
    presenting reality. They too were fascinated by recent discoveries

in science and experimented with new techniques for capturing the effects of light. Often they used tiny dabs of complementary colors, relying on the viewer's eyes and mind to bring them together and form the desired effect. The Postimpressionist painters of the late 19th and early 20th centuries worked out new ways of seeing that were highly personal. They scorned the old emphasis on reproducing reality as accurately as possible. Instead, they sought to express their own innermost visions and emotions (Harris, 1989, pp. 173–175).

In passages 27 and 28, circle all of the *conjunctions*:

27. A woman of many gifts, Margaret Fuller (1810–1850) is most aptly remembered as America's first true feminist. In her brief yet fruitful life, she was variously author, editor, literary and social critic, journalist, poet, and revolutionary. She was also one of the few female members of the prestigious Transcendentalist movement, whose ranks included Ralph Waldo Emerson, Henry David Thoreau, Elizabeth Palmer Peabody, Nathaniel Hawthorne, and many other prominent New England intellectuals of the day. As coeditor of the transcendentalist journal, *The Dial*, Fuller was able to give voice to her groundbreaking social critique on woman's place in society (Fuller, 1845/1999), the genesis of the book that was later to become *Woman in the Nineteenth Century* (Pine, 1999, p. 133).

28. When people started to analyze English grammar in the eighteenth century, it seemed logical to look at the language using the terms and distinctions which had proved so useful in studying Latin. English had no word-endings, it seemed. Therefore, it had no "grammar." But of course there is far more to grammar than word-endings. Some languages (such as Chinese) have none at all. English has less than a dozen types of regular ending (and a few irregular ones) (Crystal, 2002, p. 22).

Exercise 9–2. Word Classes

For each word that is in bold, indicate its class—noun, pronoun, verb, adjective, adverb, conjunction, or preposition. Write the word next to the class on the lines following the passage.

Many trees **on** campus are not **native to** the **local** area. Eugene can **support** a greater **variety** of trees than many **places because its** **climate** is **moderate** enough to **easily** accommodate **trees** from colder **and** warmer **areas**. This **led** to the **campus** becoming an **arboretum**. However, planting nonnative trees **displaces** local trees. For **future** tree selections on campus, a **stronger emphasis** on native **species** would **eventually** turn the campus **into** a **richer learning environment**. One student commented **thoughtfully** that **her favorite** tree was the **Eastern black walnut**, near Gerlinger Hall.

Nouns: (11) Walnut, places, climate, trees areas, campus, emphasis, species, environment, arboretum ~~moderate~~ moderate variety

Pronouns: (2) Its, her

Verbs: (3) support, led, displaces

Adjectives: (10) black, future, stronger, richer, favorite, native, local, variety Eastern, learning, moderate

Adverbs: (3) easily, eventually, thoughtfully

Conjunctions: (2) and, because

Prepositions: (3) on, to, into

Exercise 9–3. Pronouns

1. Circle the *reflexive* pronouns: me   you   us   we   ourselves   him   her   himself

2. Circle the *demonstrative* pronouns: the   it   that   those   these   their   this

3. Circle the *interrogative* pronouns: he   on   under   what   her   who   why   must

4. Circle the *possessive* pronouns: her   that   his   their   any   only   ourselves

5. Circle the *relative* pronouns: who   his   that   their   which   them   they

Exercise 9–4. Particles Versus Prepositions

Circle the *particles*:
1. She threw down the pen.
2. He ran down the hill.
3. They sat on the bench.
4. He filled up his plate.
5. She ran to the door.
6. He took off the brace.

Circle the *prepositions*:
7. He gave away his books.
8. She sat by the river.
9. They moved to Portland.
10. He ate with a fork.
11. She looked at the sea.
12. He ran from the dog.

Exercise 9–5. Adverbs

1. Circle the adverbs of *manner*:   quietly   happily   somewhere   forever   dreamy

2. Circle the adverbs of *time*:   later   pleasantly   lonely   now   everyone   always

3. Circle the adverbs of *place*:   wherever   whenever   forever   somewhere   anywhere

4. Circle the adverbs of magnitude: gleefully   definitely   unusually   slightly

5. Circle the adverbs of *likelihood*:   possibly   joyously   probably   cleverly

Exercise 9–6. Conjunctions

1. Circle the *subordinate* conjunctions: forever   anyway   unless   while   before

2. Circle the *coordinate* conjunctions: and   until   whenever   why   so   but   off

3. Circle the *adverbial conjuncts*:   consequently   because   while   wherever   thus   moreover

Exercise 9–7. Review: Word Classes

Read the following fable. Then identify each type of word listed below by filling in the blanks. List each word only once.

The Lion and the Mouse (Grosset & Dunlap, 1947, pp. 137–138)

A lion was asleep in his den one day, when a mischievous mouse for no reason at all ran across the outstretched paw and up the royal nose of the king of beasts, awakening him from his nap. The mighty beast clapped his paw upon the now thoroughly frightened little creature and would have made an end of him.

"Please," squealed the mouse, "don't kill me. Forgive me this time, O King, and I shall never forget it. A day may come, who knows, when I may do you a good turn to repay your kindness." The lion, smiling at his little prisoner's fright and amused by the thought that so small a creature ever could be of assistance to the king of beasts, let him go.

Not long afterward the lion, while ranging the forest for his prey, was caught in the net which the hunters had set to catch him. He let out a roar that echoed through the forest. Even the mouse heard it, and recognizing the voice of his former preserver and friend, ran to the spot where he lay tangled in the net of ropes.

"Well, your majesty," said the mouse, "I know you did not believe me once when I said I would return a kindness, but here is my chance." And without further ado he set to work to nibble with his sharp little teeth at the ropes that bound the lion. Soon the lion was able to crawl out of the hunter's snare and be free.

Application: No act of kindness, no matter how small, is ever wasted.

Proverb: One good turn deserves another.

List each type of word (list each word only once):

1. List the *nouns*: _____

   _____

   _____

   _____

   _____

2. List the *adjectives* (but not the participles): _____

   _____

   _____

3. List the *participles*: _____

   _____

4. List the *verbs*: _____

   _____

   _____

   _____

   _____

5. List the *adverbs*: _____

   _____

Exercise 9–8. Phrases

In each sentence below, indicate the type of phrase that is bolded. Use the following codes:

NP = noun phrase

VP = verb phrase

PP = prepositional phrase

AJP = adjective phrase

AVP = adverb phrase

_PP_ 1. The ball rolled **under the apple tree**.

AVP 2. The ranger told the ghost story **more enthusiastically** to the teenagers.

AVP _VP_ 3. The hikers **had not yet arrived** back at camp by nightfall.

AJP _AVP_ 4. The two friends sat down together **very cheerfully** to enjoy their dinner.

_NP_ 5. **The charming old village** overlooked the river.

_PP_ _AVP_ 6. Marty missed school **because of a stomachache**.

AVP _VP_ 7. They **may have eaten** fish tonight for dinner.

_PP_ 8. The resort specializes **in outdoor entertainment**.

_VP_ 9. The lion **had been watching** the sparrows peck at the corn cobs.

AJP _NP_ 10. **The dry, old bread crumbs** had been left by a group of

AVP picnickers.

_NP_ 11. **Ever since Christmas**, Eva has been happy.

AJP 12. There are **several year-round, modernized, and attractive** inns in town.

_NP_ 13. **Magnetic and electrical fields** may be present.

_PP_ 14. The French have a holiday entitlement **of five weeks a year**.

AJP 15. There are **many long, steep, and winding** stretches of trail nearby.

NP   16. **The curious and persistent geologists** discovered large ice crystals.

AVP   17. The actor, tired and sick, struggled **rather mightily** to remember his lines.

NP   18. **The densely wooded mountainside** was a familiar friend to all.

AVP ~~AVP~~ VP   19. Two crows **were fighting furiously** in the old corn field.

AJP   20. The poem was written in **flowery Victorian** language.

AJP   21. ~~AJ~~ AVP The children knocked on their new neighbor's door **somewhat shyly**.

VP   22. The athletes **were running** around the track to warm up before the meet.

?   23. AVP **Before the race**, she double-knotted her track shoes.

AJP   24. Jimmy was thrilled with the **brand new, shiny, red** bicycle.

NP   25. **The rain-soaked graduation picnic** was a memorable event.

Exercise 9–9. Verb Tenses

For each of the sentences below, indicate the *verb tense* from the following choices:

A. Past perfect tense

B. Future progressive tense

C. Simple past tense

D. Present perfect tense

E. Simple future tense

F. Past progressive tense

G. Simple present tense

H. Present progressive tense

I. Future perfect tense

C   1. Yesterday, the Jones family arrived at Heathrow Airport around 2:00 p.m.

A   2. The direct flight from San Francisco had taken over 11 hours.

_F_ 3. By 4:00 p.m., they were checking into their hotel in London.

_F_ 4. Understandably, by early evening, all were feeling tired and hungry.

_?_ 5. So they went out to a nearby pub for a delicious dinner of fish and chips.

_A_ 6. By nine o'clock that evening, the family had settled into their room for the night.

_____ 7. It is now six o'clock in the morning, their first full day in the UK.

_B_ 8. Today, the travelers will be taking the train from England to Wales.

_I_ 9. They will have reached Llandudno, their final destination, by 11:30 a.m.

_H_ 10. Now on the train, their son Liam is playing chess with his sister Jessie.

11. Jessie will eventually win the match, much to Liam's chagrin.

12. The children's mother, Martha, has just finished reading a short story.

13. And their father, Bruce, is ordering coffee from the trolley cart.

14. By two o'clock this afternoon, the Jones family will be enjoying the beach.

15. By that time, Liam will have forgotten about his loss to Jessie.

16. And Jessie will be searching for seashells and colorful rocks.

17. Liam has just learned the Welsh name for Wales, "Cymu."

18. Suddenly, Jessie wants a red tee shirt with "Cymu" on the front.

19. Dad will buy it for her and one for Liam, too.

20. Soon the Jones family will be walking back to their B & B after a fun-filled day.

CHAPTER 10

Main and Subordinate Clauses

A *clause* is a group of words that expresses a specific meaning. Every clause has a subject and a verb. However, the subject is not always stated in the clause, as in the case of nonfinite clauses (e.g., *swimming across the lake*, the dog grew weary) or coreferential coordinated main clauses (e.g., Patricia enjoyed basketball *but preferred football*). Major types of clauses are main and subordinate.

THE MAIN CLAUSE

A *main* clause [MC] has one verb and can stand by itself as a complete sentence as in the following examples, in which the verb is italicized:

People *interact* with their environment.

Pollution *is* harmful to the atmosphere.

The main clause is often called the *independent* clause or the *matrix* clause. Sometimes a sentence contains two or more main clauses, linked by a coordinate conjunction (e.g., *and, but, so*), as in the following examples of compound sentences:

The Spaniards brought new animals to Mexico *and* they also introduced new trades.

Peru has many resources *but* it also has many economic challenges.

John ran out of peanut butter *so* he went to the store.

When transcribing a language sample, compound sentences such as these should be broken into two (or more) utterances to avoid inflating the mean length of C-unit or the mean length of T-unit, as follows:

The Spaniards brought new animals to Mexico. And they also introduced new trades.

Peru has many resources. But it also has many economic challenges.

John ran out of peanut butter. So he went to the store.

Sometimes, when two main clauses contain the same subject, the subject is mentioned in the first clause but is deleted in the next one. This is called *ellipsis*:

John made cookies, (John) cleaned up the kitchen, and (John) took a nap.

These are called coordinated main clauses. The coordinated main clauses of a sentence are on equal footing with each other, such that one clause does not dominate the other.

THE SUBORDINATE CLAUSE

A *subordinate* (dependent) clause is of "lesser status" than the main clause and must be attached to the main clause. There are three primary types of finite subordinate clauses: adverbial, relative, and nominal.

Adverbial Clauses

Adverbial [ADV] clauses perform a variety of functions within a sentence by expressing different meanings such as conditionality, reason (cause), manner, time, comparison, and purpose, as in the following examples:

Less gasoline is used *when more people ride bicycles.* (conditionality)

They canceled the lecture *because the professor was ill*. (reason/cause)

She performed the solo *exactly as she had practiced it*. (manner)

We bought tickets *as soon as they were available*. (time)

Some geographers study traffic flow *while others trace human movement*. (comparison)

He moved to Boston *so that he could become wealthy*. (purpose)

Adverbial clauses often begin with subordinate conjunctions (e.g., *after, although, because, before, even though, unless, until, when, whenever, while*). Examples of subordinate conjunctions that express different meanings are shown here (adapted from Crystal, 1996, p. 205):

Conditionality: *as long as, if, in case, unless, even though, although*

Reason/cause: *because, since*

Manner: *joyfully, hurriedly, happily, sadly, apprehensively, reluctantly*

Time: *after, before, since, until, when, while*

Comparison: *as if, as though, like*

Purpose: *so that, in order that*

Nominal Clauses

Nominal [NOM] clauses, often called "complement clauses," complete a thought or express an attitude, belief, or feeling that is introduced by the main clause. Nominal clauses often follow a metacognitive verb (e.g., *know, believe, think*) or a metalinguistic verb (e.g., *say, tell, ask*) that occurs in the main clause, as in the following examples:

I know *who is coming to dinner*.

James told Susan *that he would be home late*.

Some people believe *they need supplements every day*.

Nominal clauses are enclosed in quotation marks when a speaker or writer is reporting exactly what someone has said, as in the following examples:

The young boy asked, "*Why should I become a scholar?*"

The judge told Manuel, "*Put away your money.*"

The indefinite pronouns *that, how, where, whether, whoever,* and *what* often introduce nominal clauses:

She believes *that he is innocent.*

I don't know *how we will manage.*

A teenager's self-image influences *how others see him or her.*

Adolescents are interested in *how their peers perceive them.*

She could not remember *how the candlesticks got broken.*

They told the policeman *where he could find the criminal.*

I just learned *where we will be living.*

Please tell me *whether you would like pie or cake for dessert.*

I will give the book to *whoever would like it.*

Mom has asked me *what the answer is to the math question.*

Does anyone know *what day it is?*

Relative Clauses

Relative [REL] clauses add precision by describing a noun contained in another clause (usually the main clause) of a sentence. They often begin with the relative pronouns *who, whom, whose, which, in which,* and *that,* as in the following examples:

Plato was a philosopher *who studied astronomy, government, and mathematics.*

The new teacher, *whom you've met before,* will start on Monday.

I found the dog *whose owner went to the hospital.*

Shakespeare, *whose plays we've read,* was a master of words and images.

The teacher tutors students *whose math skills are weak.*

In 509 BC, Rome became a republic, *which is a special kind of nation.*

Blood cells from a cut form a clot, *which plugs the wound.*

A republic is a nation *in which power belongs to the citizens.*

Monks lived in communities *that were called monasteries.*

The Baker's Neighbor is a play *that has been around a long time.*

Note that in each of these examples, the relative clause immediately follows the noun in the *main clause* that it describes (philosopher, teacher, dog, Shakespeare, students, republic, clot, nation, communities, play). It is in this way that relative clauses provide specific information.

FINITE VERSUS NONFINITE CLAUSES

The main clause of a sentence always contains a *finite* verb, which is one that is marked for person (first, second, third), tense (present, past, future), and number (singular, plural). The three types of subordinate clauses just discussed—adverbial, nominal, and relative—also contain finite verbs in that they are marked for person, tense, and number. However, some subordinate clauses have nonfinite verbs, which are unmarked for person, tense, and number. These include infinitive, participial, and gerundive subordinate clauses.

Infinitive Subordinate Clauses

Each complex sentence below contains a subordinate clause with an infinitive [INF] verb:

> John wants *to walk home after work today.*
>
> They wanted *to go to the basketball game.*
>
> Birds need leaves and twigs *to build their nests.*
>
> Rivers, oceans, and forests continue *to change their appearance over time.*

With infinitive verbs, the word *to* is sometimes omitted, as in these examples:

> All I did was *send* him home.
>
> Rather than Ruth *do* it, I'll ask Jimmy.
>
> I saw the kitten *chase* the lizard.

Participial Subordinate Clauses

Acting like adjectives, participial [PRT] clauses describe nouns, thereby functioning much like relative clauses. Participial verbs end in *-ing, -en,* and *-ed*. Each of the following complex sentences contains a participial [PRT] subordinate clause:

Wearing a new dress, the princess spoke eloquently.

Not easily discouraged, the basketball team fought its way to victory.

Buoyed by the good news, the travelers drove through the night.

Broken by the baseball, the window was replaced.

These examples could easily be turned into full-fledged relative clauses as follows:

The princess, *who was wearing a new dress*, spoke eloquently.

The basketball team, *which was not easily discouraged*, fought its way to victory.

The travelers, *who were buoyed by the good news*, drove through the night.

The window, *which was broken by the baseball*, was replaced.

Gerundive Subordinate Clauses

Nonfinite verbs also include gerunds, which act like nouns and function like nominal clauses. The following complex sentences contain gerundive [GER] subordinate clauses:

Planting crops in mountainous regions is often unsuccessful.

Overusing certain medicines can cause serious illness.

Building roads and bridges provides jobs for many people.

Most people enjoy *going out to dinner and watching a show*.

The man's indigestion resulted from *eating too many spicy foods*.

Choosing your friends carefully will bring you much happiness.

When participles or gerunds are used in place of single words (adjectives or nouns), they are *not* considered to be clauses, as in these examples:

The *exhausted* collie swam to shore.

The *broken* toy was repaired.

Swimming is his favorite sport.

Cooking is an enjoyable hobby.

However, when participles occur with other words and act like truncated (reduced) relative clauses, they are considered to be subordinate clauses:

The fence, *broken by the severe windstorm*, was removed.

Martha, *rounding the final curve*, took the lead in the bicycle race.

The collie, *exhausted by his rescue effort*, swam to shore.

Similarly, when gerunds occur with other words and act like truncated (reduced) nominal clauses, they are considered to be subordinate clauses:

The lead runner had the job of *setting the pace for the others*.

The Smith family enjoyed *preparing Sunday dinner for the Scouts*.

Arguing against the proposal helped the candidate win the election.

EXERCISES: MAIN AND SUBORDINATE CLAUSES

Exercise 10–1

For the following sets of proverbs, fill in the clause type, using the following codes:

MC = main clause   GER = gerundive clause

ADV = adverbial clause   INF = infinitive clause

NOM = nominal clause   PRT = participial clause

REL = relative clause

After completing a set, check your answers in the appendix before proceeding to the next set. (*Sources: Category: Proverbs*, http://en.wikiquote .org/wiki; *Creative Proverbs from Around the World*, http://creativeprov erbs.com; Politis, Reich, & Sheldon, 1998; Quotations Page, http://www .quotationspage.com; Scheffler, 1997; Stewart, 1997; Williams, 2000)

African Proverbs

1. A cutting word is [~~PRT~~ MC] worse than a bowstring. A cut may heal [MC], but the cut of the tongue does [MC] not.

2. Ashes fly [MC] back into the face of him who throws [rel] them.

3. He who is being carried [rel] does not realize [MC] how far the town is [nom].

4. Quarrels end [MC] but words once spoken [adv] never die [MC].

5. Send [~~adv~~ MC] a boy where he wants [adv] to go [inf] and you see [MC] his best pace.

6. Smooth seas do not make [~~ger~~ MC] skillful sailors.

7. The lion does not turn [MC] around when a small dog barks [adv].

8. Two birds disputed [MC] about a kernel, when a third swooped [adv] down and carried [inf] it off.

9. When a needle falls [adv] into a deep well, many people will look [mc adv] into the well, but few will be [mc] ready to go [adv inf down] after it.

10. He who learns [rel] teaches [mc].

Chinese Proverbs

11. A bit of fragrance clings [mc] to the hand that gives [rel] flowers.

12. Even a hare will bite [mc] when it is [adv] cornered.

13. A good fortune may forebode [mc] a bad luck, which may in turn disguise [rel] a good fortune.

14. If you are [adv] patient in a moment of anger, you will escape [mc] a hundred days of sorrow.

15. If you do not study [adv] hard when young, you'll end [adv mc up] bewailing [rel] your failures as you grow up [mc]. adv

16. Learning is [ger mc] a treasure that will follow [rel] its owner everywhere.

17. Listen [mc] to all, plucking [prt] a feather from every passing goose, but follow [mc] no one absolutely.

18. Make [mc] happy those who are [rel] near, and those who are [rel] far will come [mc].

19. Only when all contribute [adv] their firewood can they build [mc] up a strong fire.

20. To attract [inf] good fortune, spend [mc] a new coin on an old friend, share [mc] an old pleasure with a new friend, and lift [mc ger up] the heart of a true friend by writing [ger his] name on the wings of a dragon.

Danish Proverbs

21. It is [ ] *mc* better to ask [ ] *inf* twice than to lose [ ] *inf* your way once.

22. He who builds [____] according [____] to every man's advice will have [____] a crooked house.

23. Even a small star shines [*mc*] in the darkness.

24. A slip of the foot may soon be recovered [*mc*], but that of the tongue perhaps never.

25. Kind words don't wear [*mc*] out the tongue.

26. Bad is [*mc*] never good until worse happens [*adv*].

27. Let [*mc*] deeds match [*inf*] words.

28. Speaking [*ger*] silence is [*mc*] better than senseless speech.

29. It is [*mc*] easy to sit [*inf*] at the helm in fine weather.

30. A good plan today is [*mc*] better than a perfect plan tomorrow.

German Proverbs

31. A good conscience is [*mc*] a soft pillow.

32. A single penny fairly got [*prt*] is [*mc*] worth a thousand that are [*rel*] not.

33. All are [*mc*] not asleep who have [*rel*] their eyes shut.

34. Be [*mc*] silent, or say [*mc*] something better than silence.

35. Could everything be done [*adv*] twice, everything would be done [*mc*] better.

36. If you would have the lamp burn, [*adv*], you must pour [*mc*] oil into it.

37. Instead of complaining [____] that the rosebush is [____] full of thorns, be [____] happy that the thorn bush has [____] roses.

38. It is [____] better to turn [____] back than go [____] astray.

39. It is [____] not till the cow has lost [____] her tail, that she discovers [____] its value.

40. Small undertakings give [____] great comfort.

Hebrew Proverbs

41. Admission by the defendant is [____] worth a hundred witnesses.

42. Do not confine [____] your children to your own learning, for they were born [____] in another time.

43. Happy is [____] the generation where the great listen [____] to the small, for it follows [____] that in such a generation the small will listen [____] to the great.

44. Opinions founded [____] on prejudice are always sustained [____] with the greatest violence.

45. Promise [____] little and do [____] much.

46. Rivalry of scholars advances [____] wisdom.

47. The kind man feeds [____] his cat before sitting [____] down to dinner.

48. Whoever teaches [____] his son teaches [____] not only his son but also his son's son, and so on to the end of generations.

49. Who seeks [____] more than he needs [____] hinders [____] himself from enjoying [____] what he has [____].

50. Slander slays [____] three persons: the speaker, the spoken to, and the spoken of.

Irish Proverbs

51. Don't crow [mc] until you're [adv] out of the woods.

52. Many an honest heart beats [mc] under a ragged coat.

53. The thing that is [rel] bought dear is often sold [mc] cheap.

54. Every dog is [mc] bold on its own doorstep.

55. Distant hills look [mc] green.

56. All happy endings are [mc] beginnings as well.

57. Praise [mc] the young and they will blossom [mc].

58. A handful of skill is [mc] better than a bagful of gold.

59. Time is [mc] a great storyteller.

60. It takes [mc] time to build [inf] castles.

Japanese Proverbs

61. A single arrow is easily broken [mc], but not ten in a bundle.

62. If you understand [adv] everything, you must be [mc] misinformed.

63. Laughter cannot bring [mc] back what anger has driven [nom] away.

64. One who smiles [rel] rather than rages [rel] is [mc] always the stronger.

65. We are [mc] no more than candles burning [ptt] in the wind.

66. When you're [adv] thirsty, it's [mc] too late to think [inf] about digging [ger] a well.

67. The bamboo that bends [rel] is [mc] stronger than the oak that resists [rel].

68. If money be [*adv*] not thy servant, it will be [*mc*] thy master.

69. If you believe [*adv*] everything you read [*rel*], better not read [*mc*].

70. If you want [*adv*] a thing done well, do [*mc*] it yourself.

Mexican Proverbs

71. Conversation is [*mc*] food for the soul.

72. One must learn [*mc*] how to lose [*inf*] before learning [*adv*] how to play [*inf*].

73. Tell [*mc*] me who your friends are [*nom*] and I'll tell [*mc*] you who you are [*nom*]

74. It's [*mc*] not the fault of the mouse, but of the one who offers [*rel*] him the cheese.

75. In youth we learn [*mc*], in old age we understand [*mc*].

76. Money is [*mc*] a good servant but an evil master.

77. Lions believe [*mc*] that everyone shares [*nom*] their state of mind.

78. It is [*mc*] not enough to know [*mc*] how to ride [*inf*]; you must also know [*mc*] how to fall [*inf*].

79. He who lives [*rel*] with hope dies [*mc*] happy.

80. When the river sounds [*adv*], it's [*mc*] because it carries [*adv*] water.

Russian Proverbs

81. If you travel [*adv*] more slowly, you will get [*mc*] farther.

82. A word is [*mc*] not a sparrow. If it flies [*adv*] away, you won't catch [*mc*] it.

83. Not everything that glitters [rel] is [MC] gold.

84. Once you've committed [adv] yourself to move [inf], don't say [MC] you are [nom] not up to it.

85. Any fish is [MC] good if it is [adv] on the hook.

86. All's [MC] well that ends [nom] well.

87. One who sits [rel] between two chairs may easily fall [MC] down.

88. You will reap [MC] what you will sow [nom].

89. We do not care [MC] of what we have [nom], but we cry [MC] when it is [adv] lost.

90. It is [MC] good to be [inf] visiting, but it is [MC] better at home.

Scottish Proverbs

91. A tale never loses [MC] in the telling.

92. Take care [MC] of your pennies and your dollars will take care [MC] of themselves.

93. They that dance [rel] must pay [MC] the fiddler.

94. They that will not be counseled [rel] cannot be helped [MC].

95. What may be [nom] done at any time will be [MC] done at no time.

96. Willful waste makes [MC] woeful want.

97. They that sow [rel] the wind shall reap [MC] the whirlwind.

98. When the cup is [adv] full, carry [MC] it even.

99. Confession is [MC] good for the soul.

100. Get [MC] bait while the tide is [adv] out.

Exercise 10–2

For the following quotations, fill in the clause type, using the following codes:

MC = main clause   GER = gerundive clause

ADV = adverbial clause   INF = infinitive clause

NOM = nominal clause   PRT = participial clause

REL = relative clause

After you complete a set, check your answers in the appendix before proceeding to the next set. (*Sources*: Bachelder, 1965; Benardete, 1961; Burke, 1996; Charlton, 1994; Great Quotations, 1990; Hauser, 2008; McLellan, 1996; Quotable Shakespeare, n.d.; Searls, 2009; Thankful Kids, 2009; *Who Said?*, 2003)

Set A

1. I took [*MC*] a speed-reading course and read [*MC*] *War and Peace* in 20 minutes. It's [*MC*] about Russia. (Woody Allen)

2. I was [*MC*] seldom able to see [*INF*] an opportunity until it had ceased [*ADV*] to be [*INF*] one. (Mark Twain)

3. I must say [*MC*] I find [*NOM*] television very educational. The minute somebody turns [*REL*] it on, I go [*MC*] to the library and read [*MC*] a good book. (Groucho Marx)

4. Extemporaneous speaking should be practiced [*MC*] and cultivated [*MC*]. It is [*MC*] the lawyer's avenue to the public. (Abraham Lincoln)

5. Books were [*MC*] my pass to personal freedom. I learned [*MC*] to read [*INF*] at age three, and I soon discovered [*MC*] there was [*NOM*] a whole world to conquer [*INF*] that went [*REL*] beyond our farm in Mississippi. (Oprah Winfrey)

6. Modern cynics and skeptics see [mc] no harm in paying [adv] those to whom they entrust [rel] the minds of their children a smaller wage than is [nom] paid to those to whom they entrust [rel] the care of their plumbing. (John F. Kennedy)

7. It has been said [mc] of the world's history hitherto that might makes [nom] right. It is [mc] for us and for our time to reverse [inf] the maxim and to say [inf] that right makes [nom] might. (Abraham Lincoln)

8. Most of the luxuries, and many of the so-called comforts of life, are [mc] not only not indispensable, but positive hindrances to the elevation of mankind. With respect to luxuries and comforts, the wisest have ever lived [mc] a more simple and meager life than the poor. The ancient philosophers, Chinese, Hindoo, Persian, and Greek, were [mc] a class than which none has been [rel] poorer in outward riches, none so rich in inward. (Henry David Thoreau)

9. Upon the subject of education, not presuming [inf] to dictate [prt] any plan or system respecting [prt] it, I can only say [mc] that I view [nom] it as the most important subject which we as a people can be engaged [rel] in. That every man may receive [nom] at least a moderate education, and thereby be [inf] enabled [mc] to read [inf] the histories of his own and other countries, by which he may duly appreciate [adv] the value of our free institutions, appears [mc] to be [inf] an object of vital importance. (Abraham Lincoln)

10. I always wanted [mc] to be [inf] somebody, but I should have been [mc] more specific. (Lily Tomlin)

Set B

11. Once they notice [adv] you, they never completely close [mc] the file. (Philip K. Dick)

12. I am [*nom*] invisible, understand [*MC*], simply because people refuse [*adv*] to see [*inf*] me. (Ralph Ellison)

13. Freedom is [*MC*] indivisible. (Nelson Mandela)

14. But to live [*inf*] outside the law, you must be [*MC*] honest. (Bob Dylan)

15. It ain't [*MC*] over 'til it's [*adv*] over. (Yogi Berra)

16. For the spectator even more than for the artist, art is [*MC*] a habit-forming drug. (Marcel Duchamp)

17. Though I am [*adv*] in the depths of misery, there is [*prt*] still calmness, pure harmony and music inside me. (Vincent van Gogh)

18. Never in the field of human conflict was [*MC*] so much owed [*adv*] by so many to so few. (Winston Churchill)

19. Time spent [*prt*] with a cat is [*MC*] never wasted. (Sydney Hauser)

20. Everybody talks [*MC*] about people, but nobody ever does [*MC*] anything about them. (Fran Lebowitz)

Set C

21. I want [*MC*] to bend [*inf*] this note, bend [*inf*] that note, sing [*inf*] this way, sing [*inf*] that way, and get [*inf*] all the feeling, eat [*inf*] all the good foods, and travel [*inf*] all over in one day, and you can't do [*MC*] it. (Billie Holiday)

22. Happy is [*MC*] the house that shelters [*rel*] a cat. (Sydney Hauser)

23. If I had [*adv*] to sum [*inf*] up the totality of the Woodstock experience, I would say [*MC*] it was [*nom*] the first attempt to land [*inf*] a man on the Earth. (Abbie Hoffman)

24. Never doubt [*nom*] that a small group of thoughtful, committed people can change [*nom*] the world. (Margaret Mead)

25. Let [*mc*] them eat [*inf*] cake. (Marie-Antoinette)

26. To thine own self be [*mc*] true, and it must follow [____], as the night the day, thou canst not then be [____] false to any man. (William Shakespeare)

27. The future always looks [*mc*] good in the golden land, because no one remembers [*adv*] the past. (Joan Didion)

28. In the attitude of silence, the soul finds [*mc*] the path in a clearer light, and what is [*nom*] elusive and deceptive resolves [*mv*] itself into crystal clearness. (Mahatma Gandhi)

29. Half-finished work generally proves [*mc*] to be [*inf*] labor lost. (Abraham Lincoln)

30. We have lived [*mc*] not in proportion to the number of years that we have spent [*rel*] on the Earth, but in proportion as we have enjoyed [*adv*]. (Henry David Thoreau)

Set D

31. Nothing so needs [*mc*] reforming as other people's habits. (Mark Twain)

32. Happiness lies [*mc*] in the joy of achievement and the thrill of creative effort. (Franklin D. Roosevelt)

33. Brevity is [*mc*] the soul of wit. (William Shakespeare)

34. Keep [*mc*] your face to the sunshine and you cannot see [*mc*] the shadow. (Helen Keller)

35. The time to repair [*inf*] the roof is [*mc*] when the sun is shining [*adv*]. (John F. Kennedy)

36. The only way to get [*inf*] the best of an argument is [*mc*] to avoid [*inf*] it. (Dale Carnegie)

37. California is [MC] a Garden of Eden, a paradise to live [INF] in or see [INF]. (Woody Guthrie)

38. Fair is [MC] foul, and foul is [MC] fair. (William Shakespeare)

39. Be [MC] who you are [NOM] and say [MC] what you feel [NOM]. (Dr. Seuss)

40. All philosophers must soar [MC] with unwearied passion until they grasp [ADV] the true nature of things as they really are [ADV]. (Plato)

Set E

41. The young boy asked [MC], "Why should I become [NOM] a scholar when I can make [ADV] more money in the market place?" Plato replied [MC] that, "the pursuit of wisdom and truth is [NOM] essential to our integrity as human beings."

42. Moving [ADV] the ship of state is [MC] a slow process. States are [MC] like big tankers. They're [MC] not like speedboats. (Barack Obama)

43. Good leadership requires [MC] you to surround [INF] yourself with people of diverse perspectives who can disagree [REL] with you without fear of retaliation. (Doris Kearns Goodwin)

44. Sometimes leadership is [MC] planting [ADV] trees under whose shade you'll never sit [REL]. (Jennifer M. Granholm)

45. It takes [MC] 20 years to build [INF] a reputation and five minutes to ruin [INF] it. If you think [ADV] about that, you'll do [MC] things differently. (Warren Buffett)

46. How wonderful it is [MC] that nobody need [NOM] wait [INF] a single moment before starting [ADV] to improve [INF] the world. (Anne Frank)

47. Unless someone like you cares [adv] a whole lot, nothing is going [MC] to get [inf] better. It's [MC] not. (Dr. Seuss)

48. With every good deed, you are sowing [MC] a seed, though the harvest you may not see [adv]. (Anonymous)

49. The more we study [VC] the more we discover [MC] our ignorance. (Percy Bysshe Shelley)

50. My teacher helps [MC] me out a lot and she is [MC] nice to me and she teaches [MC] me about stuff and when I first came [adv] to her classroom, I was [MC] afraid of bugs but now I'm [MC] not. (Krysten, age 8)

Set F

51. Education is [MC] what survives [nom] when what has been learned [nom] has been forgotten [adv]. (B. F. Skinner)

52. My karate teacher can break [MC] 12 bats over his head and 10 bricks with his bare hands. (Billy, age 7)

53. My teacher is [MC] fun and hard-working and never forgets [MC] to take [inf] time to talk [inf] to her students, unlike some teachers who only teach [VC] and never talk [VC]. (Sarah, age 11)

54. The mystic chords of memory, stretching [par] from every battlefield and patriot grave, to every living heart and hearthstone, all over this broad land, will yet swell [MC] the chorus of the Union, when again touched [par], as surely they will be [adv], by the better angels of our nature. (Abraham Lincoln; Wilson, 2006, p. 67)

55. I remember [MC] when my second-grade teacher pushed [nom] me and pushed me [MC] to read [inf] and when I finally started [MC] to read [inf], I liked [MC] it so much I couldn't stop [MC]. (Chris, age 8)

56. The art of teaching [GER] is [MC] the art of assisting [GER] discovery. (Mark Van Doren)

57. Human history becomes [MC] more and more a race between education and catastrophe. (H. G. Wells)

58. Leave [MC] it longer on top, so I can have [ADV] spikes. My mom wrote [MC] on the form, "no Mohawk," so I can't get [MC] that. (David, age 13)

59. I am [MC] thankful for my dad because he never yells [ADV] at me. (Victor, 2nd grade)

60. I'm [MC] thankful that the Ducks are going [NOM] to beat [INF] the Beavers. I'm [MC] thankful that I have [NOM] clothes to wear [INF] and parents who care [REL] about me. (Frankie, 7th grade)

Exercise 10–3

For the following fable, fill in the clause type, using the codes below:

MC = main clause	GER = gerundive clause
ADV = adverbial clause	INF = infinitive clause
NOM = nominal clause	PRT = participial clause
REL = relative clause	

The Lion and the Mouse (Grosset & Dunlap, 1947, pp. 137–138)

A lion was [____] asleep in his den one day, when a mischievous mouse for no reason at all ran [____] across the outstretched paw and up the royal nose of the king of beasts, awakening [____] him from his nap. The mighty beast clapped [____] his paw upon the now thoroughly frightened little creature and would have made [____] an end of him.

"Please," squealed [____] the mouse, "don't kill [____] me. Forgive [____] me this time, O King, and I shall never forget [____] it. A day may come [____], who knows, when I may do [____] you a good turn to repay

[____] your kindness." The lion, smiling [____] at his little prisoner's fright and amused [____] by the thought that so small a creature ever could be [____] of assistance to the king of beasts, let [____] him go [____].

Not long afterward the lion, while ranging [____] the forest for his prey, was caught [____] in the net which the hunters had set [____] to catch [____] him. He let [____] out a roar that echoed [____] through the forest. Even the mouse heard [____] it, and recognizing [____] the voice of his former preserver and friend, ran [____] to the spot where he lay [____] tangled [____] in the net of ropes.

"Well, your majesty," said [____] the mouse, "I know [____] you did not believe [____] me once when I said [____] I would return [____] a kindness, but here is [____] my chance." And without further ado he set [____] to work [____] to nibble [____] with his sharp little teeth at the ropes that bound [____] the lion. Soon the lion was [____] able to crawl [____] out of the hunter's snare and be [____] free.

Application: No act of kindness, no matter how small, is [____] ever wasted.

Proverb: One good turn deserves [____] another.

Exercise 10–4: Coding Child and Adolescent Language Samples

The following exercises provide additional practice coding clauses in spoken or written language samples (or excerpts of samples) that were produced by children and adolescents. For each exercise, fill in the blanks using the following codes:

MC = main clause   GER = gerundive clause

ADV = adverbial clause   INF = infinitive clause

NOM = nominal clause   PRT = participial clause

REL = relative clause

#1: *Judy, 11th Grade (TLD)* (from the Author's Files)

General Conversation Task

1. I'm [MC] a junior.

2. I think [MC] I want [nom] to go [inf] into the elementary educational field.

3. I like [MC] little kids.

4. I'm taking [MC] keyboarding, ITT, which is [rel] international trade and tourism, and a cooking class called [prt] world cooking.

5. And then I'm taking [MC] English.

6. And I have [MC] a worker's experience period where I go [rel] and work [rel] at my job (so).

7. I work [MC] for an insurance company right now.

8. So I work [MC] there doing [prt] the filing.

9. It makes [MC] the car payment.

10. (So we get) so we already have [MC] college credit.

Favorite Game or Sport Task

1. And there's [MC] foul balls, which means [rel] there's [nom] lines drawn [prt] from the home plate through the first base out to the field like to the fence like 180 feet.

2. And then there's [MC] a line drawn [prt] from the third base line that goes [rel] out.

3. And if the ball goes [adv] past the line to the left in the line not in the playing field, it's [MC] a foul ball.

4. And that's [MC] just a ball.

5. So (it) your count is [MC] still there.

6. And you have [MC] a count when you're [adv] at bat.

7. And then (four balls or yeah) four balls means [MC] you walk [nom].

8. And so when you get [adv] the base automatically, you can't make [MC] an out with that.

9. And then (the base runners) like if you're [adv] on base, you can advance [MC] as soon as the ball leaves [adv] the pitcher's hand.

10. And you can run [MC] the bases until you get [adv] out or until your coach tells [adv] you to stop [inf].

Peer Conflict Resolution Task

Examiner: What is a good way for Debbie to deal with Melanie?

1. Maybe if there's [adv] a writing part, she can do [MC] the writing part and at least be [MC] there and help [MC] them and try [MC] to say [inf] what she feels [nom] about the whole thing and see [MC] if she has [nom] any advice of what they should do [nom] better.

2. Or (like if just) basically have [MC] a session where they can just talk [rel] and (see what) split [rel] it up into teamwork, working wise.

Examiner: Why is that a good way for Debbie to deal with Melanie?

3. So she doesn't judge [MC] her.

4. Say [MC] she doesn't do [nom] what she's supposed [nom] to do [inf].

5. But if she talks [adv] to her and sees [adv] then maybe they can change [MC] some things.

6. So that will help [MC].

Examiner: What do you think will happen if Debbie does that?

7. Well, she could either say [MC] "no" and ignore [MC] her.

8. Or she could say [MC] "yes."

9. And they could work [MC] the problem out.

10. But if she says [adv] "no," then I guess [MC] she could go [nom] to the teacher and see [nom] what they could do [nom] about it, see [nom] if maybe she could get [nom] another student to help [inf] them or have [nom] more time so the two can just work [adv] on it, Debbie and the other girl.

#2: *Saeda, 2nd Grade* (Thankful Kids, 2009)

Expository Essay

I am [MC] thankful for trees because they make [adv] oxygen for me, water because it will make [adv] me not dehydrated, and books because when I read [adv], I can learn [adv] and I love [adv] to read.

#3: *Alex, 3rd Grade* (Thankful Kids, 2009)

Expository Essay

These are [MC] some things I am [rel] thankful for. I'm [MC] thankful for my food, my lunch, and everything that is [rel] in it. I'm [MC] glad that it is [nom] a good fruit. I'm [MC] thankful for all the water and milk that we have [rel]. I'm [MC] thankful for my house. My house is [MC] warm and cozy. I love [MC] my house so much. My house is [MC] special. I am [MC] thankful for my school. I'm [MC] so thankful for my teacher. I'm [MC] thankful for all the recess we get [rel]. I'm [MC] thankful for my special book. I'm [MC] so lucky for all these things.

#4: *Kyra, 5th Grade* (Thankful Kids, 2009)

Expository Essay

I'm [MC] so thankful for my pets to be [inf] a part of my family. Every single day, I wake up [MC] with warmth on my legs from my dog Toby sleeping [inf] on my legs. When Toby hears [adv] my bus, he will wait [MC] at the door until I come [adv] home. Right when Toby sees [adv] me, he will lick [MC] me until I can't feel [adv] my face and all I can taste [rel] is [adv] slobber. I am [MC] so happy and thankful to have [inf] a dog like Toby.

#5: *Paris, 7th Grade* (Thankful Kids, 2009)

Expository Essay

I am [MC] very thankful to have [inf] a mom that can be [rel] around me, even if I don't always want [adv] her around. She comforts [MC] me when I'm [adv] sad or sick. She helps [MC] me through the bad times. She cooks [MC] and provides [MC] for me even if there's [adv] barely anything in the bank. She is [MC] my mother. And her name is [MC] Pam. But don't you wear [MC] it out. That's [MC] my job. I'm [MC] very thankful for a mother that cares [rel].

#6: *Roberto, 8th Grade* (Thankful Kids, 2009)

Letter to a Former Teacher

There are [MC] many people in my life for whom I'm [rel] thankful for. But you are [MC] the only person that comes [rel] to mind when I think [adv] of it. Through help and guidance, you are [MC] the one who helped [rel] me through sixth grade. I remember [MC] when you gave [nom] me the Honor Society application sheet. You told [MC] me to get [inf] every teacher to sign [inf] my recommendation sheets and to write [inf] the essay to tell [inf] why I should be [nom] in the Honor Society. You made [MC] sure that I got [nom] my essay done and my recommendation sheets in. You made [MC] sure I was doing [adv] it because you knew [adv] that I would have [MC] a chance to be [inf] in the Honor Society. I truly believe [MC] that without you, I would have never gotten [MC] to where I am [MC] today. I will never forget [MC] the things you did [MC] for me. And that's [MC] why I wanted [MC] to say [MC] "Thank you."

#7: *Emily, 3rd Grade (TLD)* (from the Author's Files)

Narrative Essay: "The Swan"

Once upon a time, there was [MC] a swan. She was going [MC] to have [inf] some babies. But she had never had [MC] babies before. She was [MC] nervous! So she asked [MC] the falcon for some advice. But *she* [the falcon] was asking [MC] that same question. So they went [MC] to look [inf] for someone to help [inf] them. So they asked [MC] the raven for her advice. She said [MC], "Ask [MC] the ostrich. She knows [MC]." They went [MC] to the ostrich. She said [MC] she thought [MC] and thought [MC]. At last, she said [MC], "Why don't you try [MC] laying [MC] on the nest and wait [MC] a while. And they will hatch [MC]. That's [MC] what I would do [MC]." So they went [MC] to their nests and sat [MC] and sat [MC]. And then they said [MC], "I feel [MC] something wiggling." "It must be [MC] the babies," said [MC] the swan and raven. And that was [MC] it. And of course they were [MC] very excited. The end.

#8: *Ryan, 5th Grade (TLD)* (from the Author's Files)

Expository Essay: The Nature of Friendship

Do you have [MC] a friend? I do [MC]. What do you think [MC] friendship means [MC]? I think [MC] it means [MC] someone you can trust [MC], someone you can depend [MC] on, someone you have [MC] a lot in common with, and somebody who keeps [MC] secrets. Sometimes people feel [MC] lonely and have [MC] no one to talk [inf] to. That can lead [MC] to sadness. That is [MC] some reasons why friendship is [adv] important. Sometimes friendship comforts [adv] you and makes [MC] you feel [MC] less alone. Me and my friends like

[МС] to play [ІnF] lots and lots of video games together. Some advice for good friendship is [МС] to not annoy [ІnF] the person, be [МС] nice to the person. Do not tell [МС] secrets that they have told [МС] you.

#9: Mark, 8th Grade (TLD) (from the Author's Files)

Expository Essay: The Nature of Friendship

Friendship is [____] basically an understanding between two people who share [____] common interests or beliefs. Friendship is [____] about being [____] able to trust [____] that person and being [____] able to spend [____] time with them. Friendship is [____] important to people because it gives [____] them a chance to do [____] things that they like [____] with someone they enjoy [____] spending [____] time with. Having [____] friends makes [____] life more enjoyable because you have [____] someone you can talk [____] to and that you like [____] to do [____] things with. Friends do [____] all kinds of things together from going [____] on hikes to going [____] to the movies. Friends can talk [____] to each other and go [____] places together. People who generally become [____] friends are [____] those who have [____] common interests. If someone had [____] completely different opinions about what is [____] fun to do [____] than someone else, then they probably won't become [____] very good friends. The kinds of things that can harm [____] a friendship are [____] things like arguing and fighting. If you intentionally do [____] something that you know [____] they won't like [____], it will damage [____] a friendship. A way to maintain [____] a friendship is [____] to continually spend [____] time with them. That way you can still talk [____] to each other even if they live [____] a long ways away. That can help [____] people remain [____] friends. There are [____] always ways to maintain [____] friendships. Sometimes it is [____] just hard to figure [____] out how.

#10: *Willow, 8th Grade* ("Teachers Need to Be Healthy," 2009)

Letter to the Editor (Persuasive Essay)

We think [____] that the ban of junk foods in schools should include [____] teachers. Sodas and other junk foods are [____] just as unhealthy for teachers as they are [____] for students. The teachers need [____] to set [____] a good example for the students. If students see [____] that the ban on junk food includes [____] teachers as well as themselves, they might be [____] more willing to go [____] along with the ban. To have [____] a mind and body that functions [____] the best they can [____], you need [____] to eat [____] the proper amount of nutrients. You do not get [____] these nutrients from junk foods and soda. Because of this, you do not function [____] as well as you could [____]. We think [____] it is [____] important for teachers to have [____] healthy bodies and minds, so that they will teach [____] the students better than otherwise. If teachers eat or drink [____] junk food or soda, they will not teach [____] as well.

If the teachers really cannot live [____] without the junk food, they can very easily just eat [____] it at their homes. It should not be [____] that hard for them to wait [____] the seven or eight hours that their jobs take [____] up to eat [____] junk food if they need [____] it that badly. After all, students can [____].

#11: *Trevor, 5th Grade (TLD)* (from the Author's Files)

Persuasive Essay: The Circus Controversy

I think [____] it is [____] a bad idea to have [____] animals in the circus because animals should be [____] free to do [____] what they want [____]. They're [____] stuck in small cages. So there is [____] barely enough room to get [____] their adequate exercise. People don't like [____] to be [____] imprisoned. So we should let [____] them go [____]. Then they won't be [____] forced to do [____] tricks. I think [____] it is [____] cruel to train [____] animals to do [____] a trick because if they don't do [____] it right, the trainers will hit [____] them. These are [____]

the reasons why I think [____] circuses should not be [____] allowed. For the animals' sake.

#12: *Carl, 11th Grade (TLD)* (from the Author's Files)

Persuasive Essay: The Circus Controversy

A common controversy is [____] often whether or not circuses are [____] good or bad for the community. I like [____] the clowns because often times they are [____] also animal trainers. However, there is [____] a downside to all these beneficial factors. Frequently, the animals are [____] underfed and are kept [____] in small cages. This alone infuriates [____] animal enthusiasts everywhere. Circuses can be [____] cruel to animals. Therefore, they should be closed [____] down. If animals feel [____] threatened, they could be [____] dangerous when they fight [____] back. What I believe [____] is [____] that a circus could hire [____] more people and have them go [____] to clown school. Everybody likes [____] clowns, right? The hardest part of this would be [____] training [____] all those clowns. Still, with a little creativity and some ingenuity, I think [____] a clown school could be [____] possible. Overall, I think [____] animals should not be [____] in circuses.

In summary, there are four basic sentence types: simple, complex, compound, and compound–complex. Can you identify the sentence types in Exercise 11–1?

A sentence is a grammatical construction that can stand by itself and make sense (Crystal, 1996). By definition, every sentence contains a subject and a main verb (finite verb) and expresses a complete thought. There are four basic types of sentences: *simple, complex, compound*, and *compound–complex*.

A simple sentence consists of one main clause (e.g., a duckbill platypus *lays* eggs; it is a mammal; there was a tornado watch). A complex sentence, however, contains one or more subordinate clauses in addition to the main clause (e.g., because the duckbill platypus *produces* milk for its young, scientists *call* it a mammal). A sentence that contains an infinitive verb in addition to a main clause is also complex:

> Because of the tornado watch, the teachers required all students *to stay* inside.

> The students and their teachers wanted *to go* home.

> *To prepare* for the tornado, families stored dry foods.

Sentences that contain participles (that act like truncated relative clauses) and gerunds (that act like truncated nominal clauses), in addition to a main clause, also are complex:

> Complaining [PRT] about the service, Mary wrote [MC] a letter to the manager.

> Building [GER] strong customer relationships was [MC] the manager's primary goal.

A compound sentence contains at least two main clauses that are joined by coordinate conjunctions that include *but*, *and*, *so*, and *or*:

Ice cream contains lots of sugar *but* it sure tastes good!

Cherries are fruit *and* artichokes are flowers.

We enjoy cakes *so* we bake them every week.

Fluffy will stay home *or* he will go to the park.

Compound sentences with ellipsis: Sometimes a compound sentence will delete one of the subjects, usually the second one, because it is redundant. This is called ellipsis. In the following sentence, the subject of the second main clause, *they*, is deleted:

The family packed [MC] up their car and drove [MC] to the mountains.

A *compound–complex* sentence contains at least two main clauses and one or more subordinate clauses:

Today, the major environmental concern *is* [MC] global warming, and many scientists *believe* [MC] that excess carbon dioxide *is raising* [NOM] the temperature of the atmosphere.

ACTIVE VERSUS PASSIVE SENTENCES

It is important to distinguish between sentences in the active versus the passive voice. Sentences in the active voice express ideas in a direct and straightforward manner, with the subject clearly stating who performed the main action of the sentence. The following sentences are in the active voice:

John kicked the football.

Mary wrote a letter.

Herman cut the birthday cake.

I expected that Jim would be late.

In contrast, sentences in the passive voice express ideas in an indirect, wordy, and sometimes confusing manner, as in the following examples:

The football was kicked by John.

The letter was written by Mary.

The birthday cake was cut by Herman.

It was expected (by me) that Jim would be late.

Most of the time, the active voice is preferred because it expresses ideas more efficiently. However, sometimes the passive voice is desired when the speaker or writer is attempting to avoid blaming someone for an undesirable act or even to avoid taking responsibility for such an act, for example:

Mistakes were made (by the president of the company who actually knew better).

A motorcycle was parked illegally (by its owner who was late for work).

The house was left unlocked (by its occupant who was tired and distracted).

When coding clauses in sentences that are in the passive voice, it is important to remember that the main verb is still the same verb as in the active voice, and that the code would be placed immediately after that verb, as in these examples:

Mistakes were made [MC] (by the president of the company).

The president of the company made [MC] mistakes.

The motorcycle was parked [MC] illegally (by the owner).

The owner parked [MC] the motorcycle illegally.

The house was left [MC] unlocked (by its occupant).

The occupant left [MC] the house unlocked.

It was expected [MC] that Jim would be [NOM] late.

I expected [MC] that Jim would be [NOM] late.

SUBJECTLESS SENTENCES: COMMAND AND ELLIPSIS

Although every sentence has a subject, command sentences (or imperatives) do not explicitly state the subject, which is understood by the listener. Command sentences commonly occur when someone is giving directions (e.g., eat your soup; be patient; try your best). In the following paragraph, all sentences except one ("Sauce should be fairly thick") are commands, and the subject is "you." The finite verbs have been italicized:

Soak mushrooms in warm water for 30 minutes. *Squeeze* dry and *cut* into thin strips. In a large nonstick frying pan, *heat* oil and gently *sauté* the chicken. *Add* garlic and onion. *Discard* garlic as it *begins* to brown. *Continue* cooking until onion *is* limp. *Add* remaining ingredients. *Season* with salt and pepper if desired. *Simmer* 30 minutes, or until chicken *is* tender. Sauce *should be* fairly thick. *Add* water to thin if necessary (Oliva-Rasbach & Schmidt, 1994, p. 364).

Sentences with ellipsis also omit the subject, as in the following examples:

Wish you were here.

Had a great time yesterday.

Told you so.

Looks like rain today.

Want a sandwich?

Hafta go now.

For the preceding sentences, respectively, the subjects are I, I, I, it, you, and I. Ellipsis also can occur when answering a question:

Q: Do you like baseball?

A: Depends on who's playing.

Q: What else happened at the party?

A: Can't remember.

Q: Where'd you go?

A: To the track meet.

Q: Who shall help bake this bread?

A: Don't look at me!

SENTENCE FRAGMENTS

Sentence fragments do not meet the definition of a sentence because they lack a subject and/or a main verb. However, they are acceptable in spoken and written contexts when they make a statement, express meaning, function as if they were complete, and are free of grammatical errors, as with the following examples:

And now for the star of our show . . . Bob Hope!

One for all and all for one. (English proverb)

Far from the eye, far from the heart. (Maltese proverb)

To sleep . . . perchance to dream. (Shakespeare)

Sentence fragments also occur in the context of notes such as those presented in field guides. In the following examples of sentence fragments, note the many adjectives in italics used to describe the native birds of Oregon (Tekiela, 2001):

Brewer's blackbird: An *overall grayish brown* bird (female)

Great horned owl: A *robust brown "horned"* owl with *bright yellow* eyes and *V-shaped white* bib (male)

Northern pintail: A *slender, elegant* duck with a *brown* head, *white* neck, *gray* body, and extremely *long, narrow, black* tail (male); *mottled brown* body with a *paler* head and neck, *long* tail, *gray* bill (female)

Red-winged blackbird: Jet *black* bird with *red* and *yellow* patches on *upper* wings (male); heavily *streaked brown* bird with *white* eyebrows (female)

Another type of sentence fragment is one in which a subordinate clause occurs in isolation:

When I am fit

However hard we tried

So that I arrived with no fuss, never a minute too soon or too late

Sometimes this type of fragment occurs in natural communication to answer a question or to make a comment. However, to turn them into complete sentences, they must be attached to a main clause as in the following examples (Bannister, 2004):

When I am fit, my running feels effortless.

However hard we tried, it did not seem possible to meet our target of 60 seconds.

They often drove me to athletics meetings so that I arrived with no fuss, never a minute too soon or too late.

HIERARCHICAL COMPLEXITY

Complex sentences often contain more than one subordinate clause. When one subordinate clause is embedded into another subordinate clause, which is embedded into the main clause, a complex hierarchy of clauses occurs (Quirk & Greenbaum, 1973; Scott, 2009). This can be seen in the following sentence:

I think [MC] you will succeed [NOM] if you try [ADV].

With this sentence, the ADV is embedded into the NOM, which is embedded into the MC. With these types of sentences, it is possible to count the levels of embedding that occur. The following sentence contains only one subordinate clause:

Earthworms are [MC] shredders that can break [REL] large pieces of dead material into smaller pieces.

Because it has only one subordinate clause, the sentence has only one level of embedding (or complexity); the relative clause modifies the noun, *shredders*. In contrast, the following sentence has two levels of embedding, in which the second relative clause modifies the second instance of the noun *pieces*.

Earthworms are [MC] shredders

that can break [REL] large pieces of dead material into smaller pieces,

which are [REL] processed by fungi and bacteria

In determining levels of embedding, all verbs in a sentence represent a clause, at least in the deep structure of the sentence. Now consider a quote from Oprah Winfrey:

Books were [MC] my pass to personal freedom. I learned [MC] to read [INF] at age three, and I soon discovered [MC] there was [NOM] a whole world to conquer [INF] that went [REL] beyond our farm in Mississippi.

The first sentence does not contain any embedding; it is a simple sentence. However, the second sentence, which is compound–complex, contains two levels of embedding:

I learned

> to read at age three, (level one)

and I soon discovered

> there was a whole world (level one)

>> to conquer (level two)

> that went beyond our farm in Mississippi (level two)

For another interesting example, consider the following complex sentence:

> If you are complaining [ADV] about a service you received [REL], describe [MC] the service and who performed [NOM] it.

How many levels of embedding do you think it has? To determine this, answer the following questions:

1. What is the main clause? (describe the service)*
2. What nominal clause completes it? (and who performed it)**
3. What adverbial clause introduces the main clause? (if you are complaining about a service)
4. What relative clause modifies the adverbial clause? (you received)

In this sentence, the main clause has two subordinate clauses, the adverbial and the nominal, which are on equal footing. Together, they create one level of complexity. However, the adverbial clause is modified by a relative clause. This adds another level of complexity, so the entire sentence has two levels of embedding. This can be visualized when, as shown here, each level of embedding is indented:

> If you are complaining [ADV] about a service

>> you received [REL],

> describe [MC] the service and

>> who performed [NOM] it.

For an even more interesting example, consider the following complex sentence of 44 words, written by Henry David Thoreau (2004, p. 88), which contains five levels of embedding:

---

*Note that the subject of this imperative main clause is the unstated *you*.
**Note that the metalinguistic verb *describe* calls for a nominal clause.

I went [MC] to the woods because I wished [ADV] to live [INF] deliberately, to front [INF] only the essential facts of life, and see [INF] if I could not learn [NOM] what it had [NOM] to teach [INF], and not, when I came [ADV] to die [INF], discover [INF] that I had not lived [NOM].

I went to the woods

    because I wished (level one)

        to live deliberately (level two)

        to front only the essential facts of life (level two)

        and see (level two)

            if I could not learn (level three)

                what it had (level four)

                    to teach (level five)

            and not, when I came (level three)

                to die (level four)

        discover (level two)

            that I had not lived (level three)

EXERCISES: SENTENCE TYPES

Exercise 11–1

For each quotation, indicate whether the sentence is:

A. Simple   C. Compound

B. Complex   D. Compound-complex

1. _____ All philosophers must soar with unwearied passion until they grasp the true nature of things as they really are. (Plato)

2. _____ Education is not filling a pail but the lighting of a fire. (William Butler Yeats)

3. _____ If you bungle raising your children, I don't think whatever else you do well matters very much. (Jacqueline Kennedy Onassis)

4. _____ A little learning is a dangerous thing. (Alexander Pope)

5. _____ Never give up and never give in. (Hubert H. Humphrey)

6. _____ Life is a festival only to the wise. (Ralph Waldo Emerson)

7. _____ No one can make you feel inferior without your consent. (Eleanor Roosevelt)

8. _____ To talk in public, to think in solitude, to read and to hear, to inquire and answer inquiries, is the business of the scholar. (Samuel Johnson)

9. _____ My teacher is special because she never yells at me. (Rebecca, age 8)

10. _____ There's something about taking a plow and breaking new ground. (Ken Kesey)

11. _____ The more we study, the more we discover our ignorance. (Percy Bysshe Shelley)

12. _____ My teacher helps me out a lot and she is nice to me and she teaches me about stuff and when I first came to her classroom, I was afraid of bugs but now I'm not. (Krysten, age 8)

13. _____ Education is what survives when what has been learned has been forgotten. (B. F. Skinner)

14. _____ My karate teacher can break 12 bats over his head and 10 bricks with his bare hands. (Billy, age 7)

15. _____ My teacher is fun and hard-working and never forgets to take time to talk to her students, unlike some teachers who only teach and never talk. (Sarah, age 11)

16. _____ Mix with your sage counsels some brief folly. (Cicero)

17. _____ I remember when my second-grade teacher pushed me and pushed me to read and when I finally started to read, I liked it so much I couldn't stop! (Chris, age 8)

18. _____ The art of teaching is the art of assisting discovery. (Mark Van Doren)

19. _____ Leave it longer on top, so I can have spikes. (David, age 13)

20. _____ My mom wrote on the form, "no Mohawk," so I can't get that. (David, age 13)

Exercise 11–2. Hierarchical Complexity

For each of the following sentences, indicate the number of levels of embedding it contains. Begin by coding each sentence for each type of clause it contains:

MC = main clause   GER = gerundive clause

ADV = adverbial clause   INF = infinitive clause

NOM = nominal clause   PRT = participial clause

REL = relative clause

1. Even if you're [_____] on the right track, you'll get run [_____] over if you just sit [_____] there. Levels: _____

2. With every good deed, you are sowing [_____] a seed, though the harvest you may not see [_____]. Levels: _____

3. Use [_____] a small paintbrush and a paper cup with the smaller beetles because you can damage [_____] them if you pick [_____] them up in your hand. Levels: _____

4. Jason's little sister Amanda has [_____] an ear infection for which her pediatrician prescribed [_____] a liquid antibiotic that must be kept [_____] refrigerated. Levels: _____

5. Every miler knows [_____], in the way a sailor knows [_____] the middle of the ocean, that it is [_____] not the first lap but the third that is [_____] farthest from the finish line. (Parker, 2009, p. 246) Levels: _____

6. As Jim and I went [_____] over to see [_____] what was going [_____] on, someone crawled [_____] out of the closet. (Boy, age 13) Levels: _____

7. Before you take [_____] a piece, like if there was [_____] a rook right here, you kind of make [_____] sure because there is [_____] a strategy that you can do [_____] to try [_____] to get [_____] a king in checkmate with two rooks. (Boy, age 11) Levels: _____

8. I hated [_____] him on sight and sound and would be [_____] about to put [_____] my dog whistle to my lips and blow [_____] him off the face of Christmas when suddenly he, with a violet wink, put [_____] *his* whistle to *his* lips and blew [_____] so stridently, so high, so exquisitely loud, that gobbling faces, their cheeks bulged [_____] with goose, would press [_____] against their tinseled windows, the whole length of the white echoing street. (Thomas, 1954, p. 22) Levels: _____

Exercise 11–3

Code the following sentences. Then rewrite each sentence in the active voice and code it again.

1. It was promised [_____] by Mozart that the duets would be completed [_____] soon.

   Active: _____

2. The missing duets, which had been misplaced [_____] by Frederick, were presented [_____] by Mozart to his friend Joseph Haydn.

   Active: _____

3. It was known [_____] by all patrons that a symphony could be written [_____] by Mozart in minutes.

   Active: _____

4. An amazing tonal richness was achieved [_____] by the string quartet, which was led [_____] by a new cellist from Philadelphia.

   Active: _____

5. The miniature trio for three strings was created [_____] by the new composer who was paid [_____] handsomely by the king's court.

   Active: _____

6. The young musician was supported [_____] by a generous scholarship funded [_____] by a wealthy elderly patron, to attend [_____] the Juilliard School of Music.

   Active: _____

7. The composer's status of nobility was implied [_____] by the "von" inserted [_____] before his last name, which was preferred [_____] by some over the plainer "Ernst Dohnanyi."

   Active: _____

8. The flute quartet was performed [_____] by four young musicians who had been hired [_____] by a royal family to educate [_____] its children in the finer things in life.

   Active: _____

9. A dramatic conclusion to the Christmas play was anticipated [_____] by members of the audience, many of whom had been coerced [_____] into attending [_____] the performance.

   Active: _____

10. The rock concert, sold out [_____] for months, had to be canceled [_____] by the vendor because the band's lead singer had been delayed [_____] by inclement weather in Chicago.

    Active: _____

CHAPTER 12

Units of Measurement

This chapter describes units of measurement or analysis that are commonly used when examining language samples, establishing goals, and monitoring a client's progress as a result of language intervention. They include (1) mean length of utterance (MLU), (2) the finite verb morphology composite (FVMC), (3) percentage grammatical utterances (PGU), (4) the communication unit (C-unit) and the terminable unit (T-unit), (5) mean length of C-unit (MLCU) and mean length of T-unit (MLTU), (6) words, (7) mazes, and (8) clausal density (CD).

MEAN LENGTH OF UTTERANCE IN MORPHEMES OR WORDS

Mean length of utterance is frequently used to measure syntactic development in speakers of all ages, including preschool children, school-age children, and adolescents. To offer a classic definition, MLU is the average number of morphemes or words produced per utterance in a language sample (Miller, 2009). When calculating MLU, an utterance may consist of a full sentence or a shorter production. To determine the MLU of a language sample, the total number of morphemes or words produced is divided by the total number of utterances produced.

When used with preschool children, MLU is usually calculated in morphemes (MLU-m), which includes lexical and grammatical morphemes (not derivational). Lexical morphemes are words that can stand on their own and make sense, such as *dog, tree, cat,* and *house.* Grammatical morphemes are word endings such as past tense *-ed*, plural *-s*, possessive *-s*, and third person singular *-s*. Also counted as grammatical morphemes are the copula and auxiliary verbs *is* and *are*. Grammatical morphemes add meaning and help ensure the grammatical accuracy of an utterance, as in the following examples: "She kicked the ball," "I have two cats," "I see Bill's car," "He walks to school," "She is late," and "They are walking." When a lexical morpheme (*dog*) has a grammatical morpheme attached to it (*-s*), the resulting word (*dogs*) is counted as having two morphemes. Other examples of words containing two morphemes each include *kicked*, *cats*, *Bill's*, *walks*, and *walking*. Contracted words (e.g., *she's*, *they're*, *let's*) are also two morphemes each.

If grammatical morphemes are omitted in *obligatory context*, those utterances are considered to be grammatically incorrect and should be noted as such. For example, each of the following productions has omitted a grammatical morpheme in an obligatory context: "She kick the ball yesterday," "I have two cat," "I see Bill car," "He walk to school," "She late," and "They walking." This assumes, of course, that the child speaks Standard American English rather than another dialect such as African American English (AAE), which follows different morphosyntactic rules (see Chapter 3). Thus, if a child speaks AAE, variations in these grammatical morphemes would not be considered errors but would simply reflect the child's use of his or her home or community language.

It also should be noted that certain words always occur in the plural form (e.g., *upstairs*, *pants*, *trousers*, *clothes*, *bangs*, *binoculars*). In those cases, the plural *–s* is not counted as a grammatical morpheme because children seem to learn these words as giant lexical units and it is assumed they are not using the plural marker productively in those contexts. Similarly, words that have internal pluralization (e.g., *children*, *deer*, *feet*, *geese*, *men*, *mice*, *sheep*, *teeth*, *women*) are not considered to have an additional plural marker and are counted as one morpheme each.

In contrast, derivational morphemes are suffixes that can change the part of speech of a word, resulting in a so-called "derived word." For example, by adding the suffix *-ly*, the adjective *clear* becomes the adverb *clearly*; by adding the suffix *-ness*, the adjective *happy* becomes the noun *happiness*; and by adding the suffix *-tion*, the verb *act* becomes the noun *action*. Because the production of derived words reflects lexical development, not grammatical development, derivational morphemes are not counted when calculating MLU. Therefore, derived words such as *clearly*, *happiness*, and *action* are counted as one morpheme each.

When MLU is used to analyze language samples from school-age children and adolescents, it is usually calculated in words (MLU-w) rather than morphemes. This is because most children older than age 5 years have mastered key grammatical morphemes. Therefore, the use of these morphemes no longer serves as an index of grammatical development. However, if a child older than age 5 years has a developmental language disorder and continues to struggle with the accurate production of grammatical morphemes, then MLU-m should be used.

MLU-m and MLU-w are based on all utterances contained in a language sample with the exception of *mazes*, which are false starts, hesitations, repetitions, and revisions (see the description of mazes later in this chapter). Generally, when calculating MLU, compound sentences are broken into two or more utterances, each having its own main clause. However, if the second main clause has an unstated subject that is co-referential with the subject of the first clause and that subject has been deleted via ellipsis, then both clauses are combined and are considered a single utterance. For example, the following sentence is one utterance: "The bear wanted her cub to be safe and nudged her into the cave." However, the compound sentence, "The bear left her cub in the cave and then she went to look for berries" would be broken into two utterances because it restates the subject (she):

The bear left her cub in the cave. And then she went to look for berries.

THE FINITE VERB MORPHOLOGY COMPOSITE

Designed by Bedore and Leonard (1998) for preschool language assessment, the FVMC consists of four grammatical morphemes that children with specific language impairment (SLI) who speak Standard American English frequently omit or otherwise produce inaccurately in obligatory contexts. These morphemes include the third person present singular *–s* (He walk*s* to school); the regular past tense *-ed* (She kick*ed* the ball), the copula *be* (Tom *is* here), and the auxiliary *be* (Tom *is* running). In their study, Bedore and Leonard elicited play-based conversational language samples from 19 children who had SLI and 19 age-matched peers who had typical language development (TLD), ages 3 to 5 years. Each sample was transcribed and analyzed for the use of those four grammatical morphemes in obligatory contexts, and all errors were noted. For each child, a composite score was obtained by dividing the total number of correct productions of those four morphemes by the total number of obligatory contexts that occurred, and the result was multiplied by 100. Bedore and Leonard reported that the mean FVMC was 45.86 for the SLI group and 97.50 for the TLD group, with the TLD group performing significantly better than the SLI group. Using discriminant analysis, they also reported that the FVMC was an accurate predictor of SLI or TLD group membership. Thus, the FVMC could be used to measure grammatical accuracy in the play-based conversational language samples of preschool children who have developmental language disorders.

PERCENTAGE GRAMMATICAL UTTERANCES

Also for use with preschool children, the PGU, designed by Eisenberg and Guo (2013, 2015), allows the speech-language pathologist (SLP) to determine how well the child uses standard English grammar. Rather than eliciting a play-based conversational language sample, however, with PGU, the examiner displays a set of 15 pictures (e.g., a dog eating a cake, children watching a cat stuck in a tree) and prompts the child to talk about each one (e.g., "What is happening in this picture?" "Tell me something else about the picture") to elicit a language sample. The child's sample is then transcribed, entered into the Systematic Analysis of Language Transcripts (SALT) program, and broken into C-units or smaller utterances if they express a complete thought. Only utterances that are intelligible and relevant to the pictures are included. If an utterance contains one or more grammatical errors, it is marked as ungrammatical. Thus, PGU is calculated by subtracting the number of utterances that contain one or more grammatical errors from the total number of utterances produced to obtain the number of grammatically correct utterances. Then, the total number of grammatically correct utterances is divided by the total number of utterances, and the result is multiplied by 100 to obtain the percentage of grammatically correct utterances. Eisenberg and Guo (2013) examined PGU in 3-year-old English-speaking children and found that it accurately distinguished those with SLI from age-matched peers with TLD.

C-UNITS AND T-UNITS

A C-unit or consists of one main clause and any attached subordinate clauses (Hunt, 1970). C-units, unlike T-units, may include answers to questions that are incomplete sentences (Loban, 1976). For example, if the examiner asked the child, "What did you have for breakfast?" and the child responded, "Blueberry pancakes," the child's response would count as a two-word C-unit. In general, C-units are used when examining spoken language samples and T-units are used when examining written language samples. Each of the following sentences is a C-unit or a T-unit, depending on if it is spoken or written:

Cats have been kept as domestic animals for thousands of years.

There are undoubtedly many reasons for the cat's popularity.

Many cat lovers like to attribute it to the cat's personality and beauty.

Cats have many advantages when it comes to choosing a household pet.

When a sentence contains two or more main clauses—each with its own stated subject—it is broken into at least two C-units (or T-units), as indicated by the slash (/) in the following examples:

> Cats require less care and attention than many other pets, while providing excellent companionship, love, and loyalty / but a cat's love has to be earned /

> Cats can become attached to their home territory / and most dislike travel /

> With any adult cat, you should remember that some time may be required for it to become attached to its new owner and home / and if allowed outside, it may try to return to its old home or neighborhood / (Wright & Walters, 1980)

However, sometimes a sentence will contain a second main clause whose subject is the same as that of the first main clause, but the second subject has been deleted via ellipsis. In such cases, the entire sentence is considered to be one C-unit (or T-unit) that contains two coordinated main clauses, as in the following example in which the subject of both clauses is *people*:

> Many people moved [MC] to America and entered [MC] at Ellis Island.

MEAN LENGTH OF C-UNIT AND MEAN LENGTH OF T-UNIT

The MLCU and MLTU are general indices of syntactic development for children and adolescents (Hunt, 1970; Loban, 1976). To calculate MLCU or MLTU, the total number of words produced in a sample is summed and then divided by the total number of C-units or T-units it contains. For example, if a sample contains 250 words and 15 C-units, the MLCU is 16.67 words. Alternatively, if the sample contains 360 words and 40 T-units, the MLTU is 9.0 words. MLCU and MLTU are appropriate for use with children and adolescents who speak African American English (AAE) because these metrics focus on the number of words produced, not morphemes (Ivy & Masterson, 2011). Therefore, they do not consider morphosyntactic variations that are characteristic of AAE (see Chapter 3) to reflect linguistic deficits (Washington, 2019).

In addition to reporting MLCU or MLTU, it is useful to report the total number of words and C-units or T-units contained in a sample. Each of these measures can serve as an index of language productivity (Nippold, 2009). Often, the SLP will notice that a child or adolescent talks more (e.g., produces a greater number of words and C-units) about certain topics and less about others, a pattern that could stem from factors such as knowledge of the topic, interest in the topic, and motivation to talk about it. With additional investigation into the factors underlying verbal productivity, the SLP might be able to use that information to design an intervention program that encourages the child or adolescent to tap into his or her language competencies more fully.

WORDS

What is a word? Although this may seem like a simple question, it is *not*; when transcribing language samples, SLPs often ask what constitutes a word. For example, is *Professor Virginia Finley* one, two, or three words? What about contractions such as *doesn't, wouldn't*, and *don't*? Are they one or two words each? And what about catenatives such as *gonna, wanna, lemme*, and *hafta*? When transcribing language samples, the following guidelines will help the SLP decide what constitutes a word:

1. Proper names are one word (and one morpheme) even when their spelling suggests otherwise. For example, the following proper names are each one word (and one morpheme): Mrs. Jones, David Tompkins, Home Town Buffet, Stratford-Upon-Avon, Smoke-N-Hot Coffee. To ensure that SALT counts each of these names as one word, insert the underscore (_) between each part with no spaces (e.g., Mrs._Jones, David_Tompkins, Home_Town_Buffet, Stratford_Upon_Avon, Smoke_N_Hot_Coffee).

2. Compound and hyphenated words are each one word and one morpheme (e.g., baseball, playground, sidewalk, sandbox, mid-valley, runner-up, self-esteem, word-of-mouth).

3. Interjections are one word and one morpheme (e.g., Oh! OK! Shh! Ugh! Whew!).

4. Diminutives (e.g., mommy, kitty, duckie) are one word and one morpheme each.

5. Casual variations of words that have meaning (e.g., Mmm = yes; Uhhuh = yes; Yep = yes; Nah = no) are counted as one word and one morpheme each.

6. Indefinite pronouns are one word and one morpheme each (e.g., anybody, somebody, everyone, something).

7. Contractions are two words (e.g., shouldn't, won't, couldn't, let's, we're). To ensure that SALT counts them as two words, insert a

space between them. For example, they should be typed as follows: should n't, wo n't, could n't, let 's, we 're.

8. Catenatives are two words [e.g., hafta (have to), lemme (let me), kinda (kind of), sorta (sort of)]. To ensure that they are counted as two words, insert a space between them, for example: haf ta, sor ta, kin da. However, SALT takes a different approach to catenatives and recommends they be treated as single words. Hence, according to SALT conventions, these catenatives would be transcribed as hafta, lemme, kinda, and sorta and counted as one word each. Either way, be consistent in treating them as one or two words throughout the sample, depending on personal preference.

9. Fillers such as *um*, *uh*, and *er* are not counted as words, but are mazes, and they should be enclosed in parentheses.

MAZES

Mazes are "linguistic tangles" (Loban, 1976) such as false starts, hesitations, and revisions that do not contribute to the clear expression of an idea. When a speaker is in the middle of a maze, he or she is having difficulty finding a clear path forward and is producing verbalizations that are unwanted, rejected, and replaced by others. Most of the time, the speaker will find a way out of the maze and eventually express a clear thought. Other times, the speaker may abandon the maze and the intended meaning and will move on to a new idea.

Sometimes mazes consist of fillers such as "um," "uh," and "well" used in order to buy time to formulate a clear utterance. Although most speakers produce a certain amount of maze behavior, an excessive number of mazes may reflect utterance formulation or word retrieval difficulties and should therefore be considered a red flag for a language disorder.

When mazes occur in a language sample, they are not considered to be part of the speaker's intended message. Therefore, when transcribing a language sample, all verbalizations that constitute maze behavior are enclosed in parentheses so that what is left over expresses a coherent idea and is presumed to be the speaker's intended meaning. In other words, the final reformulation is allowed to stand, and all maze behavior that preceded it is placed within parentheses. Appropriate parenthesizing of mazes can be seen in the following examples:

(The only other thing . . . um . . . uh . . . well, what I mean is) the only thing left to do is (to) to clean up this mess!

(Uh um well I mean) the other day when (I) we went to the coast, it was storming.

When calculating MLCU or MLTU, SALT will not count any words in parentheses. So, for example, after parenthesizing all mazes, the following sentence would be a 14-word C-unit:

> His dog ran after him (and so uh and and the the), got in the jeep, and rode (it in a) around with him.

Here is another example of how to handle maze behavior in an 11-year-old girl:

> I like Uno. It's kind of challenging. (Um all right need about) you can play it with two players or more. You deal out your cards. And I think you get five cards per person. And you look at your cards. And (you flip over it) you have a stack of cards. And you flip over the first card. And (you try to) if you have the card (you have) you lay down the color.

When maze behavior is parenthesized in this manner, SALT will automatically tabulate the total number of mazes in the sample, as well as the total number of words that constitute maze behavior. These totals can then be used to analyze the speaker's maze behavior in spoken language, possibly leading to additional assessment that involves administering a norm-referenced standardized language test such as the Test of Word Finding–Third Edition (German, 2014) for school-age children or the Test of Adolescent/Adult Word Finding–Second Edition (German, 2016) for adolescents.

CLAUSAL DENSITY

During childhood and adolescence, sentences increase in length because they contain a greater number of subordinate clauses, which often are embedded within other subordinate clauses. This phenomenon, which builds hierarchical complexity (clauses within clauses), increases the density of a sentence. To capture this aspect of development, a metric called *clausal density* is reported. Clausal density is calculated by summing all main and subordinate clauses in a language sample and dividing by the total number of C-units (or T-units) produced (Hunt, 1970; Loban, 1976). The following example is from a hypothetical language sample:

Total main clauses = 58

Total subordinate clauses = 52 (11 relative, 16 adverbial, 10 nominal, 8 infinitive, 4 participial, 3 gerundive)

Total clauses (main and subordinate) = 110

Total C-units = 60

Clausal density = 1.83 (110/60 = 1.83)

ANALYZING A SAMPLE OF WRITTEN LANGUAGE USING SALT

To review some of the principles discussed in this chapter, examine the following passage, an excerpt from a 2009 menu at Antoine's Restaurant in New Orleans, Louisiana. The passage has been broken into T-units and coded for the use of main and subordinate clauses. There are 159 total words and 12 T-units. Therefore, MLTU = 13.25 words. In addition, the passage contains 12 main clauses and 6 subordinate clauses (ADV = 3, INF = 2, REL = 1), for a total of 18 clauses. Therefore, CD = 1.5. Note how the underscore is used to segment words.

There is [MC] only one Antoine's.

It has become [MC] as much a part of New_Orleans as Jackson_Square and Saint_Louis_Cathedral, a restaurant that has been operated [REL] continuously by the same family since 1840.

That is [MC] now over 169 years.

Antoine's has seen [MC] the history of New_Orleans through the Civil_War, World_Wars_I_and_II, the Great_Depression, epidemics, and storms.

It all started [MC] when Antoine_Alciatore arrived [ADV] here from Marseilles, France, in 1840, and became [ADV] immediately a culinary notable.

He was [MC] 16 years old.

Young Antoine had been apprenticed [MC], since the age of eight, to the Great French Chef, Coffient, of the Hotel_de_Noailles in Marseilles.

His parents' wavering fortunes as cloth merchants required [MC] that the young boy learn [INF] a trade and help [INF] the family himself.

By the time he left [ADV] France, Antoine had served [MC] kings and royalty and the aristocracy of that country.

But the voice of opportunity in the new America cried [MC] louder than all else.

He followed [MC] that call.

And it took [MC] him to New_Orleans.

EXERCISES: UNITS OF MEASUREMENT

Exercise 12–1. Calculating MLU-m and MLU-w

The following is an excerpt from a play-based conversational language sample elicited from a 3-year-old boy, "Billy" (not his real name), adapted from Fletcher and Garman (1988). The child, C, and examiner, E, were playing with a doll house. For each utterance produced by the child, count the number of morphemes and words, and put the totals in the blank spaces. Then calculate MLU-m and MLU-w for the sample. Do not count morphemes or words for the examiner.*

	Morphemes	Words
C That doggie is woof/ing.	_____	_____
C He bite/3s you.	_____	_____
E Oh, he bit me!		
C That/'s a baby lady.	_____	_____
C Look, this got/3s trousers.	_____	_____
C He/'s got a milkman.	_____	_____
E Show me another one.		
C Let me see.	_____	_____
C I want that black one.	_____	_____
E What's that thing?		
C A tie.	_____	_____
C All the children/z.	_____	_____
E What's she doing?		
C She runn/ing.	_____	_____
C There she mummy.	_____	_____
E What next?		

---

*Note that contracted words were separated by a slash and grammatical morphemes were marked using SALT conventions (/3s = third person singular verb, /z = possessive -s, /ing = present progressive marker, /s = plural). Also following SALT conventions, these words were counted as one morpheme, one word each: *doggie, trousers, milkman, children, mummy, oh, gotta, football.*

	Morphemes	Words
C The mummy/z pram.	____	____
C A blue pram.	____	____
E What's in the pram?		
C A baby.	____	____
E And there's another little girl.		
C That/'s blue.	____	____
C That/'s gotta go in the middle.	____	____
C Oh, whose is that football for?	____	____
C Think (he's) him/z.	____	____
C What/'s that girl do/ing?	____	____
C I want a green one.	____	____
Total:	____	____

Total C utterances: ____

MLU-m: ____

MLU-w: ____

Exercise 12–2. Calculating the FVMC

Tommy, age 4;6, has specific language impairment. Use the data obtained from a play-based conversational language sample to calculate his FVMC.

	Accurate Productions	Obligatory Contexts
3rd person singular -*s*	2	8
Past tense -*ed*	2	6
Copula *be*	3	10
Auxiliary *be*	3	7
Total:	____	____

(Accurate productions/obligatory contexts) × 100 = FVMC: ____

Exercise 12–3. Calculating PGU

Each child below has specific language impairment. The clinician used a set of 15 pictures to prompt each child to talk about the pictures to elicit a language sample. For each child, use the following results to calculate the PGU.

(Grammatically correct utterances/total utterances) × 100 = PGU

	Grammatically Correct Utterances	Total Utterances	PGU
1. Jason, age 3;8	14	30	_____
2. Tyler, age 4;2	16	28	_____
3. Jenna, age 5;0	12	27	_____
4. Amy, age 3.6	10	25	_____
5. Lucas, age 4;7	18	32	_____

Exercise 12–4. Identifying C-Units and T-Units

For passages 1 through 5, indicate with a slash (/) the end of each *C-unit*. Then write the total number of C-units in the blank space.

1. Upon the subject of education, not presuming to dictate any plan or system respecting it, I can only say that I view it as the most important subject which we as a people can be engaged in that every man may receive at least a moderate education, and thereby be enabled to read the histories of his own and other countries, by which he may duly appreciate the value of our free institutions, appears to be an object of vital importance (Abraham Lincoln, cited by Bachelder, 1965, p. 7)

   How many C-units are contained in this passage? _____

2. I have been the whole day without eating and the whole night without sleeping, occupied with thinking it was no use the better plan is to learn learning without thought is labor lost and thought without learning is perilous (Confucius, 6th century bc, Peter Pauper Press, 1963, p. 42)

   How many C-units are contained in this passage? _____

3. The critical habit of thought, if usual in a society, will pervade all its mores, because it is a way of taking up the problems of life men educated in it cannot be stampeded by stump orators and are never deceived by dithyrambic oratory they are slow to believe they can hold things as possible or probable in all degrees, without certainty and without pain they can wait for evidence and weigh evidence, uninfluenced by the emphasis or confidence with which assertions are made on one side or the other they can resist appeals to their dearest prejudices and all kinds of cajolery education in the critical faculty is the only education of which it can be truly said that it makes good citizens (William Graham Sumner, 1906, p. 633)

    How many C-units are contained in this passage? _____

4. Inside England, as we have seen, one form of the language, basically an East_Midland dialect, became accepted as a literary standard in the late Middle_Ages and with this went a prestige accent based on that of the court in Westminster this does not mean that dialect differences disappeared in England / Standard_English was the language of a small minority most speakers used a nonstandard form of the language and in each area there was a speech hierarchy corresponding to the class hierarchy, differing from Standard_ English not only in accent but also in grammar and vocabulary the higher the socioeconomic level of the speakers, the nearer their speech was likely to be to Standard_English, though the degree of formality of the situation also influenced the level of speech used (Barber, 1993, p. 232)

    How many C-units are contained in this passage? _____

5. We are a nation of Christians and Muslims, Jews, and Hindus, and nonbelievers we are shaped by every language and culture, drawn from every end of this Earth and because we have tasted the bitter swill of civil war and segregation, and emerged from that dark chapter stronger and more united, we cannot help but believe that the old hatreds shall someday pass, that the lines of tribe shall soon

dissolve, that as the world grows smaller, our common humanity shall reveal itself, and that America must play its role in ushering in a new era of peace (Barack Obama, 2009)

How many C-units are contained in this paragraph? _____

For passages 6 through 10, indicate with a slash (/) the end of each T-unit. Then write the total number of T-units in the blank space.

6. Once Oregon was thought to be immune to earthquakes today we know that we have them in three different flavors—devastating subduction earthquakes like the 1700 catastrophe, deep intraplate earthquakes like the Puget_Sound temblors of 1949 and 2001, and sharp local jolts like the Spring_Break_Quake of 1993 (Sullivan, 2008, p. 67)

   How many T-units are contained in this passage? _____

7. Beatrix_Potter was a Londoner, born there in 1866 but her family had connections with Lancashire cotton and she spent her holidays from the age of 16 in the Lake_District, in rented, but rather grand houses, round Windermere and Derwentwater her parents were genteel, upper middle class Edwardians and she was educated at home and expected to devote her life to her parents or get married she found an outlet for artistic talents in drawing and painting "little books for children" and encouraged by the family's Lakeland friend, Canon_Rawnsley, her first book, *Peter_Rabbit*, was published in 1901 (Davies, 1989, p. 179)

   How many T-units are contained in this passage? _____

8. I have become a little more skillful in guessing right explanations and in devising experimental tests but this may probably be the result of mere practice, and of a larger store of knowledge I have as much difficulty as ever in expressing myself clearly and concisely and this difficulty has caused me a very great loss of time but it has

had the compensating advantage of forcing me to think long and intently about every sentence and thus I have been often led to see errors in reasoning and in my own observations or those of others (Charles Darwin, 1958, pp. 136–137)

How many T-units are contained in this passage? _____

9. Some birds, such as most eagles, hawks, ospreys, falcons, and vultures, migrate during the day larger birds can hold more body fat, go longer without eating, and take longer to migrate these birds glide along on rising columns of warm air, called thermals, which hold them aloft while they slowly make their way north or south they generally rest at night and hunt early in the morning before the sun has a chance to warm up the land and create good soaring conditions birds migrating during the day use a combination of landforms, rivers, and the rising and setting sun to guide them in the right direction (Tekiela, 2001, p. xv)

How many T-units are contained in this passage? _____

10. In the morning I watched the geese from the door through the mist, sailing in the middle of the pond, fifty rods off, so large and tumultuous that Walden appeared like an artificial pond for their amusement but when I stood on the shore they at once rose up with a great flapping of wings at the signal of their commander, and when they had got into rank circled about over my head, twenty_nine of them, and then steered straight to Canada, with a regular *honk* from the leader at intervals, trusting to break their fast in muddier pools a "plump" of ducks rose at the same time and took the route to the north in the wake of their noisier cousins (Thoreau, 2004, pp. 301–302)

How many T-units are contained in this passage? _____

Exercise 12–5. Counting Words and Calculating MLCU and MLTU

For each of the following language samples, calculate MLCU (spoken language) or MLTU (written language). First determine the number of words in each C-unit or T-unit for the child C, not the examiner E. Then, add up the total number of words produced by the child and divide by the total number of C-units/T-units produced. Write the result in the blank space.

#1: *Play-Based Conversational Sample from a 5-Year-Old Boy, Playing with a Doll House and Furniture* (Fletcher & Garman, 1988)

Words

_____   1. C That's a big one. E The table you mean?

_____   2. C Where does that go anyway? E Where do you think is the kitchen in that house?

_____   3. C Must be there. E So where shall we put the pot?

_____   4. C Take that little boy there.

_____   5. C And put that one. E OK, I take that out.

_____   6. C Bike for the baby. E Have you got a bike at home?

_____   7. C Uhhuh, a big one. E Uhhuh, you've got a big one.

_____   8. C My brother's got a motorbike. E Is he older than you?

_____   9. C Uhhuh.

_____ 10. C That might (be) go in there. E Uhhuh, it could probably go in there.

_____ 11. C This is a long one. E It's a long one indeed.

_____ 12. C Goes up there.

_____ 13. C Must be in there. E Where's your sofa at home?

_____ 14. C It's in mum's.

_____ 15. C So I move it upstairs. E Look, there's nothing in that room so far.

_____ 16. C I put it there then.

_____ 17. C That needs to be up there so that somebody can walk past.

Total child C-units: _____

Total child words: _____

Child's MLCU: _____

#2: *Narrative Essay, Boy, Age 11* (from the Author's Files)

Words

_____ 1. One day at the mall, me and my friend went to the Home_Town_Buffet.

_____ 2. I towered three to four plates of food, one dessert plate, and two sundaes.

_____ 3. On the other hand, my friend had very little.

_____ 4. Little did I know that we had to walk all over the mall.

_____ 5. So every time I saw a bench, I would lay down for as long as I could.

_____ 6. Then we went to Harry_Richie's, Game_Crazy, Radio_Shack, Target, and to another video game store.

_____ 7. My stomach was aching the whole time.

_____ 8. Me and my friend both agreed I ate way too much.

_____ 9. Then we had to walk way down and around the whole outside of the whole huge mall.

_____ 10. Then we went to the other mall and walked around.

_____ 11. I learned never to eat that much again.

Total child T-units: _____

Total child words: _____

Child's MLTU: _____

Exercise 12–6. Counting Words

For each of the following sentences, indicate the number of words it contains. Be sure to follow conventions for counting proper names, compound and hyphenated words, contractions, catenatives, interjections, fillers, etc. as described in this chapter.

_____ 1. Miss Jane Hudson was the principal of the school, Foxwood Glen.

_____ 2. The school's special cat and mascot was named Terry the Tiger.

_____ 3. Let's have Aunt Bessy's cherry cobbler for dessert tonight.

_____ 4. I'm gonna get me a giant box of Cracker Jack.

_____ 5. Lemme have a taste of your chicken a la king.

_____ 6. When we go to New York, let's go to the top of the Empire State Building.

_____ 7. After that, we'll go visit the Statue of Liberty and take photos.

_____ 8. Remember when we went to Disneyland and rode Dumbo the Flying Elephant?

_____ 9. We planned to take the steps to the top of the Eiffel Tower.

_____ 10. The Great Wall of China, one of the seven wonders of the world, is amazing!

_____ 11. We went downstairs for lunch in the new cafeteria with Mary Cohen-Smith.

_____ 12. The oatmeal at breakfast was flavored with maple syrup, vanilla, and dates.

Exercise 12–7. Identifying Mazes

The following utterances were produced by adolescents who were talking about sports and conflicts. For each utterance, use parentheses to enclose the maze behavior. What is left should be a clean, coherent utterance, presumably the speaker's final formulation. Be sure to parenthesize the verbalizations (mazes) that come *before* the final version.

Speaker #1:

1. and um you need to serve when you serve, you need to serve behind the line, not over it.

2. and then um in order to um in order to score over there you in or ok when you serve and it goes over the net, and if the other players do not hit it or if they can't get it and it's in the in the lines, then it's a point.

Speaker #2:

1. but usually the stadiums cost maybe thirty or a lot of dollars a lot of millions of dollars to put into it.

2. and they can play in any kind of weather even except for snow because they don't play in the snow.

3. and a baseball game should last a major league baseball game should last three hours.

Speaker #3:

1. and and then there's I don't know how many people play in pro.

2. but I we usually play five on five like at school like in sports for school.

3. and um that's about it.

Speaker #4:

1. and he asks Peter if he would if Mike to switch jobs with him because his sh uh shoulder was sore.

2. and he was like, "No, I don't wanna lose take a chance on losing my turn on the grill."

Speaker #5:

1. he could say, "Bob um you know you were supposed to help us with this project and when you don't participate in the group, it frustrates me because it makes our group look bad and I'd appreciate it if you'd participate in the group."

2. um he unless Bob's an absolutely nasty person, he should get some kind of good results because he was pretty polite about it and yeah.

Exercise 12–8. Calculating CD

Solve the following problems using the information that is provided.

1. 45 main clauses; 24 subordinate clauses; 45 C-units. CD = _____

2. 82 main clauses; 68 subordinate clauses; 82 C-units. CD = _____

3. 47 main clauses; 43 subordinate clauses; 42 C-units. CD = _____

4. 35 main clauses; 31 subordinate clauses; 25 C-units. CD = _____

5. 60 main clauses; 56 subordinate clauses; 60 C-units. CD = _____

6. 24 main clauses; 10 adverbial clauses; 6 relative clauses; 9 nominal clauses; 4 infinitive clauses; 5 gerundive clauses; 5 participial clauses; 24 C-units. CD = _____

7. 16 main clauses; 9 adverbial clauses; 0 relative clauses; 4 nominal clauses; 2 infinitive clauses; 0 gerundive clauses; 0 participial clauses; 16 C-units. CD = _____

8. 12 main clauses; 4 adverbial clauses; 2 relative clauses; 2 nominal clauses; 4 infinitive clauses; 0 gerundive clauses; 0 participial clauses; 12 C-units. CD = _____

9. 68 main clauses; 16 adverbial clauses; 12 relative clauses; 8 nominal clauses; 9 infinitive clauses; 4 gerundive clauses; 5 participial clauses; 70 C-units. CD = _____

10. 45 main clauses; 24 adverbial clauses; 12 relative clauses; 14 nominal clauses; 7 infinitive clauses; 2 gerundive clauses; 3 participial clauses; 45 C-units. CD = _____

CHAPTER 13

Analyzing Conversational Language Samples

This chapter consists of language samples that were elicited from children and adolescents with typical language development. They include both play-based and interview-based conversational language samples. Each sample was entered into the Systematic Analysis of Language Transcripts (SALT) software program and broken into C-units by the author. All mazes were placed within parentheses, allowing the final reformulation to stand. To allow SALT to count the number of words accurately, all contractions were separated by one space.

For each sample, fill in the clause type, using the codes shown here. Then check your answers in Appendix E of this book.

MC = main clause   GER = gerundive clause

ADV = adverbial clause   INF = infinitive clause

NOM = nominal clause   PRT = participial clause

REL = relative clause

E = examiner; C = child or adolescent

CONVERSATIONAL LANGUAGE SAMPLES

Play-Based Conversational Samples

Sample #1: Boy, Age 3 Years (Fletcher & Garman, 1988)
MLCU = 3.58   CD = 0.68

E This lady's sweeping the floor.

E This lady's holding a baby.

E This is the lady with the green coat on.

E Which one do you want first?

C Green one.

E Put her on.

C On like that.

E Who next?

C A blue one.

E Good.

C That 's [_____] a baby lady.

E What's that one?

C Green lady.

E Who shall we have first?

C A green one.

E There isn't a green one.

C Let [_____] me see [_____].

C There.

C There 's [_____] a green one.

C Look, this gots [_____] trousers.

E What's he holding?

C Do n't know [_____].

E Yes you do.

C He 's got [_____] a milkman.

E Tell me another one.

C Let [_____] me see [_____].

C I want [_____] that black one.

E What's that thing?

C A tie.

C All the childrens.

E What's she doing?

C Do n't know [_____].

C She running [_____].

C There she mummy.

E Who next?

C A pram.

C A blue pram.

E What's in the pram?

C A baby.

E And there's another little girl.

C That 's [_____] blue.

C That 's got [_____] ta go [_____] in the middle.

E Which one first?

C The ball.

E The ball.

C The red one.

C Oh, whose is [_____] that football for?

C Think [_____] (he's) him's.

E And there's one more.

C A girl.

E What's she doing?

C What 's that girl doing [_____]?

E What's she holding?

C Balls.

C Move [_____] this over here.

C She 's sleeping [_____].

E Who?

C That 's [_____] a big pussy cat.

E I like pussy cats.

C Oh, there 's [_____] lots of people.

E This is the dog that's jumping up.

E This dog is lying down.

C I want [_____] the black one.

C Where 's it go [_____]?

E And there's another one.

C There some more.

E Which dog is it?

C Do n't know [_____].

E What's she doing?

C She eating [_____] her dinner.

E Yeah.

C No, she trying [_____] to make [_____] it.

E What's happening there?

C He 's got [_____] a television.

E What's that?

C A television.

C Oh no, it 's [_____] a bus driver.

E It is.

C Oh, he's might cross [_____] over a car.

E What's inside that bus?

C I don't know [_____].

C What 's [_____] in there?

E People.

E What's happening in that picture?

C Some boys.

E Have you got any brothers and sisters?

C No.

C That boy xxx.

E We've had that one.

C This is [_____] for the radio.

Sample #2: Girl, Age 5 Years (Fletcher & Garman, 1988)

MLCU = 5.35   CD = 1.00

E Have you seen this before?

C No, have n't seen [_____] the game.

E I think it's a farm.

C Yes, I think [_____] it 's [_____] a farm.

E Do you?

C I seen [_____] farms on television.

C So I have n't been [_____] to a farm.

E What did you get for Christmas?

E Did you get any games?

C Well, (I) I love [_____] this very big one.

C (I love) I love [_____] that Sindy house.

C I had [_____] a Sindy house.

E Did you?

C Yeah, always wanted [_____] one of them.

E For Christmas?

C And I got [_____] (um) for my birthday.

E When was your birthday?

C (Um) my (birthday) birthday was [_____] before Christmas.

C And do you know [_____] what happened [_____]?

E No.

C I have [_____] this lovely, lovely (um) yacking dog.

C And I loved [_____] it.

E What's that?

C A yacking dog.

C You know [_____], one of them (um) little doggies.

C And when you switch [_____] it on, (it goes), you got [_____] to say
[_____] go [_____].

C And it goes [_____] yak_yak_yak.

E How do you stop it then?

C You (go go) clap [_____] your hands like that.

E How big is it?

C Well, about that {shows in inches}.

C Now I think [_____] (tho) these sacks, they 're [_____] very tired.

C (so I think he's um) I think [_____] he left [_____] them there.

C (that's) That 's [_____] the back door where they come [_____].

E Think that's a little hut, isn't it?

C Yeah, I think [_____] it 's [_____] a little hut.

E What do you think they keep in there?

C I do n't know [_____].

C Horsie.

E Can't get a horsie in there.

E Too little.

C What could we have [_____]?

E Maybe that's where the chickens sleep.

C Oh yeah.

C That 's [_____] a good idea.

C And they fly [_____] out there.

E Yeah.

C Uhhuh, think [_____] it may be [_____] that.

C (got) Need [_____] another pig.

C The mummy pig.

E How do you know it's a mummy pig?

C Because that 's [_____] dad.

C And that 's [_____] mummy.

E Oh, I see.

C Might be [_____] a little baby.

E There isn't one though.

C That little baby could be [_____] in that truck.

C He jumped [_____] into that truck.

E Okay.

C Like that.

E Okay.

C In the truck.

E There's no one driving that tractor.

C Oh yeah.

C We must put [_____] a man on it, must we [_____]?

C He 's driving [_____] the tractor.

E That's a good idea.

C What?

E To put him underneath like that.

E So it looks like he's inside.

C Uhhuh.

E Where's he going in that tractor do you think?

C I do n't know [_____].

E What do you think this could be?

C I think it 's [_____] a gate.

E How can it be a gate?

E Show me how.

C But I think [_____] it 's [_____] a log.

C A log.

C (xxx) a log this way.

C That way.

E I've got a cold.

C I 've got [_____] a little bit of a cold.

C I have n't got [_____] any colds.

C I have [_____] n't.

C My cold 's [_____] gone away.

E Have you had a cold already?

C Yeah.

C (I had it when it was) I had [_____] it when it was [_____] in the middle of winter.

E Still quite cold outside though.

C Yeah.

C What do you think [_____] that could be [_____]?

E I think that's where the farmer keeps his tools and things.

C I know [_____] jolly well (xxx).

E What?

C Jolly well could be [_____].

C Well, you know [_____] this little bit of hay.

E It's to keep it dry.

C Expect it is [_____].

E What do you think will happen if the hay gets wet?

C The horses wo n't eat [_____] it.

E Yeah.

E What else can we put on?

C Think [_____] we can put [_____] on.

C Oh yes, we must have [_____] a seat.

C That for the farmer.

E What is it?

C A seat, I think [_____].

C Look [_____].

E It's difficult to see what it is.

C Yeah.

E Yeah.

C I think [_____] it 's [_____] a seat.

C There 's [_____] a little seat for the farmer.

E But he's in the tractor now so he can't sit in it.

C Yeah, I know [_____].

E There's another man on there as well.

C No, I think [_____] it 's [_____] a little boy.

E Oh, a little boy.

C (Um) a little girl.

C That 's [_____] a little girl.

C It could be [_____] another little girl, could [_____] n't it?

E Do you think it's another little girl?

C Oh!

C Poor little girl!

C Dropped [_____] her!

E Dropped her on her head.

C Or maybe it 's [_____] a lady.

C Must be [_____] a lady because it 's got [_____] a apron.

C No, I know [_____].

C If there 's [_____] another bucket she could carry [_____] it.

C Maybe she picking [_____] up the bottle.

E Ok, milk bottle that the milkman left for her.

C I think [_____] it 's [_____] a bottle the milkman left [_____] for the babies, like these and them.

C Think [_____] that 's [_____] a house on the farm where all their animals sleep [_____].

C And that 's [_____] where all the hay is [_____].

C (And that) and that 's [_____] where the hay 's being made [_____].

C Where shall we put [_____] this?

E It's getting a bit full.

C Maybe here.

E Okay.

C Where all the animals are gone [_____] now?

C (xxx) a bit full.

C Maybe here.

E There are some more logs there.

C Uhhuh, except I wo n't put [_____] them on.

E You gonna put that little boy on or not?

C Yeah.

C Maybe (he's) he 's walking [_____] down (and).

C Maybe he 's (going) going [_____].

E Where?

C Do n't know [_____].

C (um) Up to see [_____] the horsie.

E Okay.

C (Going) think [_____] he 's going [_____] round there and up to horsie.

C Or maybe he 's walking [_____] over there and up there down there and round the tractor and down here and see [_____] the horsie.

C Except got [_____] a long way to go [_____].

E Have you ever been on a horsie?

C No, yeah.

E Where?

E At the fairgrounds?

C No, at the Isle_of_Wight.

E Yeah?

E Is that where you go on holidays?

C Yeah, last year.

E What did you do there?

C And we 're going [_____] to the Isle_of_Wight.

C Well, we 're going [_____] on somebody's caravan.

E Are you?

C To somewhere.

C But I do n't know [_____] where.

Interview-Based Conversational Language Samples

Sample #3: Girl, Age 7 Years (Fletcher & Garman, 1988)
MLCU = 6.32   CD = 0.93

E Margaret, you had your birthday not long ago, didn't you?

C Uhuh.

E Did you get some nice presents for your birthday?

E Do you remember what you got?

C Yes.

E What did you get?

C (um I got I got) I got [_____] a farm snap.

C And from my brother.

E Uhhuh.

C (And) and I got [_____] some (Barbie) Barbie (clothes) clothes (but) which Barbie and Sindy could wear [_____].

E Which Barbie and Sindy could wear, uhhuh.

C Uhhuh.

E So you have even more clothes for your Barbies and Sindys.

C (Um and) and I 've [_____] lots of clothes.

E Really?

E So you can dress them differently every day?

C Uhhuh.

E Did you have a birthday party?

C Yes.

E Really?

C And that cake was [_____] lovely.

E You had a lovely birthday cake?

C (I) and what was [_____] left of it was [_____] Mickey_Mouse that you could n't eat [_____].

E (um) That sounds nice.

C (And then and I) and I have [_____] (a pup) a puppet Mickey_Mouse.

E What else was left of the cake?

C A ribbon.

E A ribbon?

C A pink ribbon.

E What did you do with that?

C I have n't done [_____] anything with it yet.

C It was [_____] on the top.

C Sposta be [_____] getting washed [_____] soon.

E Is it dirty because it was on the cake?

C (um) It was [_____] n't really dirty.

C But it had [_____] lots of bits of icing on.

E Did you do anything nice last weekend?

C I went [_____] to the Forest_Park zoo.

C And there was [_____] one thing.

C There 's [_____] two things that is [_____] my favorite rides.

E What is that?

C There was [_____] this boat ride that went [_____] far up.

C (and then) and then it could go [_____] far up there.

E Uhhuh.

E It's sort of a swing.

C Uhhuh and what lots of people can go [_____] on it.

E Uhhuh, I know that.

C But I went [_____] at the back.

E You went in the back?

C And that 's [_____] really scary.

C And I went [_____] with my brother.

E How old is your brother?

C Eleven.

E Eleven.

E Were you scared?

C No.

E No.

C (And then there's my f) there is [_____] really better than that other
  ride that I told [_____] you about.

C Well, you started [_____] from this little (xxx).

C And it went [_____] round (xxxx).

C It was [_____] a boat thing.

E It was a boat thing, uhuh.

C And then it went [_____] on the lake.

E Yes.

C And then it went [_____] up this water hill.

E Right.

C Right?

C And then down and splashed [_____].

E Oh dear!

C And me and Andy went [_____] on it two times.

E Uhuh.

C And my mum and dad went [_____] (it) on it once.

E Did they like it?

C Well, (it wasn't) they were [_____] n't in favor of it when it was going [_____] up and down.

C But it was [_____] fun.

E Uhuh.

C (One time, I the boat I went on it) on the second time, I was [_____] right at the front of the boat.

C and I got [_____] soaking.

E Oh dear!

C But was [_____] a very big splash at the end.

E That sounds very lovely.

C And then it goes [_____] round the lake.

C And (then) then my mum (said) said [_____] "stay [_____] there and we'll come [_____] on with you."

E Uhuh.

C So we stayed [_____] in.

C And then it was [_____] on the next (move move) ride.

C And then (mum) my mum and dad got [_____] in.

E Yes.

C And then it went [_____] along the lake again.

E Uhuh.

C Up the hill, down the hill, splash.

C (And) and then round a (bit) bit.

C And then we got [_____] off.

E Oh dear!

C (But) but (my mum) my mum took [_____] a photograph.

E She took a photograph of you in the boat?

C Uhhuh, me and Andy (with) with the water going [_____] on.

C (My dad) but my mum and dad didn't wan [_____] na go [_____] in that boat thing.

E Um.

C A little bit of a scary cats.

E But they did in the end obviously.

C No.

E No?

C They never would go [_____] on it.

Sample #4: Boy, Age 14 Years (from the author's files)

MLCU = 9.93   CD = 1.76

E What would you like to tell me about yourself?

E For example, what could you tell me about school, or your family or friends or pets?

C (Um) at school I try [_____] to stay [_____] inclined.

C But I kind of get [_____] bored because I find [_____] it somewhat boring.

C At home I try [_____] to do [_____] my chores.

C But I do n't [_____] because (I don't really need any) I do n't have
     [_____] anything to do [_____] with the money after I get [_____] it.

C And (um) I hang [_____] out with (a) a pretty tight group of friends.

E Are they all in cross-country?

C (Um) one of them is [_____].

C And one of them is thinking [_____] about it.

C But they have n't really decided [_____] yet.

E How long have you been in cross-country?

C (Um) sixth grade.

E So two years.

E This is your second year?

C (Yes) no, this is [_____] my third.

C Started [_____] in sixth.

E Okay.

E And do you like it?

C (Um) It 's [_____] a nice warmup for track, which I 'm [_____] more
     into 'cause I 'm [_____] (kind of) better at track.

E Okay.

E What's your favorite track event?

C (Um) pole vault.

E No way!

E Isn't that when you launch yourself over a tall pole?

C Yeah.

E You do that?

C {nods}.

E Wow.

E Do you go to competitions for it?

C (Um) Well you 're not allowed [_____] to do [_____] pole vault as a track event at other middle schools because I think [_____] McArthur (is the only) has [_____] the only (pole vault for like a) pole vault coach for middle school.

E So you can't compete with anyone.

C No.

E But you have a head start on competing.

C Yeah, I have [_____] a really big head start since I 'm [_____] (like) the best person in my grade right now.

C There 's [_____] not really a lot of other people who do [_____] it, just two of my friends.

E What do you have to know to do pole vault well?

C (Um) you have [_____] to have [_____] good timing.

C (Uh) you have [_____] to be [_____] able to relax [_____] because if you (like) tighten [_____] your abs when you 're trying [_____] to turn [_____] upside down to go [_____] over the pole, you 'll end [_____] up pulling [_____] on the bar and you might stretch [_____] a muscle in your shoulder, which hurts [_____].

C I 've done [_____] that.

E You have?

E You stretched the muscle in your shoulder in pole vault?

C Yeah.

E Have you had any other track injuries?

C (Um well like) Yes, most of them are [_____] just (like) twisting [_____] ankles in long jump and stuff, though.

C They do n't hurt [_____] as bad.

C It really hurts [_____].

E How long does a twisted ankle take to recover?

C Like a day or two.

E Oh cool.

E But then you're back running full speed?

C I actually normally run [_____] with a twisted ankle.

C It kind of helps [_____] stretch [_____] it out I think [_____].

C But I try [_____] not to put [_____] a whole bunch of weight on it.

E That's really cool.

Sample #5: Girl, Age 14 Years (from the author's files)
MLCU = 9.61   CD = 1.63

E I am going to ask you a little bit about yourself.

C Well, I wish [_____] I worked [_____].

C But I do n't [_____].

C I have been trying [_____] to find [_____] a job this summer.

C But it appears [_____] no one is hiring [_____] (um) inexperienced 14-year-olds.

C (Um) I baby sit [_____] for a kid named [_____] Jacob.

C And he 's [_____] really nice.

C He 's [_____] ten and pretty mature.

C So it 's [_____] kind of like being [_____] paid [_____] (like) six dollars an hour to (um) play [_____] video games and watch [_____] TV with him and stuff.

C (Um my school) my school is [_____] Westminster_Middle_School.

C (Um it's uh) it 's [_____] an okay school.

C I think [_____] that it 's [_____] a better fit for me than Southampton (but um it's).

E Why do you think that?

C (Uh) well (we just) because (um) I was made [_____] fun of a lot when I was [_____] in fifth and sixth grades.

C So at Southampton (I would have had) I feel [_____] like there is [_____] just a more unfriendly atmosphere there.

C I 'm [_____] not sure that I really like [_____] the friends I have [_____] at my school (um).

C But I 'm going [_____] into Woodbury_High_School.

C And (um) that 's going [_____] to be [_____] a new experience for me (you know) because I 've never been [_____] to high school before.

C (Um) actually, I 'm [_____] quite familiar with one part of Woodbury_High_School.

C (I um) I am [_____] a theatre person.

C So (like um) I 've been [_____] in a summer camp where they basically use [_____] the entire (like) theatre and choir wing of Woodbury_High_School.

C And (I've been up) I 've performed [_____] on that stage at least three times.

C (Um) I 'm [_____] really into theatre and acting and stuff.

C In fact, (I was) my (uh) first professional role was [_____] in Sleeping_Beauty.

C (Um) It 's [_____] the only professional role I 've had [_____] yet because there 's [_____] just nothing up for kids although I am auditioning [_____] for My_Fair_Lady.

C (Um uh) So we 'll see [_____] how that goes [_____].

C (But um) I was [_____] in Sleeping_Beauty as a fairy.

C And (uh) over a hundred kids tried [_____] out.

C So I was [_____] pretty unprofessional.

C So I 'm [_____] not quite sure how I got [_____] in.

C But (uh) it was [_____] pretty fun.

C But so yeah.

C I performed [_____] on the Community_Center stage (um).

E When was that?

C That was [_____] when I was [_____] in fifth grade.

C I think [_____] I was going [_____] into fifth grade.

C Yeah, I was going [_____] into fifth grade.

C And (um) I was [_____] just a fairy (but).

E And did you speak?

C (Um) I sang [_____] on stage.

C But I did n't have [_____] any solos or anything.

C (Yeah I was) Yeah (uh) I ate [_____] like a mountain load of candy
   before every performance, which was [_____] not good for my voice
   I 'm [_____] sure (still but).

Sample #6: Boy, Age 14 Years (from the author's files)
MLCU = 7.76 CD = 1.21

E What would you like to tell me about yourself?

E For example, what could you tell me about school, or your family or
   friends or pets?

C (Well I have) My family is [_____] really close to me.

C Like (um) all my cousins and uncles and aunts live [_____] in
  Roseburg with me.

C And I see [_____] most of them almost every day.

C (Um).

E How many do you have?

C (I have) both my grandma and grandpas live [_____] in Roseburg.

C I have [_____] I think [_____] three aunts that live [_____] here and
  two uncles maybe.

E Do any of your aunts and uncles live elsewhere?

C (Uh) yeah, actually I have [_____] an aunt and uncle in Bend.

C But I see [_____] them like five or six times a year.

E So you have a lot of cousins?

C Yeah, I have [_____] a lot of cousins.

E That sounds fun to me.

C (Um) well (like) most of my family is [_____] (like) teachers or
  doctors.

C And then (my) one of my uncles that lives [_____] in Bend is [_____]
  an engineer.

E Oh cool.

C (Um) what else.

E Do you have pets?

C (Yeah I have) my sister has [_____] a turtle.

C And I have [_____] a dog.

E A turtle and a dog!

E Does the dog get along with the turtle?

C Well I guess [_____].

C He does n't try [_____] to bite [_____] him or anything.

E That's good.

E At least the turtle will be able to crawl into its shell.

E Does it live in a cage?

C Yeah, but (he like) sometimes my sister will let [_____] him out in the back yard to walk [_____] around in the summer.

E Is it big?

C Yeah, (it's like) well when we got [_____] it, it was [_____] like that small.

C But now it 's [_____] like that big.

E It's amazing how they grow!

C And it 's [_____] supposed to be [_____] (like) like four feet by four feet when it gets [_____] older.

C And they live [_____] like one hundred years.

E No way!

E How old is it now?

C (Um) like three?

E Wow!

E It seems like it has grown a lot in three years.

C Uhhuh, yeah.

E So it will be really big, like one of those Galapagos Islands turtles.

E And so what is your dog like?

E What do you like to do with your dog?

C Well my dog is [_____] very small.

C He 's [_____] a Chihuahua.

C He is n't [_____] really active.

C He just sits [_____] around all day.

E Is it a puppy or is it older?

C Well it 's [_____] like six I think [_____] now.

C But he is [_____] I think [_____] a teacup Chihuahua.

C I 'm [_____] not sure.

E Really!

E What 's your favorite thing about him?

C (Um) I do n't know [_____].

C Probably how (like) one second he can be [_____] like totally calm.

C But the other he will be [_____] very playful.

E He's unpredictable?

C And he listens [_____] pretty well.

E That's nice.

CHAPTER 14

Analyzing Narrative, Expository, and Persuasive Language Samples

This chapter consists of language samples that were elicited from children and adolescents with typical language development. They include samples of narrative, expository, and persuasive discourse. Each sample was entered into the Systematic Analysis of Language Transcripts (SALT) software program and broken into C-units (spoken language) or T-units (written language) by the author. All mazes were placed within parentheses, allowing the final reformulation to stand. To allow SALT to count the number of words accurately, all contractions were separated by one space.

For each sample, fill in the clause type, using the codes shown below. Then check your answers in Appendix F of this book.

MC = main clause   GER = gerundive clause

ADV = adverbial clause   INF = infinitive clause

REL = relative clause   PRT = participial clause

NOM = nominal clause

E = examiner; C = child or adolescent

NARRATIVE LANGUAGE SAMPLES

Spoken Narratives

Sample #7: Girl, Age 5 Years, retelling *Frog, Where Are You?* (Mayer 1969; sample borrowed from Miller, Andriacchi, & Nockerts 2019 and used with their permission)

MLCU = 7.21   CD = 1.21

C (Well a) when the boy was sleeping [_____], the frog crept [_____] out of the window.

C And (um) then when the boy was going [_____] to say [_____] good morning to the frog, he was [_____] gone.

C And then (th) the dog went [_____] to look [_____] for the frog in the jar.

C And then his head got stuck [_____].

C And then he looked [_____] out the window.

C And he fell [_____] down to the ground.

C The glass jar broke [_____].

C And then they were looking [_____] in the woods.

C And (um) then (th th th um he f) he found [_____] other animal.

C (Th) but it was [_____] n't his frog.

C And then he found [_____] a deer.

C He got [_____] on it.

C And it took [_____] him (t) off a cliff.

C And (um) the little boy heard [_____] this croaking sound.

C And (um he) he thought [_____] it was [_____] the frog.

C And it was [_____].

C And so he looked [_____] over a dead tree.

C And he found [_____] a mother frog and his pet frog.

C And then they found [_____] eight children and a frogs.

C And then.

E What happened at the end, anything?

C And (then they f) then they found [_____] (the) the (xxx).

C (Then they) then they got [_____] to keep [_____] a frog.

E Mmm.

C And then that was [_____] his new pet.

E Are you finished?

E Or is there anything more you wanna add?

C That 's [_____] the end.

Sample #8: Boy, Age 7 Years, retelling *Frog, Where Are You?* (Mayer 1969; sample borrowed from Miller, Andriacchi, & Nockerts 2019 and used with their permission)

MLCU = 7.64   CD = 1.26

C (Um) there was [_____] a boy.

C (Um) he had [_____] a frog and a dog.

C And (um) when they woke [_____] up the frog was [_____] gone.

C They were looking [_____] everywhere.

C And he was looking [_____] for (his d) the (um) frog.

C And he looked [_____] in his hat.

C It was [_____] n't there.

C The dog was looking [_____] for the (um) frog.

C And it was [_____] in a jar.

C And he stuck [_____] his head in it.

C And then the dog was looking [_____] out the window.

C And then the boy, he was looking [_____] out the window and calling [_____] for his frog.

C And then the dog fell [_____] down as he was leaning [_____] over.

C And then the boy picked [_____] up his dog.

C (So it) and the dog looked [_____] at him because they were [_____] really worried.

C He was [_____] really worried.

C That was [_____] their house they lived [_____] in.

C It looks [_____] kind of like a farm though.

C And he was still calling [_____].

C And there were [_____] some bees.

C So the bees were coming [_____] out of a beehive.

C And the dog was barking [_____] at the beehive.

C And then a bee must have stung [_____] the kid.

C And then there 's [_____] a little (um) mole.

C And a dog was going [_____] up.

C And he was still barking [_____] up the tree.

C And the bees' hive fell [_____] down.

C And they worked [_____] on it so hard.

C And {audible inhale} (and um) it broke [_____].

C And the bees went [_____] chasing [_____] the dog.

C (They were) they were almost going [_____] to chase [_____] him.

C And the mole is still looking [_____], like staring.

C (And he) the boy (um) climbed [_____] up the tree.

C Owl scared [_____] him.

C And the bees (um) went [_____] (whe where) all the way there chasing [_____] the dog.

C And then there 's [_____] a owl who did n't let [_____] them go anywhere because he was getting [_____] scared.

C So he looked [_____] back (and) so it would n't fall [_____] on his head.

C And (um) he did n't want [_____] to go [_____] anywhere because of the owl.

C And the owl is [_____] still there.

C And he did n't know [_____] this.

C (x) right there.

C And (um) the boy (went) was calling [_____] for his frog still.

C And his dog was sneaking [_____] around so the bees would n't come [_____].

C And (um) he wanted [_____] to see [_____] if that was [_____] a branch.

C But he climbed [_____] up it.

C But it was [_____] (really) really (a) like a reindeer or a deer or something.

C And the dog was going [_____] down there because (the reindeer the reindeer or the doe or) the deer was running [_____] and chasing [_____] the dog.

C And bad things are happening [_____] to the dog all the time.

C And (the um kid was still stuck on the) the (boy) kid, he was [_____] still stuck on the (um reindeer) doe.

C And then the boy and the dog fall [_____] down.

C They were falling [_____] down.

C But they did n't (fa) fall [_____] yet.

C And now they (fall) fell [_____] down right there.

C And {C laughs} the dog was [_____] on the boy.

C (The boy heard um) the boy heard [_____] (th) a sound going [_____] "ribbit_ribbit."

C And the dog was [_____] on top of his head.

C And he heard [_____] it too.

C And then the kid said [_____], "Shh."

C Now he comes [_____].

C And he looks [_____] under a dead old tree.

C And then he sees [_____] some frogs.

C And then he sees [_____] just two frogs.

C But now he sees [_____] more than two frogs.

C (He) So he says [_____] "Goodbye."

C And then they keep [_____] a frog instead of the old frog.

C (And the) these two frogs are [_____] (a) happily_ever_after with frogs.

Sample #9: Boy, Age 14 Years, retelling *The Mice in Council* (from the author's files)

MLCU = 9.69   CD = 2.0

E Can you retell the story?

C (Uh) I could try [_____], yes.

C So (uh) these mice are living [_____] in fear of the cat.

C That ('s uh) happens [_____] a lot (I guess).

C And so (um) they decided [_____] to make [_____] a council because of the name of the story to try [_____] and figure [_____] out a way to (uh) solve [_____] this problem.

C Because (you know) they 're losing [_____] a lot of people getting [_____] eaten [_____] up by the cat.

C So they keep [_____] talking [_____] and talking [_____].

C And nothing seems [_____] (to work) to work [_____] (that would work).

C And one (mice) mouse was [_____] (uh) smart (I guess).

C (To uh) mice decided [_____] to (uh) make [_____] it so that the cat could be heard [_____] by putting [_____] a bell around his neck.

C They thought [_____] it was [_____] an amazing idea.

C So they applauded [_____].

C And he gave [_____] a couple bows.

C And then (uh the) it was passed [_____] that they would do [_____] this 'cause they have [_____] a little council.

C But (uh) then one old mouse that 's [_____] wise (uh, uh) was (uh) congratulating [_____] him and thought [_____] of a question.

C (Uh) who would put [_____] the bell around the (mouse or) cat.

C And (uh) that 's [_____] a good question.

E Awesome, nicely retold.

Sample #10: Girl, Age 14 Years, retelling *The Mice in Council* (from the author's files)

MLCU = 12.13   CD = 2.53

C (So) the mice were [_____] always in fear of this cat because (they'd always) he 'd always approach [_____] them and try [_____] and eat [_____] them.

C And he 'd toy [_____] with them and torture [_____] them.

C So the mice called [_____] together a council meeting.

C And they discussed [_____] many plans.

C But none of them seemed [_____] (to work or) like they were going [_____] to work [_____].

C And then a very small young mouse (um) approached [_____] and said [_____] that his idea was [_____] to put [_____] a bell around the cat's neck so that whenever the cat came [_____] they would hear [_____] the bell tinkle [_____] and then they would know [_____] he was coming [_____] so they could escape [_____].

C And everyone thought [_____] it was [_____] a really great idea.

C And so (um) they applauded [_____] him.

C And he took [_____] a few bows.

C And then (um) a wise older mouse stood [_____] up.

C And (said) this is [_____] basically what he said [_____].

C This is [_____] truly a great plan.

C And (um) only a genius could figure [_____] out a plan so simple (that we could) that we would have overlooked [_____].

C And he says [_____] so now the question is [_____] who 's going [_____] to put [_____] the bell on the cat.

C So basically things are [_____] easier said [_____] than done [_____].

Sample #11: Boy, Age 14 Years, retelling *The Monkey and the Dolphin* (from the author's files)

MLCU = 9.74   CD = 1.84

E Can you tell that story back to me?

C (Uh) so (uh) I guess [_____] it was [_____] a custom to bring [_____] monkeys and other creatures along with them to amuse [_____] the (sailor) sailors.

C So one guy brought [_____] a monkey onto his boat.

C And they were sailing [_____] around somewhere (Uh) by (Greek) Greece (I guess).

C And (uh) there was [_____] a storm.

C The ship crashed [_____].

C And everyone was [_____] in the water.

C And they were swimming [_____] towards shore.

C And so was [_____] the monkey.

C And then a dolphin, who must have [_____] bad eyesight to mistake [_____] a monkey for a man, (uh) swam [_____] up and grabbed [_____] the monkey with his back.

C And so the monkey had gotten [_____] onto him.

C And they 're swimming [_____] there.

C And he asked [_____] him if he was [_____] (a uh citizen) a Athenian.

C And the monkey said [_____] "yes" (you know) trying [_____] to trick [_____] this dolphin because he 's trying [_____] to live [_____] on.

C And the dolphin asked [_____] him if he knew [_____] something or someone.

C And the monkey, (you know) thinking [_____] that oh yeah this must be [_____] (uh) someone.

C Like oh yeah I know [_____] him.

C He 's [_____] a dear friend.

C And the dolphin knew [_____] that he was lying [_____].

C So instead of saving [_____] him, he plunged [_____] down to the bottom to leave [_____] the monkey to his fate.

E Very nice.

Sample #12: Girl, Age 14 Years, retelling *The Monkey and the Dolphin* (from the author's files)

MLCU = 13.29   CD = 2.21

C (Um) so it used [_____] to be [_____] (um) a custom that sailors would take [_____] on with them animals like a monkey or a dog to keep [_____] them entertained [_____] on their long voyage.

C So on one particular (um) voyage, they took [_____] with them a monkey.

C And when they were [_____] off the coast of Sunium, there was [_____] a terrible shipwreck.

C And everyone was turned [_____] overboard, including [_____] the monkey.

C So a nearby dolphin (mis) mistook [_____] the monkey for a man.

C And so he came [_____] to his rescue.

C And then the dolphin asked [_____] him if he knew [_____] Piraeus, which was [_____] also the name of the harbor off of Athens.

C And (um) he said [_____] yes I 'm [_____] (a) an Athenian.

C I 'm [_____] from one of the first families that was [_____] here.

C And he said [_____] yes I knew [_____] Piraeus.

C He 's [_____] one of my oldest friends.

C And the dolphin knew [_____] then that he was (uh) not telling [_____] the truth, that he was lying [_____].

C And so he dove [_____] deep into the water and left [_____] the monkey to his fate.

C And so the moral of the story would be [_____] people who pretend [_____] (uh) to be [_____] someone else basically end [_____] up in deep water.

Written Narratives

Sample #13: Girl, Age 9 Years, imaginary story (Nippold, 2007, pp. 344–345)

MLTU = 13.27   **CD = 2.36**

C Today was [_____] the day that my Aunt Jane was coming [_____] to town from Pennsylvania.

C As soon as the plane landed [_____], Aunt Jane stepped [_____] out followed [_____] by a mysterious figure and a few other passengers.

C The mysterious figure walked [_____] over to a newsstand and bought [_____] a paper.

C He took [_____] one quick look at the headline and threw [_____] the paper away.

C The headline read [_____], "Sweet_Heart_Lumber_Co Orders [_____] 10,000 Wooden Stakes."

C We took [_____] Aunt Jane home.

C As soon as we got [_____] home, my sister Braeden told [_____] me she saw [_____] the mysterious man and what he did [_____].

C I invited [_____] my friends Lia and Bethany over and told [_____] them what had happened [_____] at the airport.

C We looked [_____] at the headline on the paper.

C "I do n't get [_____] it."

C "Why would he throw [_____] away a newspaper that said [_____], 'Sweet_Heart_Lumber_Co orders [_____] 10,000 Wooden Stakes,'" asked [_____] Lia, "unless he was [_____] a vampire."

Sample #14: Boy, Age 11 Years, excerpt from imaginary story titled "The Blue Beyond" (Nippold, 2007, p. 350)

MLTU = 8.94   CD = 1.82

C We climbed [_____] into the spaceship.

C Then we heard [_____] the countdown, 10_9_8_7_3_2_1 BOOM!

C The engines fired [_____] up.

C We were going [_____] up_up_up faster than I ever imagined [_____].

C It was [_____] then dark.

C But soon the stars began [_____] to appear [_____], then planets, then moons.

C "Oh no," I looked [_____] over and saw [_____] my dad struggling [_____] with the controls.

C "They 're [_____] jammed," he said [_____] worriedly.

C I looked [_____] out the window to see [_____] the Milky_Way disappearing [_____].

C We were being [_____] swept [_____] into a different galaxy.

C Boom_crash_bang!

C We made [_____] a crash landing on something hard.

C After a long time of struggling [_____], we finally managed [_____] to climb [_____] out of the damaged spaceship.

C We stopped [_____] to look [_____] at our surroundings.

C We were [_____] on a strange blue planet.

C Everything was [_____] blue.

C The ground was [_____] covered [_____] with enormous stones and boulders that made [_____] flashes of blue when the sunlight hit [_____] them.

C There was [_____] a little bit of grass here and there that was [_____] a beautiful shade of blue that made [_____] the planet sparkle [_____].

C The planet was [_____] like an ocean.

C It was [_____] gorgeous with its different shades of blue.

C There was [_____] neon blue, navy blue, royal blue, and sky blue.

C "Let [_____] 's call [_____] this planet The_Blue_Beyond," my dad suggested [_____].

C "Can we go [_____] exploring," I asked [_____].

C "Maybe we 'll find [_____] some life."

C As we were walking [_____] around, my dad jerked [_____] me behind a rock.

C "What was [_____] that for," I asked [_____].

C ("Shhhhh") {sound effects from his dad}.

C He pointed [_____] to a clearing.

C In that clearing was [_____] a little creature with big bug eyes.

C Its blue skin perfectly matched [_____] its surroundings.

C Its sharp piranha-like teeth sparkled [_____] in the sunlight.

C And its pointed little ears bobbed [_____] up and down as it ran [_____].

C It screeched [_____] as it approached [_____] a dead little animal.

C And the rest of the troop came [_____] running [_____] to help [_____].

C As they fought [_____] over the animal, my dad whispered [_____], "You never want [_____] to mess [_____] with those guys!"

Sample #15: Boy, Age 17 Years, essay titled "What Happened One Day" (from the author's files)

MLTU = 13.68   CD = 2.58

C One day a long time ago, my friend Jack and I went [_____] on a camping trip all by ourselves.

C We set [_____] up camp and went [_____] fishing to try [_____] and catch [_____] our dinner.

C I caught [_____] two fish while Jack caught [_____] three.

C We were getting [_____] ready to leave [_____] when I looked [_____] up the river and saw [_____] this big dark blurry figure run [_____] off into the bushes.

C I did n't think [_____] anything of it.

C I just thought [_____] it was [_____] an elk.

C On our way back to the camp, Jack started [_____] taunting [_____] me and bragging [_____] about how he was [_____] a better fisherman than I was [_____] because he caught [_____] three fish while I only caught [_____] two.

C We got [_____] back to camp.

C And I started [_____] a fire to cook [_____] the fish.

C I always started [_____] the fires.

C I was [_____] the best fire starter.

C We cooked [_____] some of our fish and put [_____] the rest in the ice chest for breakfast.

C We made [_____] our beds and went [_____] to sleep [_____].

C Jack was still bragging [_____] about his fish.

C When I woke [_____] in the morning, I opened [_____] my eyes to see [_____] Bigfoot eating [_____] our fish.

C As I leaned [_____] over to wake [_____] up Jack, it looked [_____] at me and ran [_____] off into the forest.

C Just like that, our camping trip turned [_____] into a hunt for rock solid proof of Bigfoot.

C After three days trying [_____] and failing [_____] to find [_____] Bigfoot anywhere, we gave [_____] up and went [_____] home.

C Ever since that day, I always have been [_____] sure to bring [_____] three things camping with me, a gun, a camera, and a better type of fishing bait.

EXPOSITORY LANGUAGE SAMPLES

Spoken Language

Sample #16: Boy, Age 13 Years, Favorite Game or Sport task (from the author's files)

MLCU = 10.06   CD = 1.67

E What is your favorite game or sport?

C My favorite sport in school would be [_____] wrestling.

E Why is wrestling your favorite sport?

C Well the (uh) coaches are [_____] really nice and everything.

C (We got got uh) we started [_____] out doing [_____] these (like uh) extra things.

C And (then uh and) then eventually I did [_____] everything and got [_____] good at it.

C So started [_____] getting [_____] gold medals and stuff.

E I'm not too familiar with the sport of wrestling, so I would like you to tell me all about it.

E For example, tell me what the goals are, and how many people may play a match.

E Also, tell me about the rules that players need to follow.

E Tell me everything you can think of about the sport of wrestling so that someone who has never played before would know how to play.

C (We) you start [_____] on a mat.

C You warm up [_____].

C You go [_____] over to the mat.

C You shake [_____] hands.

C And the ref blows [_____] the whistle.

C And when you wrestle [_____], you start [_____] out neutral.

C And (you have to um you have to) you take [_____] the guy down by getting [_____] control of him while their hands or their feet are [_____] on the mat.

C And if you 're taking [_____] a guy down (you can't like if you come around the back), you can 't just pick [_____] them up and slap [_____] them on the mat.

C Otherwise, it 's [_____] unnecessary roughness.

C You get docked [_____] off a point.

C And if they are [_____] (uh) too injured to wrestle [_____] then they win [_____] the match.

C And (um) it 's [_____] really big on sportsmanship.

C So you can 't go [_____] over and yell [_____] at the ref or yell [_____] at (the) them.

C Otherwise you 'll get kicked [_____] for the next tournament.

C And (um yeah you also you have um you have to) you have [_____] to shake [_____] hands because it 's [_____] pretty much sportsmanship to do [_____] that.

C And once you get [_____] the take down on them, you (um) try [_____] to break [_____] them down to their back.

C And you get [_____] them past a 45-degree angle.

C And you get [_____] near full points.

C Then (uh) for 3 points, it 's [_____] like 2 points.

C And (uh 5 points it's like 3 poin er uh) 5 seconds it 's [_____] 3 points.

C And then after that, (you uh for how long) you hold [_____] them down.

C And it 's [_____] about a 2-second pin.

C And if you get [_____] both their shoulders down and (uh them you uh) if you pin [_____] them, you get [_____] to shake [_____] hands.

C And you win [_____].

C But there 's [_____] also points.

C Like for college, there 's [_____] advantage time which is [_____] where (like somebody if) somebody was riding [_____] a person for a long time.

C And they get [_____] points.

C (But once they go neutral then the timing down and stuff).

C (So uh they have to kinda like) that 's [_____] how it goes [_____] with the advantage time.

C They get [_____] certain amount of points at the end for advantage time and stuff.

C (uh) it 's [_____] pretty much big on sportsmanship.

C And it 's [_____] pretty easy to learn [_____].

C Also you can 't lock [_____] hands while they 're [_____] down around their waist (but) like around the leg (or around the ar).

C But around the arm is [_____] okay.

C And stuff like that (and can't like uh).

C In freestyle you can do [_____] that because it 's [_____] a big part of freestyle.

E Now I would like you to tell me what a player should do in order to win the sport of wrestling.

E In other words, what are some key strategies that every good player should know?

C You just try [_____] to turn [_____] them so you get [_____] back points.

C And (uh once second) once both their shoulders touch [_____] the mat, they 're [_____] pinned.

E Do they have to go all the way down?

C No you just have [_____] to get [_____] their shoulders to touch [_____].

E How long is a match?

C (um matches are usually like in reg) I think [_____] they 're [_____] the same in everyone.

C So (they) for middle school, it 's [_____] (like) about (like uh) three minutes or maybe four minutes or something like that.

C For high school it 's [_____] six minutes.

C And college I 'm [_____] not sure.

C I think [_____] it 's [_____] about the same as high school or (like) 30 seconds more or something.

E So a match isn't all that long.

C Yeah it 's [_____] not too hard (it's just) if you 're [_____] conditioned well and you have [_____] a good work ethic.

C Then you 'll probably do [_____] well in wrestling.

C But if you do n't try [_____] your hardest, you 're never going [_____] to get [_____] anywhere.

C Yeah it 's [_____] pretty much you can beat [_____] guys that are [_____] strong as long as you have [_____] a good technique.

C But (strength is kinda like) some people can just do [_____] bad technique and just knock [_____] you down and (um) then pin [_____] me and stuff.

C But most of the time, you can get [_____] them.

E What about freestyle?

C (Well in freestyle it's just you) I do n't know [_____] much about freestyle.

C But you just touch [_____] (their both) their shoulders on the mat.

C And you win [_____].

C Or you win [_____] by points at the end of the match.

C Same with collegiate except in collegiate it (like) 2 points pin.

C And (then like you'll uh and) if you do n't pin [_____] through the whole match, then you win [_____] by a certain amount of points.

C And then you get [_____] a certain amount of points for your team.

C But you can also technical [_____] them which is [_____] (like) when (you uh if) you (get) gain [_____] (like) 15 points more than them.

C Then they stop [_____] the match.

C And you win [_____].

Sample #17: Girl, Age 17 Years, Peer Conflict Resolution Science Fair task* (from the author's files)

MLCU = 15.45   CD = 3.40

E Now I'd like you to tell the story back to me, in your own words.

E Try to tell me everything you can remember about the story.

C The teacher gave [_____] the four girls an assignment to work [_____] together on a science project.

C And they decided [_____] they were going [_____] to make [_____] a model airplane that could actually fly [_____].

C And everyone worked [_____] on it except for one girl named [_____] Melanie.

C And (it made Debbie angry or um) it made [_____] her indifferent because she would n't do [_____] the work.

E What is the main problem here?

C (Um) not everyone was participating [_____] equally or helping [_____] participating [_____].

E Why is that a problem?

C Well if one person does n't do [_____] anything and they 're [_____] still in the group, they 're still going [_____] to get [_____] the same grade.

C Or they 're still going [_____] to be [_____] in that group as all the people that worked [_____] as hard.

C But they did n't contribute [_____] to it at all.

C So the other people may feel [_____] like they did n't deserve [_____] it.

E What is a good way for Debbie to deal with Melanie?

---

*Note: This task involves briefly retelling a story before moving into expository discourse.

C (um) I guess [_____] Debbie could ask [_____] Melanie why she did
   n't want [_____] to help [_____] or maybe she wanted [_____] to do
   [_____] something different than what they wanted [_____] to do
   [_____].

C Maybe that 's [_____] the reason she did n't want [_____] to help [_____].

C (Or) and if that did n't work [_____], then she could ask [_____] the
   teacher to help [_____] them.

E Why is that a good way for Debbie to deal with Melanie?

C Because it 's [_____] calm.

C She 's not going [_____] to be [_____] like yelling [_____] at her.

C They 're going [_____] to try [_____] to compromise [_____] about it
   so that the three girls can do [_____] what they want [_____] to do
   [_____].

C But Melanie can also help [_____] since they 're all contributing
   [_____] to it.

E What do you think will happen if Debbie does that?

C (um) Maybe Melanie will say [_____] that she did n't want [_____] to
   make [_____] an airplane or (she um) she wanted [_____] to do [_____]
   something different.

C And so maybe they could interact [_____] that way and find [_____]
   out what the problem was [_____] so Melanie could help [_____] do
   [_____] something.

E How do you think they both will feel if Debbie does that?

C I think [_____] that they would kind of feel [_____] more relaxed and
   not so uptight about her not helping [_____] or maybe Melanie not
   getting [_____] to do [_____] what she wants [_____] to do [_____].

C Maybe they would both feel [_____] more comfortable about the
   problem or talking [_____] about it.

Sample #18: Girl, Age 17 Years, Peer Conflict Resolution Fast Food Restaurant task** (from the author's files)

MLCU = 11.63   CD = 2.21

E Now I'd like you to tell the story back to me, in your own words.

C (um Jane and Kathy) Jane is going [_____] to cook [_____] the food on the grill.

C And Kathy is going [_____] to take [_____] out the garbage.

C But her arm really hurts [_____].

C And she wants [_____] to switch [_____] jobs.

C But Jane does n't want [_____] to lose [_____] her spot at the grill.

E What is the main problem here?

C The main problem is [_____] that (maybe) maybe Jane does n't want [_____] to give [_____] up her spot.

C Maybe they could just switch [_____] for a minute for her to take [_____] out the garbage.

C Or maybe she could help [_____] Kathy take [_____] out the garbage.

C The main problem is [_____] that (they don't want to) Jane does n't want [_____] to switch [_____] jobs.

C But maybe she can just help [_____] Kathy instead do [_____] the grill.

E Why is that a problem?

C Because she said [_____] that she did n't want [_____] to give [_____] up her spot at the grill.

C So obviously she did n't want [_____] to give [_____] up her spot at the grill.

C And (maybe) I do n't know [_____] why.

E What is a good way for Jane to deal with Kathy?

**Note: This task involves briefly retelling a story before moving into expository discourse.

C Well Jane could help [_____] Kathy take [_____] the garbage out.

C Or someone else could do [_____] it.

E Why is that a good way for Jane to deal with Kathy?

C Because they could both get [_____] their jobs done and help [_____] each other.

E What do you think will happen if Jane does that?

C I think [_____] that Kathy would really appreciate [_____] it if Jane helped [_____] her (and) and maybe in turn Kathy would help [_____] Jane if she wanted [_____] it.

C (Or um) then they could both get [_____] their jobs done.

E How do you think they both will feel if Jane does that?

C They 'll both feel [_____] (like) happy that everything got done [_____] or happy (that they solved) that they could help [_____] each other and solve [_____] the problems.

Written Language

Sample #19: Girl, Age 17 Years, the Nature of Friendship expository essay (from the author's files)

MLTU = 12.10   CD = 2.20

C To me, friendship is [_____] a relationship between two or more people that like [_____] spending [_____] time with each other.

C A friend is [_____] someone you can talk [_____] to when there is [_____] no other.

C You can tell [_____] them your secrets.

C And they will always have [_____] your back.

C If the world did n't have [_____] friendship, then relationships and social status would n't mean [_____] a thing.

C The world would be [_____] full of people that do n't like [_____] each other.

C And most of all, there would n't be [_____] anyone to talk [_____] with.

C Friends mostly keep [_____] you occupied.

C If I did n't have [_____] friends, then my life would lack [_____] the excitement everyone needs [_____].

C I would just wake [_____] up, go [_____] to school, come home [_____] and either watch [_____] TV or do [_____] nothing.

C With friends, it 's [_____] like our lives are [_____] all intertwined.

C And if one of us is doing [_____] something exciting, then the rest should be [_____] in on it as well.

C Living [_____] a boring life is n't [_____] worth it.

C Usually friends share [_____] common interests.

C Either it being [_____] culture, neighborhood, or personalities, they are [_____] usually like the other.

C Friendship to children is [_____] having [_____] someone to play [_____] with.

C Usually it 's [_____] a person from school or a neighbor.

C For teenagers like me, friendship means [_____] someone to talk [_____] to when we get [_____] in a fight with our parents, boyfriend, or girlfriends.

C Adults see [_____] friendship as more of a companionship.

C If they have [_____] common interest in things, then they are [_____] more than likely to become [_____] friends.

C Or they have just been [_____] friends for a really long time.

C Usually people are [_____] friends one year then just are [_____] n't the next.

C People grow [_____] up and change [_____] and make [_____] new friends every day.

C Sometimes friends just drift [_____] apart over the years.

C Other times, friends can do [_____] or say [_____] something that does n't make [_____] them trustworthy.

C The usual result is [_____] a misunderstanding or someone gets [_____] hurt.

C The best of friends are [_____] the ones that stay [_____] in touch for a really long time.

C There have been [_____] cases of people being [_____] friends since they were [_____] three.

C And now at age sixty they are [_____] still together.

C Friendships come [_____] and go [_____], and depending [_____] on what kind of friendship it is [_____], can last [_____] a lifetime.

PERSUASIVE LANGUAGE SAMPLES

Spoken Language

Sample #20: Girl, Age 15 Years, arguing for later school start time (Miller, Andriacchi, & Nockerts, 2019; borrowed with permission from the authors)

MLCU = 14.67   CD = 2.61

C (Um) I think [_____] (that the time in school) that school should start [_____] later in the morning.

C (Um) It can help [_____] students focus [_____] more because students come [_____] in so early.

C And (they) some of them do n't go [_____] to sleep [_____] until later at night anyways, especially for people that have [_____] after school sports because (you_know, like) having [_____] to stay [_____] out later.

C And if you got [_____] more sleep at home, you would n't necessarily have [_____] to worry [_____] about students sleeping [_____] in class (so) which is [_____] probably a big problem because I see [_____] a lot of kids sleeping [_____] in class.

C (Um) transportation could be [_____] another reason because the kids (um) get [_____] up late.

C They oversleep [_____] and have [_____] no way to the bus in the mornings.

C Or they have [_____] no way to school.

C Or they are [_____] too far to walk [_____].

C So most students miss [_____] the bus because they have [_____] to get [_____] up so early.

C And (um) students are failing [_____] classes mostly because they can't focus [_____] or because they (um) are sleeping [_____] in class and kind a missing [_____] (the) the details that they need [_____] to learn [_____].

C And (um they could um) it 'll be [_____] better grades, I think [_____], if they can just focus [_____] more.

C It 'll be [_____] better grades.

C And (kind a like because) here we have [_____] like MASH and stuff.

C So it 'll be [_____] better grades for them and less of that.

C And some kids they skip [_____] school not necessarily because they (like) are [_____] sick or something, just really because they just need [_____] the time off.

C Most of them do [_____] it for sleep (but).

C And (um) if we can 't necessarily come [_____] into school later, we could get [_____] out of school earlier (which) or (you_know) get [_____] a free time in between school to kind a just give [_____] the kids just a minute to get [_____] theirselfs together.

C Or (um) we need [_____] shorter classes because like long classes, and sitting [_____] in the same spot for a long time, kind a gets [_____] boring (so).

C And (um) I want [_____] later school hours (um) because then (it w) it 'll be [_____] easier for me and for more students because they would n't be [_____] so sleepy.

C It could cause [_____] more focus.

C And (um) you could ask [_____] more students (if you know) if you were [_____] n't too sure on what I was saying [_____] (so).

E Good.

E Is there anything else you can tell me?

C (Um probably that) I 'm trying [_____] to think [_____].

C I do n't know [_____] because (like) some kids they (like) do n't go [_____] to bed until like twelve or like one.

C And so (i) it 's [_____] really hard to get [_____] up (you_know) at six.

C Most kids get [_____] up at six (because the bus) around bus (x) times.

C So it 's [_____] really hard.

C Like I, personally, get [_____] up at six and have [_____] to get [_____] my little sisters up at six.

C And (like) especially, it 's [_____] (hard for) harder for people that 's [_____] not morning people to (you_know) get [_____] dressed and get [_____] your stuff together.

C And it 's [_____] really hard to focus [_____] because you wake [_____] up so late.

C And (you wanna) you do n't wan [_____] na have [_____] to (like) rush [_____] (so).

C And then you rush [_____].

C And you forget [_____] things or (you_know) forget [_____] things you might need [_____] for school or classes.

C And that could also lead [_____] to a bad day, not having [_____] what you need [_____] (so).

Written Language

Sample #21: Boy, Age 17 Years, the Circus Controversy persuasive essay (from the author's files)

MLTU = 15.50   CD = 2.93

C Should animals perform [_____] in circuses?

C I believe [_____] that being [_____] trained to do [_____] tricks and to entertain [_____] audiences is [_____] a very good use for animals.

C There are [_____], however, a couple of sides on this subject.

C Some people think [_____] only of the entertainment with no concern for the animals' needs.

C Circuses may not feed [_____] the animals well or give [_____] them adequate space to live [_____] just for a little extra profit.

C It 's [_____] also possible that they use [_____] dangerous training techniques.

C These are [_____] all negative aspects on animals performing [_____] in circuses.

C There is [_____] also a good side to having [_____] circus animals.

C They can provide [_____] much entertainment for both adults and children, performing [_____] stunts, tricks, and acrobatics, jumping [_____] through fiery hoops, walking [_____] on hind legs, things you do n't usually see [_____] your pets doing [_____].

C This can also help [_____] to eliminate [_____] any fears children might have [_____] of the performing animals.

C Looking [_____] back at this reasoning and the impressions it gives [_____] us, I can see [_____] that there is [_____] an easy solution to get [_____] rid of the negative aspects.

C Allow [_____] for the animals to perform [_____] in circuses, but only if they are [_____] treated well, given [_____] enough food, large ugh living areas, and trained [_____] without using [_____] too harsh punishment.

C Using [_____] this method, there are [_____] only positive reasons.

C So why not have [_____] animals perform [_____] in circuses?

Sample #22: Girl, Age 18 Years, the Circus Controversy persuasive essay (from the author's files)

MLTU = 11.69   CD = 2.44

C I feel [_____] that animals performing [_____] for our entertainment is [_____] a bad idea!

C We have [_____] many other forms of entertainment in this day and age.

C We do not need [_____] to force [_____] wild animals to do [_____] things for our entertainment.

C The animals that are [_____] part of circuses do not have [_____] the proper habitat that they need [_____].

C They do not have [_____] space that they need [_____].

C And they have been known [_____] to become [_____] violent.

C I do not have [_____] a problem with people performing [_____], with cats and dogs, even horses.

C But all of these are [_____] domestic animals.

C Tigers, bears, and elephants should not be [_____] locked [_____] in small cages, forced [_____] to do [_____] tricks, and be [_____] poorly treated [_____].

C There is [_____] no reason that people and domestic animals could not give [_____] just as good of a performance.

C Wild animals are [_____] just that, wild.

C They need [_____] to be [_____] in habitats that are [_____] suitable for them.

C They need [_____] to be [_____] fed [_____] right and let [_____] to use [_____] their instincts.

C Malnutrition, small confined areas, and entertainment for people is [_____] not what these creatures are [_____] on this earth for.

C They are [_____] animals, not actors.

C And we need [_____] to remember [_____] this.

APPENDIX A

Answer Key for Chapter 9

WORDS AND PHRASES

Exercise 9–1. Identifying Words in Passages

In passages 1 through 6, circle all of the *nouns* including *gerunds* and *proper nouns* (but not pronouns).

1. **Computers** can do **lots** of **things**. They can add **millions** of **numbers** in the **twinkling** of an **eye**. They can outwit chess **grandmasters**. They can guide **weapons** to their **targets**. They can book you onto a **plane** between a guitar-strumming **nun** and a nonsmoking physics **professor**. Some can even play the **bongos**. That's quite a **variety**! So if we're going to talk about **computers**, we'd better decide right now which of them we're going to look at, and how (Feynman, 1996, p. 1).

2. Most of the **luxuries**, and many of the so-called **comforts** of **life**, are not only not indispensable, but positive **hindrances** to the **elevation** of **mankind**. With **respect** to **luxuries** and **comforts**, the **wisest** have ever lived a more simple and meager **life** than the **poor**. The ancient **philosophers**, Chinese, Hindoo, Persian, and Greek, were a

class than which none has been poorer in outward **riches**, none so rich in inward (Thoreau, 2004, p. 14).

3. For a French **parent**, **education** is everything. The **child** must have as many and as important **certificates** of academic **attainment** as possible. In American and British business **life**, **experience** counts. In French **life**, the right **education** and the right **certificates** count. This is why some experienced American and British **teachers** wishing to work in **France** are horrified to find their **experience** downgraded because they do not have the equivalent degree **certificate** to the French one (Tomalin, 2003, p. 93).

4. There are two **kinds** of **knowledge**. One is the everyday **kind** of **knowledge** we have of the **world**, which we get through our **senses** (usually called "empirical" **knowledge**). **Plato** thought that this **kind** of **knowledge** was useful enough for ordinary **people** to go about their everyday **lives**. But it wasn't the real **thing**. Like **Heraclitus**, **Pythagoras**, and maybe **Socrates**, **Plato** thought that the empirical **world** was a **kind** of **illusion**, a **veil** that hid the real **truth** from us (Robinson & Groves, 2005, p. 62).

5. **Plato** was probably the greatest **philosopher** of all **time**, and the first to collect all **sorts** of different **ideas** and **arguments** into **books** that everyone can read. He wanted to know about everything and constantly pestered his fellow **philosophers** for **answers** to his disturbing **questions**. He also had resolute **ideas** of his own, some of which seem sensible enough, and some of which now seem extremely odd. But, from the **start**, he knew that "**doing philosophy**" was a very special **activity** (Robinson & Groves, 2005, p. 3).

6. I propose that **educationalists** should no longer conceive of **children** as passive, empty jam **jars** who need to be stuffed with **information**, but as independently-minded problem **solvers** who

need to be continually challenged (John Dewey; Robinson & Groves, 2004, p. 111).

In passages 7 through 12, circle all of the *adjectives* including the *participles*:

7. The legacy of **Scotland's tumultuous** and often **violent** history can be found in its **extraordinary** array of **prehistoric** sites, **religious** ruins, and other **historic** attractions. Today these relics offer visitors **intriguing** insights into **some** of the **defining** battles, heroes, and **forgotten** worlds of the country's **rich** and **turbulent** past (Wilson & Murphy, 2008, p. 274).

8. Once Oregon was thought to be **immune** to earthquakes. Today we know that we have them in **three different** flavors—**devastating subduction** earthquakes like the **1700** catastrophe, **deep intraplate** earthquakes like the **Puget Sound** temblors of 1949 and 2001, and **sharp local** jolts like the **Spring Break** Quake of 1993 (Sullivan, 2008, p. 67).

9. **Some** artists are **finite** draftsmen with **meticulous drawing** skills. **Other** artists are storytellers. A few invent a **new** lens of perception. But Sarkis Antikajian is a painter. His work is a **bodacious** celebration of brush **dipped** in paint and **spread** across canvas. While **some** painters claim they paint light, Sarkis Antikajian paints energy. He leaves his viewer **breathless** by the onslaught on his transcription. His **masterful** use of **intense** chroma ravishes the **visual** cortex in a **heady** embrace. Sarkis wields color with the **same** bravado **employed** by the trumpeter Maynard Ferguson when he plays C above **high** C (Moffet, 2006, pp. 18–19).

10. The **ancient** Greeks made **extensive** use of honey in salves and potions, in **prepared** dishes, to make perfume, as libations for the dead, and to appease the gods. Bee-keepers numbered among their ranks the philosopher Aristotle; for Hippocrates, the father of medicine, honey was a **favorite** remedy. The followers of Pythagoras

lived on a diet of bread and honey—and seemed to far outlive any of their contemporaries (Style, 1993, p. 14).

11. **French** culture once dominated **Western** civilization. From about 1650 to about 1920, the **upper** classes in **several** countries preferred French to their own **native** languages. French was the **official** language for **diplomatic** negotiations and **much government** business. The achievements of **French** writers, artists, architects, and composers were widely admired and imitated. Since then, **other** cultures have moved to the forefront. English has overtaken French as the most widely **spoken** language (Harris, 1989, p. 167).

12. Mister Fox was just about **famished** and **thirsty** too, when he stole into a vineyard where the **sun-ripened** grapes were hanging upon a trellis in a **tempting** show, but too **high** for him to reach. He took a run and a jump, **snapping** at the **nearest** bunch, but missed. Again and again he jumped, only to miss the **luscious** prize. At last, **worn** out with his efforts, he retreated, **muttering**: "Well, I never really wanted those grapes anyway. I am **sure** they are **sour**, and perhaps **wormy** in the bargain." ("The Fox and the Grapes," Grosset & Dunlap, 1947, p. 14)

In passages 13 through 17, circle all of the *finite verbs*:

13. Trieste, set on a gulf with rolling hills as a backdrop, **is** the most important seaport on the northern Adriatic. Because of its geographic position and its history, the cooking of Trieste **is** eclectic. *Gnocchetti di fegato*, liver dumplings, **are** a reminder of Austrian ties. Venezia's influence **is** apparent in its many risotto, including its own version of *risi e bisi*. It also **has** its own variation of *brodetto*, the fish stew so popular along the entire Italian coastline. Made with local fish, the sauce **contains** vinegar, wine, and sometimes tomatoes, and **is** always **served** with grilled polenta. There **are** many rich desserts. Typical **are** *strucoli*, similar to strudel, which like *preniz*, an Easter

specialty, **are made** with a variety of ingredients (Luciano et al., 1991, p. 87).

14. When first I **took** up my abode in the woods, that **is**, **began** to spend my nights as well as days there, which, by accident, **was** on Independence Day, or the fourth of July, 1845, my house **was** not finished for winter, but **was** merely a defense against the rain, without plastering or chimney, the walls being of rough weatherstained boards, with wide chinks, which **made** it cool at night (Thoreau, 2004, p. 81).

15. The only house I **had been** the owner of before, if I **except** a boat, **was** a tent, which I **used** occasionally when making excursions in the summer, and this **is** still rolled up in my garret; but the boat, after passing from hand to hand, **has gone** down the stream of time. With this more substantial shelter about me, I **had made** some progress toward settling in the world (Thoreau, 2004, p. 82).

16. Sonja Kovalevsky (1850–1891), earlier known as Sophia Korvin-Krukovsky, **was** a gifted mathematician. She **was born** in Moscow to Russian nobility. She **left** Russia in 1868 because universities **were closed** to women. She **went** to Germany because she **wished** to study with Karl Weierstrass in Berlin. It **was said** that her early interest in mathematics **was** due in part to an odd wallpaper that **covered** her room in a summer house. Fascinated, she **spent** hours trying to make sense of it. The paper **turned** out to be lecture notes on higher mathematics purchased by her father during his student days (K. Smith, 1995, p. 479).

17. In his famous laboratory school at the University of Chicago, children **were** (and still **are**) **encouraged** to solve problems by inventing hypotheses and testing them. Dewey **thought** that art **should be encouraged** because it **stimulates** imaginative "solutions" to its own unique "problems" (Robinson & Groves, 2004, p. 111).

In passages 18 through 22, circle all of the *adverbs*:

18. Western Iran extends from the border with Armenia and Azerbaijan in the north to the industrial city of Ahvaz near the Gulf. **Culturally**, it is the **most** diverse part of Iran, with Azaris, Armenians, Loris, Bakhtiaris, and Kurds among the distinct ethnic groups you'll encounter. Despite this and a wealth of historical, religious, and cultural sights, stunning mountain scenery, and great trekking possibilities, few travelers see more than Tabriz. Pity them, then take advantage of the unspoilt expanses, and go yourself (Ham et al., 2006, p. 199).

19. The Middle East is home to some of the world's **most** significant cities—Jerusalem, Cairo, Damascus, Baghdad, and Istanbul. The ruins of the **once similarly** epic cities of history—Petra, Persepolis, Ephesus, Palmyra, Baalbek, Leptis Magna, and the bounty of ancient Egypt—also mark the passage of centuries in a region where the ancient world lives and breathes. The landscapes of the region are **equally** spellbinding, from the unrivaled seas of sand dunes and palm-fringed lakes in Libya's Sahara desert to the stunning mountains of the north, and the underwater world of the Red Sea (Ham et al., 2006, p. 4).

20. Mt. Fuji is the highest mountain in Japan and **by far** the **most** splendid, but during July and August (the open season) it is not a **dauntingly** hard climb. An athlete, it is said, could leave home in Tokyo in the morning, reach the peak and be home in time for dinner. Most people prefer to take it at a **more** leisurely pace, spending a night at the top and greeting the morning sun with a cry of "*Banzai!*" (Popham, 1992, p. 159).

21. I left the woods for as good a reason as I went there. **Perhaps** it seemed to me that I had **several** more lives to live, and could not spare **any** more time for that one. It is remarkable how **easily**

and **insensibly** we fall into a particular route, and make a beaten track for ourselves. I had not lived there a week before my feet wore a path from my door to the pond-side; and though it is five or six years since I trod it, it is **still quite** distinct. It is true, I fear that others may have fallen into it, and so helped to keep it open (Thoreau, 2004, p. 313).

22. John Dewey (1859–1952) was a systematic pragmatist or "instrumentalist" who believed that being "philosophical" **really** meant being **critically** intelligent and maintaining a "scientific" approach to human problems. Pragmatists like Dewey were great enthusiasts for the successes of science and its methods of inquiry. Dewey was convinced that philosophy could **also** play a key role in a creative American democracy by contributing to all kinds of knowledge in ethics, art, education, and the **newly** emerging social sciences. Like Pierce, Dewey was a theoretical "fallibilist," but **still firmly** a believer in the real possibility of practical progress in human affairs. Society can **only** progress if its members are educated to be intelligent and flexible (Robinson & Groves, 2004, p. 111).

In passage 23, circle all of the *prepositions*:

23. The year 1877 was an important one **in** the study **of** the planet Mars. The Red Planet came unusually close **to** Earth, affording astronomers an especially good view. **Of** particular note was the discovery, **by** U.S. Naval Observatory astronomer Asaph Hall, **of** the two moons circling Mars. But most exciting was the report **of** the Italian astronomer Giovanni Schiaparelli **on** his observations **of** a network **of** linear markings that he termed *canali*. **In** Italian, the word usually means "grooves" or "channels," but it can also mean "canals" (Chaisson & McMillan, 2005, p. 140).

In passages 24 and 25, circle all of the *pronouns*:

24. **This** country, with **its** institutions, belongs to the people **who** inhabit **it**. Whenever **they** shall grow weary of the existing government, **they** can exercise **their** *constitutional* right of amending **it**, or **their** *revolutionary* right to dismember, or overthrow **it**. **I** cannot be ignorant of the fact **that** many worthy, and patriotic citizens are desirous of having the constitution amended (Emerson, 1841/2009, *Self-Reliance*, p. 41).

25. **All** the barnyard knew **that** the hen was indisposed. So **one** day, the cat decided to pay **her** a visit of condolence. Creeping up to **her** nest, the cat in **his** most sympathetic voice said, "How are **you**, **my** dear friend? **I** was so sorry to hear of **your** illness. Isn't **there** **something that I** can bring **you** to cheer **you** up and to help **you** feel like **yourself** again?" "Thank **you**," said the hen. "Please be good enough to leave **me** in peace, and **I** have no fear but **I** shall soon be well." Moral: Uninvited guests are often most welcome when **they** are gone ("The Cat and the Hen," Grosset & Dunlap, 1947, p. 133).

In passage 26, circle all of the *articles*:

26. Starting in **the** 1870s, another upheaval in **the** arts resulted from **the** development of **a** new approach to painting called Impressionism. Young artists rejected **the** long-accepted, conventional ways of presenting reality. They too were fascinated by recent discoveries in science and experimented with new techniques for capturing **the** effects of light. Often they used tiny dabs of complementary colors, relying on **the** viewer's eyes and mind to bring them together and form **the** desired effect. **The** Postimpressionist painters of **the** late nineteenth and early twentieth centuries worked out new ways of seeing that were highly personal. They scorned **the** old emphasis on reproducing reality as accurately as possible. Instead, they sought to express their own innermost visions and emotions (Harris, 1989, pp. 173–175).

In passages 27 and 28, circle all of the *conjunctions*:

27. A woman of many gifts, Margaret Fuller (1810–1850) is most aptly remembered **as** America's first true feminist. In her brief **yet** fruitful life, she was variously author, editor, literary **and** social critic, journalist, poet, **and** revolutionary. She was also one of the few female members of the prestigious Transcendentalist movement, whose ranks included Ralph Waldo Emerson, Henry David Thoreau, Elizabeth Palmer Peabody, Nathaniel Hawthorne, **and** many other prominent New England intellectuals of the day. **As** coeditor of the transcendentalist journal, *The Dial*, Fuller was able to give voice to her groundbreaking social critique on woman's place in society, the genesis of the book that was later to become *Woman in the Nineteenth Century* (Pine, 1999, p. 133).

28. **When** people started to analyze English grammar in the eighteenth century, it seemed logical to look at the language using the terms **and** distinctions which had proved so useful in studying Latin. English had no word-endings, it seemed. **Therefore**, it had no "grammar." **But** of course there is far more to grammar **than** word-endings. Some languages (such as Chinese) have none at all. English has less than a dozen types of regular endings (**and** a few irregular ones) (Crystal, 2002, p. 22).

Exercise 9–2. Word Classes

For each word that is in bold, indicate its class—noun, pronoun, verb, adjective, adverb, conjunction, or preposition. Write the word next to the class on the lines following the passage.

Many trees **on** campus are not **native to** the **local** area. Eugene can **support** a greater **variety** of trees than many **places because its climate** is **moderate** enough to **easily** accommodate **trees** from colder **and** warmer **areas**. This **led** to the **campus** becoming an **arboretum**. However, planting nonnative trees **displaces** local trees. For **future** tree selections on campus, a **stronger emphasis** on native **species** would **eventually** turn the campus **into** a **richer learning environment**. One student commented **thoughtfully** that **her favorite** tree was the **Eastern black walnut**, near Gerlinger Hall.

Nouns (11):	variety, places, climate, trees, areas, campus, arboretum, emphasis, species, environment, walnut
Pronouns (2):	its, her
Verbs (3):	support, led, displaces
Adjectives (10):	native, local, moderate, future, stronger, richer, learning, favorite, Eastern, black
Adverbs (3):	easily, eventually, thoughtfully
Conjunctions (2):	because, and
Prepositions (3):	on, to, into

Exercise 9–3. Pronouns

1. Circle the *reflexive* pronouns: me   you   us   we   **ourselves**   him   her   **himself**

2. Circle the *demonstrative* pronouns: the   it   **that**   **those**   **these**   their   **this**

3. Circle the *interrogative* pronouns: he   on   under   **what**   her   **who**   **why**   must

4. Circle the *possessive* pronouns: **her**   that   **his**   **their**   any   only   ourselves

5. Circle the *relative* pronouns: **who**   his   **that**   their   **which**   them   they

Exercise 9–4. Particles Versus Prepositions

Circle the *particles*:

1. She threw **down** the pen.
2. He ran down the hill.
3. They sat on the bench.
4. He filled **up** his plate.
5. She ran to the door.
6. He took **off** the brace.

Circle the *prepositions*:

7. He gave away his books
8. She sat **by** the river.
9. They moved **to** Portland.
10. He ate **with** a fork.
11. She looked **at** the sea.
12. He ran **from** the dog.

Exercise 9–5. Adverbs

1. Circle the adverbs of *manner*: **quietly happily** somewhere forever   dreamy

2. Circle the adverbs of *time*: **later** pleasantly   lonely   **now** everyone   **always**

3. Circle the adverbs of *place*: **wherever** whenever   forever **somewhere   anywhere**

4. Circle the adverbs of *magnitude*: gleefully   definitely   **unusually slightly**

5. Circle the adverbs of *likelihood*: **possibly** joyously   **probably** cleverly

Exercise 9–6. Conjunctions

1. Circle the *subordinate* conjunctions: forever   anyway   **unless** **while**   **before**

2. Circle the *coordinate* conjunctions: **and**   until   whenever   why to   **but**   off

3. Circle the *adverbial* conjuncts: **consequently**   because   while wherever   **thus**   **moreover**

Exercise 9–7. Review: Word Classes

Read the following fable. Then identify each type of word listed below by filling in the blanks. List each word only once.

The Lion and the Mouse (Grosset & Dunlap, 1947, pp. 137–138)

A lion was asleep in his den one day, when a mischievous mouse for no reason at all ran across the outstretched paw and up the royal nose of the king of beasts, awakening him from his nap. The mighty beast clapped his paw upon the now thoroughly frightened little creature and would have made an end of him.

"Please," squealed the mouse, "don't kill me. Forgive me this time, O King, and I shall never forget it. A day may come, who knows, when I may do you a good turn to repay your kindness." The lion, smiling at his little prisoner's fright and amused by the thought that so small a creature ever could be of assistance to the king of beasts, let him go.

Not long afterward the lion, while ranging the forest for his prey, was caught in the net which the hunters had set to catch him. He let out a roar that echoed through the forest. Even the mouse heard it, and recognizing the voice of his former preserver and friend, ran to the spot where he lay tangled in the net of ropes.

"Well, your majesty," said the mouse, "I know you did not believe me once when I said I would return a kindness, but here is my chance." And without further ado he set to work to nibble with his sharp little teeth at the ropes that bound the lion. Soon the lion was able to crawl out of the hunter's snare and be free.

Application: No act of kindness, no matter how small, is ever wasted. Proverb: One good turn deserves another.

List each type of word (list each word only once):

1. List the *nouns*: lion, den, day, mouse, reason, paw, nose, king, beasts, nap, creature, end, time, turn, kindness, fright, thought, assistance, forest, prey, net, hunters, roar, voice, preserver, friend, spot, ropes, majesty, chance, ado, teeth, snare, act, matter

2. List the *adjectives* (but not the participles): asleep, one, mischievous, royal, mighty, little, good, prisoner's, small, former, further, sharp, hunter's, free

3. List the *participles*: outstretched, awakening, frightened, smiling, amused, ranging, recognizing, tangled, wasted

4. List the *verbs*: was, ran, clapped, would have made, squealed, do kill, forgive, shall forget, may come, knows, may do, to repay, could be, let go, was caught, had set, to catch, let, echoed, heard, ran, lay, said, know, did believe, would return, is, set, to work, to nibble, bound, to crawl, be, deserves

5. List the *adverbs*: now, thoroughly, never, so (small), ever, afterward, once, soon

Exercise 9–8 Phrases

In each sentence below, indicate the type of phrase that is bolded. Use the following codes:

NP = noun phrase

VP = verb phrase

PP = prepositional phrase

AJP = adjective phrase

AVP = adverb phrase

PP 1. The ball rolled **under the apple tree**.

AVP 2. The ranger told the ghost story **more enthusiastically** to the teenagers.

VP 3. The hikers **had not yet arrived** back at camp by nightfall.

AVP 4. The two friends sat down together **very cheerfully** to enjoy their dinner.

NP 5. **The charming old village** overlooked the river.

AVP 6. Marty missed school **because of a stomachache**.

VP 7. They **may have eaten** fish tonight for dinner.

PP 8. The resort specializes **in outdoor entertainment**.

VP 9. The lion **had been watching** the sparrows peck at the corn cobs.

NP 10. **The dry, old bread crumbs** had been left by a group of picnickers.

AVP 11. **Ever since Christmas**, Eva has been happy.

AJP 12. There are **several year-round, modernized, and attractive** inns in town.

NP 13. **Magnetic and electrical fields** may be present.

PP 14. The French have a holiday entitlement **of five weeks a year**.

AJP 15. There are **many long, steep, and winding** stretches of trail nearby.

NP 16. **The curious and persistent geologists** discovered large ice crystals.

AVP   17. The actor, tired and sick, struggled **rather mightily** to remember his lines.

NP   18. **The densely wooded mountainside** was a familiar friend to all.

VP   19. Two crows **were fighting furiously** in the old corn field.

AJP   20. The poem was written in **flowery Victorian** language.

AVP   21. The children knocked on their new neighbor's door **somewhat shyly**.

VP   22. The athletes **were running** around the track to warm up before the meet.

AVP   23. **Before the race**, she double-knotted her track shoes.

AJP   24. Jimmy was thrilled with the **brand new, shiny, red** bicycle.

NP   25. **The rain-soaked graduation picnic** was a memorable event.

Exercise 9–9. Verb Tenses

For each of the sentences below, indicate the *verb tense* from the following choices:

    A. Past perfect tense
    B. Future progressive tense
    C. Simple past tense
    D. Present perfect tense
    E. Simple future tense
    F. Past progressive tense
    G. Simple present tense
    H. Present progressive tense
    I. Future perfect tense

C   1. Yesterday, the Jones family arrived at Heathrow Airport around 2:00 p.m.

A   2. The direct flight from San Francisco had taken over 11 hours.

F   3. By 4:00 p.m., they were checking into their hotel in London.

F   4. Understandably, by early evening, all were feeling tired and hungry.

C   5. So they went out to a nearby pub for a delicious dinner of fish and chips.

A   6. By nine o'clock that evening, the family had settled into their room for the night.

G   7. It is now six o'clock in the morning, their first full day in the UK.

B   8. Today, the travelers will be taking the train from England to Wales.

I   9. They will have reached Llandudno, their final destination, by 11:30 a.m.

H   10. Now on the train, their son Liam is playing chess with his sister Jessie.

E   11. Jessie will eventually win the match, much to Liam's chagrin.

D   12. The children's mother, Martha, has just finished reading a short story.

H   13. And their father, Bruce, is ordering coffee from the trolley cart.

B   14. By two o'clock this afternoon, the Jones family will be enjoying the beach.

I   15. By that time, Liam will have forgotten about his loss to Jessie.

B   16. And Jessie will be searching for seashells and colorful rocks.

D   17. Liam has just learned the Welsh name for Wales, "Cymu."

G   18. Suddenly, Jessie wants a red tee shirt with "Cymu" on the front.

E   19. Dad will buy it for her and one for Liam, too.

B   20. Soon the Jones family will be walking back to their B & B after a fun-filled day.

3. He who is being carried [REL] does [MC] realize [MC] how far the town is [NOM].

APPENDIX B

Answer Key for
Chapter 10

MAIN AND SUBORDINATE CLAUSES

Exercise 10–1

For the following sets of proverbs, fill in the clause type, using the following codes:

MC = main clause   GER = gerundive clause

ADV = adverbial clause   INF = infinitive clause

NOM = nominal clause   PRT = participial clause

REL = relative clause

(*Sources: Category: Proverbs*, http://www.en.wikiquote.org/wiki; *Creative Proverbs from Around the World*, http://www.creativeproverbs.com); Politis, Reich, & Sheldon, 1998; Quotations Page, http://www.quotationspage.com; Scheffler, 1997; Stewart, 1997; Williams, 2000)

African Proverbs

1. A cutting word is **[MC]** worse than a bowstring. A cut may heal **[MC]**, but the cut of the tongue does **[MC]** not.

2. Ashes fly **[MC]** back into the face of him who throws **[REL]** them.

3. He who is being carried **[REL]** does not realize **[MC]** how far the town is **[NOM]**.

4. Quarrels end **[MC]** but words once spoken never die **[MC]**.

5. Send **[MC]** a boy where he wants **[ADV]** to go **[INF]** and you see **[MC]** his best pace.

6. Smooth seas do not make **[MC]** skillful sailors.

7. The lion does not turn **[MC]** around when a small dog barks **[ADV]**.

8. Two birds disputed **[MC]** about a kernel, when a third swooped **[ADV]** down and carried **[ADV]** it off.

9. When a needle falls **[ADV]** into a deep well, many people will look **[MC]** into the well, but few will be **[MC]** ready to go **[INF]** down after it.

10. He who learns **[REL]** teaches **[MC]**.

Chinese Proverbs

11. A bit of fragrance clings **[MC]** to the hand that gives **[REL]** flowers.

12. Even a hare will bite **[MC]** when it is **[ADV]** cornered.

13. A good fortune may forebode **[MC]** a bad luck, which may in turn disguise **[REL]** a good fortune.

14. If you are **[ADV]** patient in a moment of anger, you will escape **[MC]** a hundred days of sorrow.

15. If you do not study **[ADV]** hard when young, you'll end **[MC]** up bewailing **[PRT]** your failures as you grow up **[ADV]**.

16. Learning is **[MC]** a treasure that will follow **[REL]** its owner everywhere.

17. Listen **[MC]** to all, plucking **[PRT]** a feather from every passing goose, but follow **[MC]** no one absolutely.

18. Make **[MC]** happy those who are **[REL]** near, and those who are **[REL]** far will come **[MC]**.

19. Only when all contribute **[ADV]** their firewood can they build **[MC]** up a strong fire.

20. To attract **[INF]** good fortune, spend **[MC]** a new coin on an old friend, share **[MC]** an old pleasure with a new friend, and lift **[MC]** up the heart of a true friend by writing **[GER]** his name on the wings of a dragon.

Danish Proverbs

21. It is **[MC]** better to ask **[INF]** twice than to lose **[INF]** your way once.

22. He who builds **[REL]** according to every man's advice will have **[MC]** a crooked house.

23. Even a small star shines **[MC]** in the darkness.

24. A slip of the foot may soon be **[MC]** recovered, but that of the tongue perhaps never.

25. Kind words don't wear **[MC]** out the tongue.

26. Bad is **[MC]** never good until worse happens **[ADV]**.

27. Let **[MC]** deeds match **[INF]** words.

28. Speaking **[GER]** silence is **[MC]** better than senseless speech.

29. It is **[MC]** easy to sit **[INF]** at the helm in fine weather.

30. A good plan today is **[MC]** better than a perfect plan tomorrow.

German Proverbs

31. A good conscience is [MC] a soft pillow.

32. A single penny fairly got [PRT] is [MC] worth a thousand that are [REL] not.

33. All are [MC] not asleep who have [REL] their eyes shut.

34. Be [MC] silent, or say [MC] something better than silence.

35. Could everything be [ADV] done twice, everything would be [MC] done better.

36. If you would have [ADV] the lamp burn, you must pour [MC] oil into it.

37. Instead of complaining [PRT] that the rosebush is [NOM] full of thorns, be [MC] happy that the thorn bush has [NOM] roses.

38. It is [MC] better to turn [INF] back than go [INF] astray.

39. It is [MC] not till the cow has lost [ADV] her tail, that she discovers [NOM] its value.

40. Small undertakings give [MC] great comfort.

Hebrew Proverbs

41. Admission by the defendant is [MC] worth a hundred witnesses.

42. Do not confine [MC] your children to your own learning, for they were born [ADV] in another time.

43. Happy is [MC] the generation where the great listen [NOM] to the small, for it follows [MC] that in such a generation the small will listen [NOM] to the great.

44. Opinions founded [PRT] on prejudice are always sustained [MC] with the greatest violence.

45. Promise **[MC]** little and do **[MC]** much.

46. Rivalry of scholars advances **[MC]** wisdom.

47. The kind man feeds **[MC]** his cat before sitting **[GER]** down to dinner.

48. Whoever teaches **[NOM]** his son teaches **[MC]** not only his son but also his son's son, and so on to the end of generations.

49. Who seeks **[NOM]** more than he needs **[REL]** hinders **[MC]** himself from enjoying **[GER]** what he has **[NOM]**.

50. Slander slays **[MC]** three persons: the speaker, the spoken to, and the spoken of.

Irish Proverbs

51. Don't crow **[MC]** until you're **[ADV]** out of the woods.

52. Many an honest heart beats **[MC]** under a ragged coat.

53. The thing that is **[REL]** bought dear is often sold **[MC]** cheap.

54. Every dog is **[MC]** bold on its own doorstep.

55. Distant hills look **[MC]** green.

56. All happy endings are **[MC]** beginnings as well.

57. Praise **[MC]** the young and they will blossom **[MC]**.

58. A handful of skill is **[MC]** better than a bagful of gold.

59. Time is **[MC]** a great storyteller.

60. It takes **[MC]** time to build **[INF]** castles.

Japanese Proverbs

61. A single arrow is easily broken **[MC]**, but not ten in a bundle.

62. If you understand **[ADV]** everything, you must be **[MC]** misinformed.

63. Laughter cannot bring **[MC]** back what anger has driven **[NOM]** away.

64. One who smiles **[REL]** rather than rages **[REL]** is **[MC]** always the stronger.

65. We are **[MC]** no more than candles burning **[PRT]** in the wind.

66. When you're **[ADV]** thirsty, it's **[MC]** too late to think **[INF]** about digging **[GER]** a well.

67. The bamboo that bends **[REL]** is **[MC]** stronger than the oak that resists **[REL]**.

68. If money be **[ADV]** not thy servant, it will be **[MC]** thy master.

69. If you believe **[ADV]** everything you read **[REL]**, better not read **[MC]**.

70. If you want **[ADV]** a thing done well, do **[MC]** it yourself.

Mexican Proverbs

71. Conversation is **[MC]** food for the soul.

72. One must learn **[MC]** how to lose **[INF]** before learning **[GER]** how to play **[INF]**.

73. Tell **[MC]** me who your friends are **[NOM]** and I'll tell **[MC]** you who you are **[NOM]**.

74. It's **[MC]** not the fault of the mouse, but of the one who offers **[REL]** him the cheese.

75. In youth we learn **[MC]**, in old age we understand **[MC]**.

76. Money is **[MC]** a good servant, but an evil master.

77. Lions believe **[MC]** that everyone shares **[NOM]** their state of mind.

78. It is **[MC]** not enough to know **[INF]** how to ride **[INF]**; you must also know **[MC]** how to fall **[INF]**.

79. He who lives **[REL]** with hope dies **[MC]** happy.

80. When the river sounds **[ADV]**, it's **[MC]** because it carries **[ADV]** water.

Russian Proverbs

81. If you travel **[ADV]** more slowly, you will get **[MC]** farther.

82. A word is **[MC]** not a sparrow. If it flies **[ADV]** away, you won't catch **[MC]** it.

83. Not everything that glitters **[REL]** is **[MC]** gold.

84. Once you've committed **[ADV]** yourself to move **[INF]**, don't say **[MC]** you are **[NOM]** not up to it.

85. Any fish is **[MC]** good if it is **[ADV]** on the hook.

86. All's **[MC]** well that ends **[REL]** well.

87. One who sits **[REL]** between two chairs may easily fall **[MC]** down.

88. You will reap **[MC]** what you will sow **[NOM]**.

89. We do not care **[MC]** of what we have **[NOM]**, but we cry **[MC]** when it is **[ADV]** lost.

90. It is **[MC]** good to be **[INF]** visiting, but it is **[MC]** better at home.

Scottish Proverbs

91. A tale never loses [MC] in the telling.

92. Take care [MC] of your pennies and your dollars will take care [MC] of themselves.

93. They that dance [REL] must pay [MC] the fiddler.

94. They that will not be counseled [REL] cannot be helped [MC].

95. What may be [NOM] done at any time will be [MC] done at no time.

96. Willful waste makes [MC] woeful want.

97. They that sow [REL] the wind shall reap [MC] the whirlwind.

98. When the cup is [ADV] full, carry [MC] it even.

99. Confession is [MC] good for the soul.

100. Get [MC] bait while the tide is [ADV] out.

Exercise 10–2

For the following quotations, fill in the clause type, using the following codes:

MC = main clause   GER = gerundive clause

ADV = adverbial clause   INF = infinitive clause

NOM = nominal clause   PRT = participial clause

REL = relative clause

(*Sources:* Bachelder, 1965; Benardete, 1961; Burke, 1996; Charlton, 1994; Great Quotations, 1990; McLellan, 1996; Quotable Shakespeare, n.d.; Searls, 2009; Thankful Kids, 2009; *Who Said?*, 2003).

Set A

1. I took **[MC]** a speed-reading course and read **[MC]** *War and Peace* in 20 minutes. It's **[MC]** about Russia. (Woody Allen)

2. I was **[MC]** seldom able to see **[INF]** an opportunity until it had ceased **[ADV]** to be **[INF]** one. (Mark Twain)

3. I must say **[MC]** I find **[NOM]** television very educational. The minute somebody turns **[REL]** it on, I go **[MC]** to the library and read **[MC]** a good book. (Groucho Marx)

4. Extemporaneous speaking should be practiced **[MC]** and cultivated **[MC]**. It is **[MC]** the lawyer's avenue to the public. (Abraham Lincoln)

5. Books were **[MC]** my pass to personal freedom. I learned **[MC]** to read **[INF]** at age three, and I soon discovered **[MC]** there was **[NOM]** a whole world to conquer **[INF]** that went **[REL]** beyond our farm in Mississippi. (Oprah Winfrey)

6. Modern cynics and skeptics see **[MC]** no harm in paying **[GER]** those to whom they entrust **[REL]** the minds of their children a smaller wage than is **[NOM]** paid to those to whom they entrust **[REL]** the care of their plumbing. (John F. Kennedy)

7. It has been said **[MC]** of the world's history hitherto that might makes **[NOM]** right. It is **[MC]** for us and for our time to reverse **[INF]** the maxim and to say **[INF]** that right makes **[NOM]** might. (Abraham Lincoln)

8. Most of the luxuries, and many of the so-called comforts of life, are **[MC]** not only not indispensable, but positive hindrances to the elevation of mankind. With respect to luxuries and comforts, the wisest have ever lived **[MC]** a more simple and meager life than the poor. The ancient philosophers, Chinese, Hindoo, Persian, and Greek, were **[MC]** a class than which none has been **[REL]** poorer in outward riches, none so rich in inward. (Henry David Thoreau)

9. Upon the subject of education, not presuming to dictate **[INF]** any plan or system respecting **[PRT]** it, I can only say **[MC]** that I view **[NOM]** it as the most important subject which we as a people can be engaged **[REL]** in. That every man may receive **[NOM]** at least a moderate education, and thereby be **[INF]** enabled to read **[INF]** the histories of his own and other countries, by which he may duly appreciate **[ADV]** the value of our free institutions, appears **[MC]** to be **[INF]** an object of vital importance. (Abraham Lincoln)

10. I always wanted **[MC]** to be **[INF]** somebody, but I should have been **[MC]** more specific. (Lily Tomlin)

Set B

11. Once they notice **[ADV]** you, they never completely close **[MC]** the file. (Philip K. Dick)

12. I am **[NOM]** invisible, understand **[MC]**, simply because people refuse **[ADV]** to see **[INF]** me. (Ralph Ellison)

13. Freedom is **[MC]** indivisible. (Nelson Mandela)

14. But to live **[INF]** outside the law, you must be **[MC]** honest. (Bob Dylan)

15. It ain't **[MC]** over 'til it's **[ADV]** over. (Yogi Berra)

16. For the spectator even more than for the artist, art is **[MC]** a habit-forming drug. (Marcel Duchamp)

17. Though I am **[ADV]** in the depths of misery, there is **[MC]** still calmness, pure harmony, and music inside me. (Vincent van Gogh)

18. Never in the field of human conflict was **[MC]** so much owed **[PRT]** by so many to so few. (Winston Churchill)

19. Time spent **[PRT]** with a cat is **[MC]** never wasted. (Sydney Hauser)

20. Everybody talks **[MC]** about people, but nobody ever does **[MC]** anything about them. (Fran Lebowitz)

Set C

21. I want **[MC]** to bend **[INF]** this note, bend **[INF]** that note, sing **[INF]** this way, sing **[INF]** that way, and get **[INF]** all the feeling, eat **[INF]** all the good foods, and travel **[INF]** all over in one day, and you can't do **[MC]** it. (Billie Holiday)

22. Happy is **[MC]** the house that shelters **[REL]** a cat. (Sydney Hauser)

23. If I had **[ADV]** to sum **[INF]** up the totality of the Woodstock experience, I would say **[MC]** it was **[NOM]** the first attempt to land **[INF]** a man on the Earth. (Abbie Hoffman)

24. Never doubt **[MC]** that a small group of thoughtful, committed people can change **[NOM]** the world. (Margaret Mead)

25. Let **[MC]** them eat **[INF]** cake. (Marie-Antoinette)

26. To thine own self be **[MC]** true, and it must follow **[MC]**, as the night the day, thou canst not then be **[NOM]** false to any man. (William Shakespeare)

27. The future always looks **[MC]** good in the golden land, because no one remembers **[ADV]** the past. (Joan Didion)

28. In the attitude of silence, the soul finds **[MC]** the path in a clearer light, and what is **[NOM]** elusive and deceptive resolves **[MC]** itself into crystal clearness. (Mahatma Gandhi)

29. Half finished work generally proves **[MC]** to be **[INF]** labor lost. (Abraham Lincoln)

30. We have lived **[MC]** not in proportion to the number of years that we have spent **[REL]** on the earth, but in proportion as we have enjoyed **[ADV]**. (Henry David Thoreau)

Set D

31. Nothing so needs [MC] reforming as other people's habits. (Mark Twain)

32. Happiness lies [MC] in the joy of achievement and the thrill of creative effort. (Franklin D. Roosevelt)

33. Brevity is [MC] the soul of wit. (William Shakespeare)

34. Keep [MC] your face to the sunshine and you cannot see [MC] the shadow. (Helen Keller)

35. The time to repair [INF] the roof is [MC] when the sun is shining [ADV]. (John F. Kennedy)

36. The only way to get [INF] the best of an argument is [MC] to avoid [INF] it. (Dale Carnegie)

37. California is [MC] a Garden of Eden, a paradise to live [INF] in or see [INF]. (Woody Guthrie)

38. Fair is [MC] foul, and foul is [MC] fair. (William Shakespeare)

39. Be [MC] who you are [NOM] and say [MC] what you feel [NOM]. (Dr. Seuss)

40. All philosophers must soar [MC] with unwearied passion until they grasp [ADV] the true nature of things as they really are [ADV]. (Plato)

Set E

41. The young boy asked [MC], "Why should I become [NOM] a scholar when I can make [ADV] more money in the market place?" Plato replied [MC] that, "the pursuit of wisdom and truth is [NOM] essential to our integrity as human beings."

42. Moving **[GER]** the ship of state is **[MC]** a slow process. States are **[MC]** like big tankers. They're **[MC]** not like speedboats. (Barack Obama)

43. Good leadership requires **[MC]** you to surround **[INF]** yourself with people of diverse perspectives who can disagree **[REL]** with you without fear of retaliation. (Doris Kearns Goodwin)

44. Sometimes leadership is **[MC]** planting **[GER]** trees under whose shade you'll never sit **[REL]**. (Jennifer M. Granholm)

45. It takes **[MC]** 20 years to build **[INF]** a reputation and five minutes to ruin **[INF]** it. If you think **[ADV]** about that, you'll do **[MC]** things differently. (Warren Buffett)

46. How wonderful it is **[MC]** that nobody need **[NOM]** wait **[INF]** a single moment before starting **[GER]** to improve **[INF]** the world. (Anne Frank)

47. Unless someone like you cares **[ADV]** a whole lot, nothing is going **[MC]** to get **[INF]** better. It's **[MC]** not. (Dr. Seuss)

48. With every good deed, you are sowing **[MC]** a seed, though the harvest you may not see **[ADV]**. (Anonymous)

49. The more we study **[REL]** the more we discover **[MC]** our ignorance. (Percy Bysshe Shelley)

50. My teacher helps **[MC]** me out a lot and she is **[MC]** nice to me and she teaches **[MC]** me about stuff and when I first came **[ADV]** to her classroom, I was **[MC]** afraid of bugs but now I'm **[MC]** not. (Krysten, age 8)

Set F

51. Education is **[MC]** what survives **[NOM]** when what has been learned **[NOM]** has been forgotten **[ADV]**. (B. F. Skinner)

52. My karate teacher can break **[MC]** 12 bats over his head and 10 bricks with his bare hands. (Billy, age 7)

53. My teacher is **[MC]** fun and hard-working and never forgets **[MC]** to take **[INF]** time to talk **[INF]** to her students, unlike some teachers who only teach **[REL]** and never talk **[REL]**. (Sarah, age 11)

54. The mystic chords of memory, stretching **[PRT]** from every battlefield, and patriot grave, to every living heart and hearthstone, all over this broad land, will yet swell **[MC]** the chorus of the Union, when again touched **[PRT]**, as surely they will be **[ADV]**, by the better angels of our nature. (Abraham Lincoln; Wilson, 2006, p. 67)

55. I remember **[MC]** when my second-grade teacher pushed **[NOM]** me and pushed me **[NOM]** to read **[INF]** and when I finally started **[ADV]** to read **[INF]**, I liked **[MC]** it so much I couldn't stop **[NOM]**! (Chris, age 8)

56. The art of teaching **[GER]** is **[MC]** the art of assisting **[GER]** discovery. (Mark Van Doren)

57. Human history becomes **[MC]** more and more a race between education and catastrophe. (H. G. Wells)

58. Leave **[MC]** it longer on top, so I can have **[ADV]** spikes. My mom wrote **[MC]** on the form, "no Mohawk," so I can't have **[MC]** that. (David, age 13)

59. I am **[MC]** thankful for my dad because he never yells **[ADV]** at me. (Victor, 2nd grade).

60. I'm **[MC]** thankful that the Ducks are going **[NOM]** to beat **[INF]** the Beavers. I'm **[MC]** thankful that I have **[NOM]** clothes to wear **[INF]** and parents who care **[REL]** about me. (Frankie, 7th grade)

Exercise 10–3

For the following fable, fill in the clause type, using the codes below:

MC = main clause

ADV = adverbial clause

NOM = nominal clause

REL = relative clause

GER = gerundive clause

INF = infinitive clause

PRT = participial clause

The Lion and the Mouse (Grosset & Dunlap, 1947, pp. 137–138)

A lion was **[MC]** asleep in his den one day, when a mischievous mouse for no reason at all ran **[ADV]** across the outstretched paw and up the royal nose of the king of beasts, awakening **[PRT]** him from his nap. The mighty beast clapped **[MC]** his paw upon the now thoroughly frightened little creature and would have made **[MC]** an end of him.

"Please," squealed **[MC]** the mouse, "don't kill **[NOM]** me. Forgive **[MC]** me this time, O King, and I shall never forget **[MC]** it. A day may come **[MC]**, who knows, when I may do **[NOM]** you a good turn to repay **[INF]** your kindness." The lion, smiling **[PRT]** at his little prisoner's fright and amused **[PRT]** by the thought that so small a creature ever could be **[REL]** of assistance to the king of beasts, let **[MC]** him go **[INF]**.

Not long afterward the lion, while ranging **[PRT]** the forest for his prey, was caught **[MC]** in the net which the hunters had set **[REL]** to catch **[INF]** him. He let **[MC]** out a roar that echoed **[REL]** through the forest. Even the mouse heard **[MC]** it, and recognizing **[PRT]** the voice of his former preserver and friend, ran **[MC]** to the spot where he lay **[REL]** tangled **[PRT]** in the net of ropes.

"Well, your majesty," said **[MC]** the mouse, "I know **[NOM]** you did not believe **[NOM]** me once when I said **[ADV]** I would return **[NOM]** a kindness, but here is **[NOM]** my chance." And without further ado he set **[MC]** to work **[INF]** to nibble **[INF]** with his sharp little teeth at the ropes that bound **[REL]** the lion. Soon the lion was **[MC]** able to crawl **[INF]** out of the hunter's snare and be **[INF]** free.

Application: No act of kindness, no matter how small, is **[MC]** ever wasted.

Proverb: One good turn deserves **[MC]** another.

Exercise 10–4. Coding Child and Adolescent Language Samples

The following exercises provide additional practice coding clauses in spoken or written language samples (or excerpts of samples) that were produced by children and adolescents. For each exercise, fill in the blanks using the following codes:

MC = main clause   GER = gerundive clause

ADV = adverbial clause   INF = infinitive clause

NOM = nominal clause   PRT = participial clause

REL = relative clause

#1: *Judy, 11th Grade (TLD)* (from the Author's Files)

General Conversation Task:

1. I'm **[MC]** a junior.

2. I think **[MC]** I want **[NOM]** to go **[INF]** into the elementary educational field.

3. I like **[MC]** little kids.

4. I'm taking **[MC]** keyboarding, ITT which is **[REL]** international trade and tourism, and a cooking class called **[PRT]** world cooking.

5. And then I'm taking **[MC]** English.

6. And I have **[MC]** a worker's experience period where I go **[REL]** and work **[REL]** at my job (so).

7. I work **[MC]** for an insurance company right now.

8. So I work **[MC]** there doing **[PRT]** the filing.

9. It makes **[MC]** the car payment.

10. (So we get) So we already have **[MC]** college credit.

Favorite Game or Sport Task:

1. And there's **[MC]** foul balls, which means **[REL]** there's **[NOM]** lines drawn **[PRT]** from the home plate through the first base out to the field like to the fence like 180 feet.

2. And then there's **[MC]** a line drawn **[PRT]** from the third base line that goes **[REL]** out.

3. And if the ball goes **[ADV]** past the line to the left in the line not in the playing field, it's **[MC]** a foul ball.

4. And that's **[MC]** just a ball.

5. So (it) your count is **[MC]** still there.

6. And you have **[MC]** a count when you're **[ADV]** at bat.

7. And then (four balls or yeah) four balls means **[MC]** you walk **[NOM]**.

8. And so when you get **[ADV]** the base automatically, you can't make **[MC]** an out with that.

9. And then (the base runners) like if you're **[ADV]** on base, you can advance **[MC]** as soon as the ball leaves **[ADV]** the pitcher's hand.

10. And you can run **[MC]** the bases until you get **[ADV]** out or until your coach tells **[ADV]** you to stop **[INF]**.

Peer Conflict Resolution Task:

Examiner: What is a good way for Debbie to deal with Melanie?

1. Maybe if there's **[ADV]** a writing part, she can do **[MC]** the writing part and at least be **[MC]** there and help **[MC]** them and try **[MC]** to say **[INF]** what she feels **[NOM]** about the whole thing and see **[MC]** if she has **[NOM]** any advice of what they should do **[NOM]** better.

2. Or (like if just) basically have **[MC]** a session where they can just talk **[REL]** and (see what) split **[REL]** it up into teamwork, working wise.

Examiner: Why is that a good way for Debbie to deal with Melanie?

3. So she doesn't judge **[MC]** her.

4. Say **[MC]** she doesn't do **[NOM]** what she's supposed **[NOM]** to do **[INF]**.

5. But if she talks **[ADV]** to her and sees **[ADV]**, then maybe they can change **[MC]** some things.

6. So that will help **[MC]**.

Examiner: What do you think will happen if Debbie does that?

7. Well, she could either say **[MC]** "no" and ignore **[MC]** her.

8. Or she could say **[MC]** "yes."

9. And they could work **[MC]** the problem out.

10. But if she says **[ADV]** "no," then I guess **[MC]** she could go **[NOM]** to the teacher and see **[NOM]** what they could do **[NOM]** about it, see **[NOM]** if maybe she could get **[NOM]** another student to help **[INF]** them or have **[NOM]** more time so the two can just work **[ADV]** on it, Debbie and the other girl.

#2: *Saeda, 2nd Grade* (Thankful Kids, 2009)

Expository Essay

I am **[MC]** thankful for trees because they make **[ADV]** oxygen for me, water because it will make **[ADV]** me not dehydrated, and books because when I read **[ADV]**, I can learn **[ADV]** and I love **[ADV]** to read.

#3: Alex, 3rd Grade (Thankful Kids, 2009)

Expository Essay

These are **[MC]** some things I am **[REL]** thankful for. I'm **[MC]** thankful for my food, my lunch, and everything that is **[REL]** in it. I'm **[MC]** glad that it is **[NOM]** a good fruit. I'm **[MC]** thankful for all the water and milk that we have **[REL]**. I'm **[MC]** thankful for my house. My house is **[MC]** warm and cozy. I love **[MC]** my house so much. My house is **[MC]** special. I am **[MC]** thankful for my school. I'm **[MC]** so thankful for my teacher. I'm **[MC]** thankful for all the recess we get **[REL]**. I'm **[MC]** thankful for my special book. I'm **[MC]** so lucky for all these things.

#4: Kyra, 5th Grade (Thankful Kids, 2009)

Expository Essay

I'm **[MC]** so thankful for my pets to be **[INF]** a part of my family. Every single day, I wake up **[MC]** with warmth on my legs from my dog Toby sleeping **[PRT]** on my legs. When Toby hears **[ADV]** my bus, he will wait **[MC]** at the door until I come **[ADV]** home. Right when Toby sees **[ADV]** me, he will lick **[MC]** me until I can't feel **[ADV]** my face and all I can taste **[REL]** is **[ADV]** slobber. I am **[MC]** so happy and thankful to have **[INF]** a dog like Toby.

#5: Paris, 7th Grade (Thankful Kids, 2009)

Expository Essay

I am **[MC]** very thankful to have **[INF]** a mom that can be **[REL]** around me, even if I don't always want **[ADV]** her around. She comforts **[MC]** me when I'm **[ADV]** sad or sick. She helps **[MC]** me through the bad times. She cooks **[MC]** and provides **[MC]** for me even if there's **[ADV]** barely anything in the bank. She is **[MC]** my mother. And her name is **[MC]** Pam. But don't you wear **[MC]** it out. That's **[MC]** my job. I'm **[MC]** very thankful for a mother that cares **[REL]**.

#6: *Roberto, 8th Grade* (Thankful Kids, 2009)

Letter to a Former Teacher

There are **[MC]** many people in my life for whom I'm **[REL]** thankful for. But you are **[MC]** the only person that comes **[REL]** to mind when I think **[ADV]** of it. Through help and guidance, you are **[MC]** the one who helped **[REL]** me through sixth grade. I remember **[MC]** when you gave **[NOM]** me the Honor Society application sheet. You told **[MC]** me to get **[INF]** every teacher to sign **[INF]** my recommendation sheets and to write **[INF]** the essay to tell **[INF]** why I should be **[NOM]** in the Honor Society. You made **[MC]** sure that I got **[NOM]** my essay done and my recommendation sheets in. You made **[MC]** sure I was doing **[NOM]** it because you knew **[ADV]** that I would have **[NOM]** a chance to be **[INF]** in the Honor Society. I truly believe **[MC]** that without you, I would have never gotten **[NOM]** to where I am **[NOM]** today. I will never forget **[MC]** the things you did **[REL]** for me. And that's **[MC]** why I wanted **[NOM]** to say **[INF]**, "Thank you."

#7: *Emily, 3rd Grade (TLD)* (from the Author's Files)

Narrative Essay: "The Swan"

Once upon a time, there was **[MC]** a swan. She was going **[MC]** to have **[INF]** some babies. But she had never had **[MC]** babies before. She was **[MC]** nervous! So she asked **[MC]** the falcon for some advice. But *she* [the falcon] was asking **[MC]** that same question. So they went **[MC]** to look **[INF]** for someone to help **[INF]** them. So they asked **[MC]** the raven for her advice. She said **[MC]**, "Ask **[NOM]** the ostrich. She knows **[NOM]**." They went **[MC]** to the ostrich. She said **[MC]** she thought **[NOM]** and thought **[NOM]**. At last, she said **[MC]**, "Why don't you try **[NOM]** laying **[GER]** on the nest and wait **[NOM]** a while. And they will hatch **[MC]**. That's **[MC]** what I would do **[NOM]**." So they went **[MC]** to their nests and sat **[MC]** and sat **[MC]**. And then they said **[MC]**, "I feel **[NOM]** something wiggling." "It must be **[NOM]** the babies," said **[MC]** the swan and raven. And that was **[MC]** it. And of course they were **[MC]** very excited. The end.

#8: Ryan, 5th Grade (TLD) (from the Author's Files)

Expository Essay: The Nature of Friendship

Do you have **[MC]** a friend? I do **[MC]**. What do you think **[MC]** friendship means **[NOM]**? I think **[MC]** it means **[NOM]** someone you can trust **[REL]**, someone you can depend **[REL]** on, someone you have **[REL]** a lot in common with, and somebody who keeps **[REL]** secrets. Sometimes people feel **[MC]** lonely and have **[MC]** no one to talk **[INF]** to. That can lead **[MC]** to sadness. That is **[MC]** some reasons why friendship is **[NOM]** important. Sometimes friendship comforts **[MC]** you and makes **[MC]** you feel **[INF]** less alone. Me and my friends like **[MC]** to play **[INF]** lots and lots of video games together. Some advice for good friendship is **[MC]** to not annoy **[INF]** the person, be **[INF]** nice to the person. Do not tell **[MC]** secrets that they have told **[REL]** you.

#9: Mark, 8th Grade (TLD) (from the Author's Files)

Expository Essay: The Nature of Friendship

Friendship is **[MC]** basically an understanding between two people who share **[REL]** common interests or beliefs. Friendship is **[MC]** about being **[GER]** able to trust **[INF]** that person and being **[GER]** able to spend **[INF]** time with them. Friendship is **[MC]** important to people because it gives **[ADV]** them a chance to do **[INF]** things that they like **[REL]** with someone they enjoy **[REL]** spending **[GER]** time with. Having **[GER]** friends makes **[MC]** life more enjoyable because you have **[ADV]** someone you can talk **[REL]** to and that you like **[REL]** to do **[INF]** things with. Friends do **[MC]** all kinds of things together from going **[GER]** on hikes to going **[GER]** to the movies. Friends can talk **[MC]** to each other and go **[MC]** places together. People who generally become **[REL]** friends are **[MC]** those who have **[REL]** common interests.

If someone had [ADV] completely different opinions about what is [NOM] fun to do [INF] than someone else, then they probably won't become [MC] very good friends. The kinds of things that can harm [REL] a friendship are [MC] things like arguing [GER] and fighting [GER]. If you intentionally do [ADV] something that you know [REL] they won't like [NOM], it will damage [MC] a friendship. A way to maintain [INF] a friendship is [MC] to continually spend [INF] time with them. That way you can still talk [MC] to each other even if they live [ADV] a long ways away. That can help [MC] people remain [INF] friends. There are [MC] always ways to maintain [INF] friendships. Sometimes it is [MC] just hard to figure [INF] out how.

#10: Willow, 8th Grade ("Teachers Need to Be Healthy," 2009)

Letter to the Editor (Persuasive Essay)

We think [MC] that the ban of junk foods in schools should include [NOM] teachers. Sodas and other junk foods are [MC] just as unhealthy for teachers as they are [ADV] for students. The teachers need [MC] to set [INF] a good example for the students. If students see [ADV] that the ban on junk food includes [NOM] teachers as well as themselves, they might be [MC] more willing to go [INF] along with the ban. To have [INF] a mind and body that functions [REL] the best they can [REL], you need [MC] to eat [INF] the proper amount of nutrients. You do not get [MC] these nutrients from junk foods and soda. Because of this, you do not function [MC] as well as you could [ADV]. We think [MC] it is [NOM] important for teachers to have [INF] healthy bodies and minds, so that they will teach [ADV] the students better than otherwise. If teachers eat or drink [ADV] junk food or soda, they will not teach [MC] as well. If the teachers really cannot live [ADV] without the junk food, they can very easily just eat [MC] it at their homes. It should not be [MC] that hard for them to wait [INF] the seven or eight hours that their jobs take [REL] up to eat [INF] junk food if they need [ADV] it that badly. After all, students can [MC].

#11: Trevor, 5th Grade (TLD) (from the Author's Files)

Persuasive Essay: The Circus Controversy

I think **[MC]** it is **[NOM]** a bad idea to have **[INF]** animals in the circus because animals should be **[ADV]** free to do **[INF]** what they want **[NOM]**. They're **[MC]** stuck in small cages. So there is **[MC]** barely enough room to get **[INF]** their adequate exercise. People don't like **[MC]** to be **[INF]** imprisoned. So we should let **[MC]** them go **[INF]**. Then they won't be **[MC]** forced to do **[INF]** tricks. I think **[MC]** it is **[NOM]** cruel to train **[INF]** animals to do **[INF]** a trick because if they don't do **[ADV]** it right, the trainers will hit **[ADV]** them. These are **[MC]** the reasons why I think **[NOM]** circuses should not be **[NOM]** allowed. For the animals' sake.

#12: Carl, 11th Grade (TLD) (from the Author's Files)

Persuasive Essay: The Circus Controversy

A common controversy is **[MC]** often whether or not circuses are **[NOM]** good or bad for the community. I like **[MC]** the clowns because often times they are **[ADV]** also animal trainers. However, there is **[MC]** a downside to all these beneficial factors. Frequently, the animals are **[MC]** underfed and are kept **[MC]** in small cages. This alone infuriates **[MC]** animal enthusiasts everywhere. Circuses can be **[MC]** cruel to animals. Therefore, they should be closed **[MC]** down. If animals feel **[ADV]** threatened, they could be **[MC]** dangerous when they fight **[ADV]** back. What I believe **[NOM]** is **[MC]** that a circus could hire **[NOM]** more people and have them go **[INF]** to clown school. Everybody likes **[MC]** clowns, right? The hardest part of this would be **[MC]** training **[GER]** all those clowns. Still, with a little creativity and some ingenuity, I think **[MC]** a clown school could be **[NOM]** possible. Overall, I think **[MC]** animals should not be **[NOM]** in circuses.

APPENDIX C

Answer Key for
Chapter 11

SENTENCE TYPES

Exercise 11–1

For each quotation, indicate whether the sentence is:

    A. Simple   C. Compound

    B. Complex   D. Compound-complex

1. __B__ All philosophers must soar with unwearied passion until they grasp the true nature of things as they really are. (Plato)

2. __B__ Education is not filling a pail but the lighting of a fire. (William Butler Yeats)

3. __B__ If you bungle raising your children, I don't think whatever else you do well matters very much. (Jacqueline Kennedy Onassis)

4. __A__ A little learning is a dangerous thing. (Alexander Pope)

5. __C__ Never give up and never give in. (Hubert H. Humphrey)

6. __A__ Life is a festival only to the wise. (Ralph Waldo Emerson)

7. __B__ No one can make you feel inferior without your consent. (Eleanor Roosevelt)

8. __B__ To talk in public, to think in solitude, to read and to hear, to inquire and answer inquiries, is the business of the scholar. (Samuel Johnson)

9. __B__ My teacher is special because she never yells at me. (Rebecca, age 8)

10. __B__ There's something about taking a plow and breaking new ground. (Ken Kesey)

11. __B__ The more we study, the more we discover our ignorance. (Percy Bysshe Shelley)

12. __D__ My teacher helps me out a lot and she is nice to me and she teaches me about stuff and when I first came to her classroom, I was afraid of bugs but now I'm not. (Krysten, age 8)

13. __B__ Education is what survives when what has been learned has been forgotten. (B. F. Skinner)

14. __A__ My karate teacher can break 12 bats over his head and 10 bricks with his bare hands. (Billy, age 7)

15. __D__ My teacher is fun and hard-working and never forgets to take time to talk to her students, unlike some teachers who only teach and never talk. (Sarah, age 11)

16. __A__ Mix with your sage counsels some brief folly. (Cicero)

17. __D__ I remember when my second-grade teacher pushed me and pushed me to read and when I finally started to read, I liked it so much I couldn't stop! (Chris, age 8)

18. __B__ The art of teaching is the art of assisting discovery. (Mark Van Doren)

19. __B__ Leave it longer on top, so I can have spikes. (David, age 13)

20. __C__ My mom wrote on the form, "no Mohawk," so I can't get that. (David, age 13)

Exercise 11–2. Hierarchical Complexity

For each of the following sentences, indicate the number of levels of embedding it contains. Begin by coding each sentence for each type of clause it contains:

MC = main clause   GER = gerundive clause
ADV = adverbial clause   INF = infinitive clause
NOM = nominal clause   PRT = participial clause
REL = relative clause

1. Even if you're **[ADV]** on the right track, you'll get run **[MC]** over if you just sit **[ADV]** there.   Levels: 1

2. With every good deed, you are sowing **[MC]** a seed, though the harvest you may not see **[ADV]**.   Levels: 1

3. Use **[MC]** a small paintbrush and a paper cup with the smaller beetles because you can damage **[ADV]** them if you pick **[ADV]** them up in your hand.   Levels: 2

4. Jason's little sister Amanda has **[MC]** an ear infection for which her pediatrician prescribed **[REL]** a liquid antibiotic that must be kept **[REL]** refrigerated.   Levels: 2

5. Every miler knows **[MC]**, in the way a sailor knows **[REL]** the middle of the ocean, that it is **[NOM]** not the first lap but the third that is **[REL]** farthest from the finish line. (Parker, 2009, p. 246)   Levels: 2

6. As Jim and I went **[ADV]** over to see **[INF]** what was going **[NOM]** on, someone crawled **[MC]** out of the closet. (Boy, age 13)   Levels: 3

7. Before you take **[ADV]** a piece, like if there was **[ADV]** a rook right here, you kind of make **[MC]** sure because there is **[ADV]** a strategy that you can do **[REL]** to try **[INF]** to get **[INF]** a king in checkmate with two rooks. (Boy, age 11)   Levels: 4

8. I hated **[MC]** him on sight and sound and would be **[MC]** about to put **[INF]** my dog whistle to my lips and blow **[INF]** him off the face of Christmas when suddenly he, with a violet wink, put **[ADV]** *his* whistle to *his* lips and blew **[ADV]** so stridently, so high, so exquisitely loud, that gobbling faces, their cheeks bulged **[PRT]** with goose, would press **[NOM]** against their tinseled windows, the whole length of the white echoing street. (Thomas, 1954, p. 22)   Levels: 3

Exercise 11–3

Code the following sentences. Then rewrite each sentence in the active voice and code it again.

1. It was promised **[MC]** by Mozart that the duets would be completed **[NOM]** soon.

    Active: Mozart promised **[MC]** that he would complete **[NOM]** the duets soon.

2. The missing duets, which had been misplaced **[REL]** by Frederick, were presented **[MC]** by Mozart to his friend Joseph Haydn.

    Active: Mozart presented **[MC]** the missing duets, which Frederick had misplaced **[REL]**, to his friend Joseph Haydn.

3. It was known **[MC]** by all patrons that a symphony could be written **[NOM]** by Mozart in minutes.

    Active: All patrons knew **[MC]** that Mozart could write **[NOM]** a symphony in minutes.

4. An amazing tonal richness was achieved **[MC]** by the string quartet, which was led **[REL]** by a new cellist from Philadelphia.

    Active: The string quartet achieved **[MC]** an amazing tonal richness under the leadership of a new cellist from Philadelphia.
    OR: The new cellist from Philadelphia led **[MC]** the string quartet as it achieved **[ADV]** an amazing tonal richness.

5. The miniature trio for three strings was created **[MC]** by the new composer who was paid **[REL]** handsomely by the king's court.

    Active: The new composer created **[MC]** the miniature trio for three strings, and the king's court paid **[MC]** him/her handsomely.

    OR: The new composer, whom the king's court paid **[REL]** handsomely, created **[MC]** the miniature trio for three strings.

6. The young musician was supported **[MC]** by a generous scholarship funded **[PRT]** by a wealthy elderly patron, to attend **[INF]** the Juilliard School of Music.

    Active: A wealthy elderly patron funded **[MC]** a generous scholarship to support **[INF]** the young musician so that he/she could attend **[ADV]** the Juilliard School of Music.

7. The composer's status of nobility was implied **[MC]** by the "von" inserted **[PRT]** before his last name, which was preferred **[REL]** by some over the plainer "Ernst Dohnanyi."

    Active: The "von" that was inserted **[REL]** before his last name implied **[MC]** the composer's status of nobility, which some people preferred **[REL]** over the plainer "Ernst Dohnanyi."

8. The flute quartet was performed **[MC]** by four young musicians who had been hired **[REL]** by a royal family to educate **[INF]** its children in the finer things in life.

    Active: To educate **[INF]** its children in the finer things in life, the royal family hired **[MC]** four young musicians who played **[REL]** the flute quartet.

9. A dramatic conclusion to the Christmas play was anticipated **[MC]** by members of the audience, many of whom had been coerced **[REL]** into attending **[GER]** the performance.

    Active: Members of the audience anticipated **[MC]** a dramatic conclusion to the Christmas play because someone had coerced **[ADV]** many of them into attending **[GER]** the performance.

10. The rock concert, sold out **[PRT]** for months, had to be canceled **[MC]** by the vendor because the band's lead singer had been delayed **[ADV]** by inclement weather in Chicago.

Active: The vendor had to cancel **[MC]** the rock concert, which had been sold out **[REL]** for months, because inclement weather in Chicago delayed **[ADV]** the band's lead singer.

APPENDIX D

Answer Key for Chapter 12

UNITS OF MEASUREMENT

Exercise 12–1. Calculating MLU-m and MLU-w

The following is an excerpt from a play-based conversational language sample elicited from a 3-year-old boy, "Billy" (not his real name), adapted from Fletcher and Garman (1988). The child, C, and examiner, E, were playing with a doll house. For each utterance produced by the child, count the number of morphemes and words, and put the totals in the blank spaces. Then calculate MLU-m and MLU-w for the sample. Do not count morphemes or words for the examiner.*

	Morphemes	Words
C That doggie is woof/ing.	5	4
C He bite/3s you.	4	3
E Oh, he bit me!		
C That/'s a baby lady.	5	5

---

*Note that contracted words were separated by a slash and grammatical morphemes were marked using SALT conventions (/3s = third person singular verb; /z = possessive –s; /ing = present progressive marker; /s = plural). Also following SALT conventions, these words were counted as one morpheme, one word each: *doggie, trousers, milkman, children, mummy, oh, gotta, football.*

		Morphemes	Words
C	Look, this got/3s trousers.	5	4
C	He/'s got a milkman.	5	5
E	Show me another one.		
C	Let me see.	3	3
C	I want that black one.	5	5
E	What's that thing?		
C	A tie.	2	2
C	All the children/z.	4	3
E	What's she doing?		
C	She runn/ing.	3	2
C	There she mummy.	3	3
E	What next?		
C	The mummy/z pram.	4	3
C	A blue pram.	3	3
E	What's in the pram?		
C	A baby.	2	2
E	And there's another little girl.		
C	That/'s blue.	3	3
C	That/'s gotta go in the middle.	7	7
C	Oh, whose is that football for?	6	6
C	Think (he's) him/z.	3	2
C	What/'s that girl do/ing?	6	5
C	I want a green one.	5	5
	Total:	83	75

Total C utterances: 20

MLU-m: 4.15

MLU-w: 3.75

Exercise 12–2. Calculating the FVMC

Tommy, age 4;6, has specific language impairment. Use the data obtained from a play-based conversational language sample to calculate his FVMC.

	Accurate Productions	Obligatory Contexts
3rd person singular -s	2	8
Past tense -ed	2	6
Copula be	3	10
Auxiliary be	3	7
Total:	10	31

(Accurate productions/obligatory contexts) × 100 = FVMC: <u>32.25</u>

Exercise 12–3. Calculating PGU

Each child below has specific language impairment. The clinician used a set of 15 pictures to prompt each child to talk about the pictures to elicit a language sample. For each child, use the following results to calculate the PGU.

(Grammatically correct utterances/total utterances) × 100 = PGU

	Grammatically Correct Utterances	Total Utterances	PGU
1. Jason, age 3;8	14	30	<u>47%</u>
2. Tyler, age 4;2	16	28	<u>57%</u>
3. Jenna, age 5;0	12	27	<u>44%</u>
4. Amy, age 3.6	10	25	<u>40%</u>
5. Lucas, age 4;7	18	32	<u>56%</u>

Exercise 12–4. Identifying C-units and T-units

For passages 1 through 5, indicate with a slash (/) the end of each *C-unit*. Then write the total number of C-units in the blank space.

1. Upon the subject of education, not presuming to dictate any plan or system respecting it, I can only say that I view it as the most important subject which we as a people can be engaged in / that every man may receive at least a moderate education, and thereby be enabled to read the histories of his own and other countries, by which he may duly appreciate the value of our free institutions, appears to be an object of vital importance / (Abraham Lincoln, cited by Bachelder, 1965, p. 7)

   How many C-units are contained in this passage? __2__

2. I have been the whole day without eating and the whole night without sleeping, occupied with thinking / it was no use / the better plan is to learn / learning without thought is labor lost / and thought without learning is perilous / (Confucius, 6th century BC, Peter Pauper Press, 1963, p. 42)

   How many C-units are contained in this passage? __5__

3. The critical habit of thought, if usual in a society, will pervade all its mores, because it is a way of taking up the problems of life / men educated in it cannot be stampeded by stump orators and are never deceived by dithyrambic oratory / they are slow to believe / they can hold things as possible or probable in all degrees, without certainty and without pain / they can wait for evidence and weigh evidence, uninfluenced by the emphasis or confidence with which assertions are made on one side or the other / they can resist appeals to their dearest prejudices and all kinds of cajolery / education in the critical faculty is the only education of which it can be truly said that it makes good citizens / (William Graham Sumner, 1906, p. 633)

   How many C-units are contained in this passage? __7__

4. Inside England, as we have seen, one form of the language, basically
    an East_Midland dialect, became accepted as a literary standard
    in the late Middle_Ages / and with this went a prestige accent
    based on that of the court in Westminster / this does not mean
    that dialect differences disappeared in England / Standard_English
    was the language of a small minority / most speakers used a
    nonstandard form of the language / and in each area there was a
    speech hierarchy corresponding to the class hierarchy, differing
    from Standard_English not only in accent but also in grammar and
    vocabulary / the higher the socioeconomic level of the speakers, the
    nearer their speech was likely to be to Standard_English, though
    the degree of formality of the situation also influenced the level of
    speech used / (Barber, 1993, p. 232)

    How many C-units are contained in this passage? __7__

5. We are a nation of Christians and Muslims, Jews, and Hindus, and
    nonbelievers / we are shaped by every language and culture, drawn
    from every end of this Earth / and because we have tasted the bitter
    swill of civil war and segregation, and emerged from that dark
    chapter stronger and more united, we cannot help but believe that
    the old hatreds shall someday pass, that the lines of tribe shall soon
    dissolve, that as the world grows smaller, our common humanity
    shall reveal itself, and that America must play its role in ushering in a
    new era of peace / (Barack Obama, 2009)

    How many C-units are contained in this paragraph? __3__

For passages 6 through 10, indicate with a slash (/) the end of each *T-unit*.
Then write the total number of T-units in the blank space.

6. Once Oregon was thought to be immune to earthquakes / today
    we know that we have them in three different flavors—devastating
    subduction earthquakes like the 1700 catastrophe, deep intraplate
    earthquakes like the Puget_Sound temblors of 1949 and 2001, and

sharp local jolts like the Spring_Break_Quake of 1993 / (Sullivan, 2008, p. 67)

How many T-units are contained in this passage? __2__

7. Beatrix_Potter was a Londoner, born there in 1866 / but her family had connections with Lancashire cotton / and she spent her holidays from the age of 16 in the Lake_District, in rented, but rather grand houses, round Windermere and Derwentwater / her parents were genteel, upper middle class Edwardians / and she was educated at home and expected to devote her life to her parents or get married / she found an outlet for artistic talents in drawing and painting "little books for children" / and encouraged by the family's Lakeland friend, Canon_Rawnsley, her first book, *Peter_Rabbit*, was published in 1901 / (Davies, 1989, p. 179)

How many T-units are contained in this passage? __7__

8. I have become a little more skillful in guessing right explanations and in devising experimental tests / but this may probably be the result of mere practice, and of a larger store of knowledge / I have as much difficulty as ever in expressing myself clearly and concisely / and this difficulty has caused me a very great loss of time / but it has had the compensating advantage of forcing me to think long and intently about every sentence / and thus I have been often led to see errors in reasoning and in my own observations or those of others / (Charles Darwin, 1958, pp. 136–137)

How many T-units are contained in this passage? __6__

9. Some birds, such as most eagles, hawks, ospreys, falcons, and vultures, migrate during the day / larger birds can hold more body fat, go longer without eating, and take longer to migrate / these birds glide along on rising columns of warm air, called thermals, which hold them aloft while they slowly make their way north or south / they generally rest at night and hunt early in the morning before the sun has a chance to warm up the land and create

good soaring conditions / birds migrating during the day use a combination of landforms, rivers, and the rising and setting sun to guide them in the right direction / (Tekiela, 2001, p. xv)

How many T-units are contained in this passage? __5__

10. In the morning I watched the geese from the door through the mist, sailing in the middle of the pond, fifty rods off, so large and tumultuous that Walden appeared like an artificial pond for their amusement / but when I stood on the shore they at once rose up with a great flapping of wings at the signal of their commander, and when they had got into rank circled about over my head, twenty_nine of them, and then steered straight to Canada, with a regular *honk* from the leader at intervals, trusting to break their fast in muddier pools / a "plump" of ducks rose at the same time and took the route to the north in the wake of their noisier cousins / (Thoreau, 2004, pp. 301–302)

How many T-units are contained in this passage? __3__

Exercise 12–5. Counting Words and Calculating MLCU and MLTU

For each of the following language samples, calculate MLCU (spoken language) or MLTU (written language). First determine the number of words in each C-unit or T-unit for the child C, not the examiner E. Then, add up the total number of words produced by the child and divide by the total number of C-units/T-units produced. Write the result in the blank space.

#1: Play-Based Conversational Sample from a 5-Year-Old Boy, Playing with a Doll House and Furniture (Fletcher & Garman, 1988)

Words

__5__   1. C That's a big one. E The table you mean?

__5__   2. C Where does that go anyway? E Where do you think is the kitchen in that house?

__3__   3. C Must be there. E So where shall we put the pot?

__5__   4. C Take that little boy there.

___4___   5. C And put that one. E OK, I take that out.

___4___   6. C Bike for the baby. E Have you got a bike at home?

___4___   7. C Uhhuh, a big one. E Uhhuh, you've got a big one.

___6___   8. C My brother's got a motorbike. E Is he older than you?

___1___   9. C Uhhuh.

___5___   10. C That might (be) go in there. E Uhhuh, it could probably go in there.

___5___   11. C This is a long one. E it's a long one indeed.

___3___   12. C Goes up there.

___4___   13. C Must be in there. E Where's your sofa at home?

___4___   14. C It's in mum's.

___5___   15. C So I move it upstairs. E Look, there's nothing in that room so far.

___5___   16. C I put it there then.

___12___   17. C That needs to be up there so that somebody can walk past.

Total child C-units: ___17___

Total child words: ___80___

Child's MLCU: ___4.71___

#2: *Narrative Essay, Boy, Age 11* (from the Author's Files)

Words

___13___   1. One day at the mall, me and my friend went to the Home_Town_Buffet.

___14___   2. I towered three to four plates of food, one dessert plate, and two sundaes.

___9___   3. On the other hand, my friend had very little.

___13___   4. Little did I know that we had to walk all over the mall.

___17___   5. So every time I saw a bench, I would lay down for as long as I could.

___14___   6. Then we went to Harry_Richie's, Game_Crazy, Radio_Shack, Target, and to another video game store.

___7___   7. My stomach was aching the whole time.

___11___   8. Me and my friend both agreed I ate way too much.

___17___   9. Then we had to walk way down and around the whole outside of the whole huge mall.

___10___   10. Then we went to the other mall and walked around.

___8___   11. I learned never to eat that much again.

Total child T-units: ___11___

Total child words: ___133___

Child's MLTU: ___12.09___

Exercise 12–6. Counting Words

For each of the following sentences, indicate the number of words it contains. Be sure to follow conventions for counting proper names, compound and hyphenated words, contractions, catenatives, interjections, fillers, etc. as described in this chapter.

___8___   1. Miss Jane Hudson was the principal of the school, Foxwood Glen.

___9___   2. The school's special cat and mascot was named Terry the Tiger.

___9___   3. Let's have Aunt Bessy's cherry cobbler for dessert tonight.

___11___   4. I'm gonna get me a giant box of Cracker Jack.

___8___   5. Lemme have a taste of your chicken a la king.

___14___   6. When we go to New York, let's go to the top of the Empire State Building.

___11___   7. After that, we'll go visit the Statue of Liberty and take photos.

___9___   8. Remember when we went to Disneyland and rode Dumbo the Flying Elephant?

___12___   9. We planned to take the steps to the top of the Eiffel Tower.

___12___ 10. The Great Wall of China, one of the seven wonders of the world, is amazing!

___11___ 11. We went downstairs for lunch in the new cafeteria with Mary Cohen-Smith.

___12___ 12. The oatmeal at breakfast was flavored with maple syrup, vanilla, and dates.

Exercise 12–7. Identifying Mazes

The following utterances were produced by adolescents who were talking about sports and conflicts. For each utterance, use parentheses to enclose the maze behavior. What is left should be a clean, coherent utterance, presumably the speaker's final formulation. Be sure to parenthesize the verbalizations (mazes) that come *before* the final version.

Speaker #1:

1. and (um you need to serve) when you serve, you need to serve behind the line, not over it.

2. (and then um in order to um in order to score over there you in or ok) when you serve and it goes over the net, and if the other players do not hit it or if they can't get it and it's (in the) in the lines, then it's a point.

Speaker #2:

1. but usually the stadiums cost (maybe thirty or a lot of dollars a lot of) millions of dollars to put into it.

2. and they can play in any kind of weather (even) except for snow because they don't play in the snow.

3. and (a baseball game should last) a major league baseball game should last three hours.

Speaker #3:

1. (and and then there's) I don't know how many people play in pro.

2. but (I) we usually play five on five (like at school) like in sports for school.

3. and (um) that's about it.

Speaker #4:

1. and he asks (Peter if he would if) Mike to switch jobs with him because his (sh uh) shoulder was sore.

2. and he was like, "No, I don't wanna (lose) take a chance on losing my turn on the grill."

Speaker #5:

1. he could say, "Bob (um you know) you were supposed to help us with this project and when you don't participate in the group, it frustrates me because it makes our group look bad and I'd appreciate it if you'd participate in the group."

2. (um he) unless Bob's an absolutely nasty person, he should get some kind of good results because he was pretty polite about it (and yeah).

Exercise 12–8. Calculating CD

Solve the following problems using the information that is provided.

1. 45 main clauses; 24 subordinate clauses; 45 C-units. CD = _1.53_

2. 82 main clauses; 68 subordinate clauses; 82 C-units. CD = _1.83_

3. 47 main clauses; 43 subordinate clauses; 42 C-units. CD = _2.14_

4. 35 main clauses; 31 subordinate clauses; 25 C-units. CD = <u>2.64</u>

5. 60 main clauses; 56 subordinate clauses; 60 C-units. CD = <u>1.93</u>

6. 24 main clauses; 10 adverbial clauses; 6 relative clauses; 9 nominal clauses; 4 infinitive clauses; 5 gerundive clauses; 5 participial clauses; 24 C-units. CD = <u>2.63</u>

7. 16 main clauses; 9 adverbial clauses; 0 relative clauses; 4 nominal clauses; 2 infinitive clauses; 0 gerundive clauses; 0 participial clauses; 16 C-units. CD = <u>1.94</u>

8. 12 main clauses; 4 adverbial clauses; 2 relative clauses; 2 nominal clauses; 4 infinitive clauses; 0 gerundive clauses; 0 participial clauses; 12 C-units. CD = <u>2.0</u>

9. 68 main clauses; 16 adverbial clauses; 12 relative clauses; 8 nominal clauses; 9 infinitive clauses; 4 gerundive clauses; 5 participial clauses; 70 C-units. CD = <u>1.74</u>

10. 45 main clauses; 24 adverbial clauses; 12 relative clauses; 14 nominal clauses; 7 infinitive clauses; 2 gerundive clauses; 3 participial clauses; 45 C-units. CD = <u>2.38</u>

APPENDIX E

Answer Key for Chapter 13

ANALYZING CONVERSATIONAL LANGUAGE SAMPLES

The following are language samples that were elicited from children and adolescents with typical language development. They include both play-based and interview-based conversational language samples. Each sample was entered into the Systematic Analysis of Language Transcripts (SALT) software program and broken into C-units by the author. All mazes were placed within parentheses, allowing the final reformulation to stand. To allow SALT to count the number of words accurately, all contractions were separated by one space.

For each sample, fill in the clause type, using the codes shown here.

MC = main clause   GER = gerundive clause

ADV = adverbial clause   INF = infinitive clause

NOM = nominal clause   PRT = participial clause

REL = relative clause

E = examiner; C = child or adolescent

CONVERSATIONAL LANGUAGE SAMPLES

Play-Based Conversational Samples

Sample #1: Boy, Age 3 Years (Fletcher & Garman, 1988)

MLCU = 3.58   CD = 0.68

E This lady's sweeping the floor.

E This lady's holding a baby.

E This is the lady with the green coat on.

E Which one do you want first?

C Green one.

E Put her on.

C On like that.

E Who next?

C A blue one.

E Good.

C That 's [**MC**] a baby lady.

E What's that one?

C Green lady.

E Who shall we have first?

C A green one.

E There isn't a green one.

C Let [**MC**] me see [**INF**].

C There.

C There 's [**MC**] a green one.

C Look, this gots [**MC**] trousers.

E What's he holding?

C Do n't know [**MC**].

E Yes you do.

C He 's got [**MC**] a milkman.

E Tell me another one.

C Let [**MC**] me see [**INF**].

C I want [**MC**] that black one.

E What's that thing?

C A tie.

C All the childrens.

E What's she doing?

C Do n't know [**MC**].

C She running [**MC**].

C There she mummy.

E Who next?

C A pram.

C A blue pram.

E What's in the pram?

C A baby.

E And there's another little girl.

C That 's [**MC**] blue.

C That 's got [**MC**] ta go [**INF**] in the middle.

E Which one first?

C The ball.

E The ball.

C The red one.

C Oh, whose is [**MC**] that football for?

C Think [**MC**] (he's) him's.

E And there's one more.

C A girl.

E What's she doing?

C What 's that girl doing [**MC**]?

E What's she holding?

C Balls.

C Move [**MC**] this over here.

C She 's sleeping [**MC**].

E Who?

C That 's [**MC**] a big pussy cat.

E I like pussy cats.

C Oh, there 's [**MC**] lots of people.

E This is the dog that's jumping up.

E This dog is lying down.

C I want [**MC**] the black one.

C Where 's it go [**MC**]?

E And there's another one.

C There some more.

E Which dog is it?

C Do n't know [**MC**].

E What's she doing?

C She eating [**MC**] her dinner.

E Yeah.

C No, she trying [**MC**] to make [**INF**] it.

E What's happening there?

C He 's got [**MC**] a television.

E What's that?

C A television.

C Oh no, it 's [**MC**] a bus driver.

E It is.

C Oh, he's might cross [**MC**] over a car.

E What's inside that bus?

C I don't know [**MC**].

C What 's [**MC**] in there?

E People.

E What's happening in that picture?

C Some boys.

E Have you got any brothers and sisters?

C No.

C That boy xxx.

E We've had that one.

C This is [**MC**] for the radio.

Sample #2: Girl, Age 5 Years (Fletcher & Garman, 1988)

MLCU = 5.35   CD = 1.00

E Have you seen this before?

C No, have n't seen [**MC**] the game.

E I think it's a farm.

C Yes, I think [**MC**] it 's [**NOM**] a farm.

E Do you?

C I seen [**MC**] farms on television.

C So I have n't been [**MC**] to a farm.

E What did you get for Christmas?

E Did you get any games?

C Well, (I) I love [**MC**] this very big one.

C (I love) I love [**MC**] that Sindy house.

C I had [**MC**] a Sindy house.

E Did you?

C Yeah, always wanted [**MC**] one of them.

E For Christmas?

C And I got [**MC**] (um) for my birthday.

E When was your birthday?

C (Um) my (birthday) birthday was [**MC**] before Christmas.

C And do you know [**MC**] what happened [**NOM**]?

E No.

C I have [**MC**] this lovely, lovely (um) yacking dog.

C And I loved [**MC**] it.

E What's that?

C A yacking dog.

C You know [**MC**], one of them (um) little doggies.

C And when you switch [**ADV**] it on, (it goes), you got [**MC**] to say [**INF**] go [**NOM**].

C And it goes [**MC**] yak_yak_yak.

E How do you stop it then?

C You (go go) clap [**MC**] your hands like that.

E How big is it?

C Well, about that {shows in inches}.

C Now I think [**MC**] (tho) these sacks, they 're [**NOM**] very tired.

C (so I think he's um) I think [**MC**] he left [**NOM**] them there.

C (that's) That 's [**MC**] the back door where they come [**REL**].

E Think that's a little hut, isn't it?

C Yeah, I think [**MC**] it 's [**NOM**] a little hut.

E What do you think they keep in there?

C I do n't know [**MC**].

C Horsie.

E Can't get a horsie in there.

E Too little.

C What could we have [**MC**]?

E Maybe that's where the chickens sleep.

C Oh yeah.

C That 's [**MC**] a good idea.

C And they fly [**MC**] out there.

E Yeah.

C Uhhuh, think [**MC**] it may be [**NOM**] that.

C (got) Need [**MC**] another pig.

C The mummy pig.

E How do you know it's a mummy pig?

C Because that 's [**ADV**] dad.

C And that 's [**ADV**] mummy.

E Oh, I see.

C Might be [**MC**] a little baby.

E There isn't one though.

C That little baby could be [**MC**] in that truck.

C He jumped [**MC**] into that truck.

E Okay.

C Like that.

E Okay.

C In the truck.

E There's no one driving that tractor.

C Oh yeah.

C We must put [**MC**] a man on it, must we [**MC**]?

C He 's driving [**MC**] the tractor.

E That's a good idea.

C What?

E To put him underneath like that.

E So it looks like he's inside.

C Uhhuh.

E Where's he going in that tractor do you think?

C I do n't know [**MC**].

E What do you think this could be?

C I think it 's [**MC**] a gate.

E How can it be a gate?

E Show me how.

C But I think [**MC**] it 's [**NOM**] a log.

C A log.

C (xxx) a log this way.

C That way.

E I've got a cold.

C I 've got [**MC**] a little bit of a cold.

C I have n't got [**MC**] any colds.

C I have [**MC**] n't.

C My cold 's [**MC**] gone away.

E Have you had a cold already?

C Yeah.

C (I had it when it was) I had [**MC**] it when it was [**ADV**] in the middle of winter.

E Still quite cold outside though.

C Yeah.

C What do you think [**MC**] that could be [**NOM**]?

E I think that's where the farmer keeps his tools and things.

C I know [**MC**] jolly well (xxx).

E What?

C Jolly well could be [**MC**].

C Well, you know [**MC**] this little bit of hay.

E It's to keep it dry.

C Expect it is [**MC**].

E What do you think will happen if the hay gets wet?

C The horses wo n't eat [**MC**] it.

E Yeah.

E What else can we put on?

C Think [**MC**] we can put [**NOM**] on.

C Oh yes, we must have [**MC**] a seat.

C That for the farmer.

E What is it?

C A seat, I think [**MC**].

C Look [**MC**].

E It's difficult to see what it is.

C Yeah.

E Yeah.

C I think [**MC**] it 's [**NOM**] a seat.

C There 's [**MC**] a little seat for the farmer.

E But he's in the tractor now so he can't sit in it.

C Yeah, I know [**MC**].

E There's another man on there as well.

C No, I think [**MC**] it 's [**NOM**] a little boy.

E Oh, a little boy.

C (Um) a little girl.

C That 's [**MC**] a little girl.

C It could be [**MC**] another little girl, could [**MC**] n't it?

E Do you think it's another little girl?

C Oh!

C Poor little girl!

C Dropped [**MC**] her!

E Dropped her on her head.

C Or maybe it 's [**MC**] a lady.

C Must be [**MC**] a lady because it 's got [**ADV**] a apron.

C No, I know [**MC**].

C If there 's [**ADV**] another bucket she could carry [**MC**] it.

C Maybe she picking [**MC**] up the bottle.

E Ok, milk bottle that the milkman left for her.

C I think [**MC**] it 's [**NOM**] a bottle the milkman left [**REL**] for the babies,
   like these and them.

C Think [**MC**] that 's [**NOM**] a house on the farm where all their animals
   sleep [**REL**].

C And that 's [**MC**] where all the hay is [**NOM**].

C (And that) and that 's [**MC**] where the hay 's being made [**NOM**].

C Where shall we put [**MC**] this?

E It's getting a bit full.

C Maybe here.

E Okay.

C Where all the animals are gone [**MC**] now?

C (xxx) a bit full.

C Maybe here.

E There are some more logs there.

C Uhhuh, except I wo n't put [MC] them on.

E You gonna put that little boy on or not?

C Yeah.

C Maybe (he's) he 's walking [MC] down (and).

C Maybe he 's (going) going [MC].

E Where?

C Do n't know [MC].

C (um) Up to see [INF] the horsie.

E Okay.

C (Going) think [MC] he 's going [NOM] round there and up to horsie.

C Or maybe he 's walking [MC] over there and up there down there and round the tractor and down here and see [INF] the horsie.

C Except got [MC] a long way to go [INF].

E Have you ever been on a horsie?

C No, yeah.

E Where?

E At the fairgrounds?

C No, at the Isle_of_Wight.

E Yeah?

E Is that where you go on holidays?

C Yeah, last year.

E What did you do there?

C And we 're going [MC] to the Isle_of_Wight.

C Well, we 're going [**MC**] on somebody's caravan.

E Are you?

C To somewhere.

C But I do n't know [**MC**] where.

Interview-Based Conversational Language Samples

Sample #3: Girl, Age 7 Years (Fletcher & Garman, 1988)
MLCU = 6.32   CD = 0.93

E Margaret, you had your birthday not long ago, didn't you?

C Uhuh.

E Did you get some nice presents for your birthday?

E Do you remember what you got?

C Yes.

E What did you get?

C (um I got I got) I got [**MC**] a farm snap.

C And from my brother.

E Uhhuh.

C (And) and I got [**MC**] some (Barbie) Barbie (clothes) clothes (but) which Barbie and Sindy could wear [**REL**].

E Which Barbie and Sindy could wear, uhhuh.

C Uhhuh.

E So you have even more clothes for your Barbies and Sindys.

C (Um and) and I 've [**MC**] lots of clothes.

E Really?

E So you can dress them differently every day?

C Uhhuh.

E Did you have a birthday party?

C Yes.

E Really?

C And that cake was [MC] lovely.

E You had a lovely birthday cake?

C (I) and what was [NOM] left of it was [MC] Mickey_Mouse that you could n't eat [REL].

E (um) That sounds nice.

C (And then and I) and I have [MC] (a pup) a puppet Mickey_Mouse.

E What else was left of the cake?

C A ribbon.

E A ribbon?

C A pink ribbon.

E What did you do with that?

C I have n't done [MC] anything with it yet.

C It was [MC] on the top.

C Sposta be [INF] getting washed [PRT] soon.

E Is it dirty because it was on the cake?

C (um) It was [MC] n't really dirty.

C But it had [MC] lots of bits of icing on.

E Did you do anything nice last weekend?

C I went [MC] to the Forest_Park zoo.

C And there was [MC] one thing.

C There 's [MC] two things that is [REL] my favorite rides.

E What is that?

C There was [**MC**] this boat ride that went [**REL**] far up.

C (and then) and then it could go [**MC**] far up there.

E Uhhuh.

E It's sort of a swing.

C Uhhuh and what lots of people can go [**REL**] on it.

E Uhhuh, I know that.

C But I went [**MC**] at the back.

E You went in the back?

C And that 's [**MC**] really scary.

C And I went [**MC**] with my brother.

E How old is your brother?

C Eleven.

E Eleven.

E Were you scared?

C No.

E No.

C (And then there's my f) there is [**MC**] really better than that other ride that I told [**REL**] you about.

C Well, you started [**MC**] from this little (xxx).

C And it went [**MC**] round (xxxx).

C It was [**MC**] a boat thing.

E It was a boat thing, uhuh.

C And then it went [**MC**] on the lake.

E Yes.

C And then it went [**MC**] up this water hill.

E Right.

C Right?

C And then down and splashed [**MC**].

E Oh dear!

C And me and Andy went [**MC**] on it two times.

E Uhuh.

C And my mum and dad went [**MC**] (it) on it once.

E Did they like it?

C Well, (it wasn't) they were [**MC**] n't in favor of it when it was going [**ADV**] up and down.

C But it was [**MC**] fun.

E Uhuh.

C (One time, I the boat I went on it) on the second time, I was [**MC**] right at the front of the boat.

C and I got [**MC**] soaking.

E Oh dear!

C But was [**MC**] a very big splash at the end.

E That sounds very lovely.

C And then it goes [**MC**] round the lake.

C And (then) then my mum (said) said [**MC**] "stay [**NOM**] there and we 'll come [**NOM**] on with you."

E Uhuh.

C So we stayed [**MC**] in.

C And then it was [**MC**] on the next (move move) ride.

C And then (mum) my mum and dad got [**MC**] in.

E Yes.

C And then it went [**MC**] along the lake again.

E Uhuh.

C Up the hill, down the hill, splash.

C (And) and then round a (bit) bit.

C And then we got [**MC**] off.

E Oh dear!

C (But) but (my mum) my mum took [**MC**] a photograph.

E She took a photograph of you in the boat?

C Uhhuh, me and Andy (with) with the water going [**PRT**] on.

C (My dad) but my mum and dad didn't wan [**MC**] na go [**INF**] in that boat thing.

E Um.

C A little bit of a scary cats.

E But they did in the end obviously.

C No.

E No?

C They never would go [**MC**] on it.

Sample #4: Boy, Age 14 Years (from the author's files)

MLCU = 9.93   CD = 1.76

E What would you like to tell me about yourself?

E For example, what could you tell me about school, or your family or friends or pets?

C (Um) at school I try [**MC**] to stay [**INF**] inclined.

C But I kind of get **[MC]** bored because I find **[ADV]** it somewhat boring.

C At home I try **[MC]** to do **[INF]** my chores.

C But I do n't **[MC]** because (I don't really need any) I do n't have **[ADV]** anything to do **[INF]** with the money after I get **[ADV]** it.

C And (um) I hang **[MC]** out with (a) a pretty tight group of friends.

E Are they all in cross-country?

C (Um) one of them is **[MC]**.

C And one of them is thinking **[MC]** about it.

C But they have n't really decided **[MC]** yet.

E How long have you been in cross-country?

C (Um) sixth grade.

E So two years.

E This is your second year?

C (Yes) no, this is **[MC]** my third.

C Started **[MC]** in sixth.

E Okay.

E And do you like it?

C (Um) It 's **[MC]** a nice warmup for track, which I 'm **[REL]** more into 'cause I 'm **[ADV]** (kind of) better at track.

E Okay.

E What's your favorite track event?

C (Um) pole vault.

E No way!

E Isn't that when you launch yourself over a tall pole?

C Yeah.

E You do that?

C {nods}.

E Wow.

E Do you go to competitions for it?

C (Um) Well you 're not allowed **[MC]** to do **[INF]** pole vault as a track
   event at other middle schools because I think **[ADV]** McArthur (is the
   only) has **[NOM]** the only (pole vault for like a) pole vault coach for
   middle school.

E So you can't compete with anyone.

C No.

E But you have a head start on competing.

C Yeah, I have **[MC]** a really big head start since I 'm **[ADV]** (like) the
   best person in my grade right now.

C There 's **[MC]** not really a lot of other people who do **[REL]** it, just two
   of my friends.

E What do you have to know to do pole vault well?

C (Um) you have **[MC]** to have **[INF]** good timing.

C (Uh) you have **[MC]** to be **[INF]** able to relax **[INF]** because if you
   (like) tighten **[ADV]** your abs when you 're trying **[ADV]** to turn **[INF]**
   upside down to go **[INF]** over the pole, you 'll end **[ADV]** up pulling
   [GER] on the bar and you might stretch **[ADV]** a muscle in your
   shoulder, which hurts **[REL]**.

C I 've done **[MC]** that.

E You have?

E You stretched the muscle in your shoulder in pole vault?

C Yeah.

E Have you had any other track injuries?

C (Um well like) Yes, most of them are **[MC]** just (like) twisting **[GER]** ankles in long jump and stuff, though.

C They do n't hurt **[MC]** as bad.

C It really hurts **[MC]**.

E How long does a twisted ankle take to recover?

C Like a day or two.

E Oh cool.

E But then you 're back running full speed?

C I actually normally run **[MC]** with a twisted ankle.

C It kind of helps **[NOM]** stretch **[INF]** it out I think **[MC]**.

C But I try **[MC]** not to put **[INF]** a whole bunch of weight on it.

E That 's really cool.

Sample #5: Girl, Age 14 Years (from the author's files)
MLCU = 9.61   CD = 1.63

E I am going to ask you a little bit about yourself.

C Well, I wish **[MC]** I worked **[NOM]**.

C But I do n't **[MC]**.

C I have been trying **[MC]** to find **[INF]** a job this summer.

C But it appears **[MC]** no one is hiring **[NOM]** (um) inexperienced 14-year-olds.

C (Um) I baby sit **[MC]** for a kid named **[PRT]** Jacob.

C And he 's **[MC]** really nice.

C He 's **[MC]** ten and pretty mature.

C So it 's **[MC]** kind of like being **[GER]** paid **[PRT]** (like) six dollars an hour to (um) play **[INF]** video games and watch **[INF]** TV with him and stuff.

C (Um my school) my school is **[MC]** Westminster_Middle_School.

C (Um it's uh) it 's **[MC]** an okay school.

C I think **[MC]** that it 's **[NOM]** a better fit for me than Southampton (but um it's).

E Why do you think that?

C (Uh) well (we just) because (um) I was made **[ADV]** fun of a lot when I was **[ADV]** in fifth and sixth grades.

C So at Southampton (I would have had) I feel **[MC]** like there is **[NOM]** just a more unfriendly atmosphere there.

C I 'm **[MC]** not sure that I really like **[NOM]** the friends I have **[REL]** at my school (um).

C But I 'm going **[MC]** into Woodbury_High_School.

C And (um) that 's going **[MC]** to be **[INF]** a new experience for me (you know) because I 've never been **[ADV]** to high school before.

C (Um) actually, I 'm **[MC]** quite familiar with one part of Woodbury_High_School.

C (I um) I am **[MC]** a theatre person.

C So (like um) I 've been **[MC]** in a summer camp where they basically use **[REL]** the entire (like) theatre and choir wing of Woodbury_High_School.

C And (I've been up) I 've performed **[MC]** on that stage at least three times.

C (Um) I 'm **[MC]** really into theatre and acting and stuff.

C In fact, (I was) my (uh) first professional role was **[MC]** in Sleeping_Beauty.

C (Um) It 's **[MC]** the only professional role I 've had **[REL]** yet because there 's **[ADV]** just nothing up for kids although I am auditioning **[ADV]** for My_Fair_Lady.

C (Um uh) So we 'll see **[MC]** how that goes **[NOM]**.

C (But um) I was **[MC]** in Sleeping_Beauty as a fairy.

C And (uh) over a hundred kids tried **[MC]** out.

C So I was **[MC]** pretty unprofessional.

C So I 'm **[MC]** not quite sure how I got **[NOM]** in.

C But (uh) it was **[MC]** pretty fun.

C But so yeah.

C I performed **[MC]** on the Community_Center stage (um).

E When was that?

C That was **[MC]** when I was **[ADV]** in fifth grade.

C I think **[MC]** I was going **[NOM]** into fifth grade.

C Yeah, I was going **[MC]** into fifth grade.

C And (um) I was **[MC]** just a fairy (but).

E And did you speak?

C (Um) I sang **[MC]** on stage.

C But I did n't have **[MC]** any solos or anything.

C (Yeah I was) Yeah (uh) I ate **[MC]** like a mountain load of candy before every performance, which was **[NOM]** not good for my voice I 'm **[REL]** sure (still but).

Sample #6: Boy, Age 14 Years (from the author's files)

MLCU = 7.76   CD = 1.21

E What would you like to tell me about yourself?

E For example, what could you tell me about school, or your family or friends or pets?

C (Well I have) My family is **[MC]** really close to me.

C Like (um) all my cousins and uncles and aunts live **[MC]** in Roseburg with me.

C And I see **[MC]** most of them almost every day.

C (Um).

E How many do you have?

C (I have) both my grandma and grandpas live **[MC]** in Roseburg.

C I have **[NOM]** I think **[MC]** three aunts that live **[REL]** here and two uncles maybe.

E Do any of your aunts and uncles live elsewhere?

C (Uh) yeah, actually I have **[MC]** an aunt and uncle in Bend.

C But I see **[MC]** them like five or six times a year.

E So you have a lot of cousins?

C Yeah, I have **[MC]** a lot of cousins.

E That sounds fun to me.

C (Um) well (like) most of my family is **[MC]** (like) teachers or doctors.

C And then (my) one of my uncles that lives **[REL]** in Bend is **[MC]** an engineer.

E Oh cool.

C (Um) what else.

E Do you have pets?

C (Yeah I have) my sister has **[MC]** a turtle.

C And I have **[MC]** a dog.

E A turtle and a dog!

E Does the dog get along with the turtle?

C Well I guess **[MC]**.

C He does n't try **[MC]** to bite **[INF]** him or anything.

E That's good.

E At least the turtle will be able to crawl into its shell.

E Does it live in a cage?

C Yeah, but (he like) sometimes my sister will let **[MC]** him out in the back yard to walk **[INF]** around in the summer.

E Is it big?

C Yeah, (it's like) well when we got **[ADV]** it, it was **[MC]** like that small.

C But now it 's **[MC]** like that big.

E It's amazing how they grow!

C And it 's **[MC]** supposed to be **[INF]** (like) like four feet by four feet when it gets **[ADV]** older.

C And they live **[MC]** like one hundred years.

E No way!

E How old is it now?

C (Um) like three

E Wow!

E It seems like it has grown a lot in three years.

C Uhhuh, yeah.

E So it will be really big, like one of those Galapagos Islands turtles.

E And so what is your dog like?

E What do you like to do with your dog?

C Well my dog is [MC] very small.

C He 's [MC] a Chihuahua.

C He is n't [MC] really active.

C He just sits [MC] around all day.

E Is it a puppy or is it older?

C Well it 's [NOM] like six I think [MC] now.

C But he is [NOM] I think [MC] a teacup Chihuahua.

C I 'm [MC] not sure.

E Really!

E What 's your favorite thing about him?

C (Um) I do n't know [MC].

C Probably how (like) one second he can be [MC] like totally calm.

C But the other he will be [MC] very playful.

E He's unpredictable?

C And he listens [MC] pretty well.

E That's nice.

APPENDIX F

Answer Key for Chapter 14

ANALYZING NARRATIVE, EXPOSITORY, AND PERSUASIVE LANGUAGE SAMPLES

The following are language samples that were elicited from children and adolescents with typical language development. They include samples of narrative, expository, and persuasive discourse. Each sample was entered into the Systematic Analysis of Language Transcripts (SALT) software program and broken into C-units (spoken language) or T-units (written language) by the author. All mazes were placed within parentheses, allowing the final reformulation to stand. To allow SALT to count the number of words accurately, all contractions were separated by one space.

For each sample, fill in the clause type, using the codes shown below.

MC = main clause   GER = gerundive clause

ADV = adverbial clause   INF = infinitive clause

REL = relative clause   PRT = participial clause

NOM = nominal clause

E = examiner; C = child or adolescent

NARRATIVE LANGUAGE SAMPLES

Spoken Narratives

Sample #7: Girl, Age 5 Years, retelling *Frog, Where Are You?* (Mayer 1969; sample borrowed from Miller, Andriacchi, & Nockerts 2019 and used with their permission)

MLCU = 7.21   CD = 1.21

C (Well a) when the boy was sleeping [**ADV**], the frog crept [**MC**] out of the window.

C And (um) then when the boy was going [**ADV**] to say [**INF**] good morning to the frog, he was [**MC**] gone.

C And then (th) the dog went [**MC**] to look [**INF**] for the frog in the jar.

C And then his head got stuck [**MC**].

C And then he looked [**MC**] out the window.

C And he fell [**MC**] down to the ground.

C The glass jar broke [**MC**].

C And then they were looking [**MC**] in the woods.

C And (um) then (th th th um he f) he found [**MC**] other animal.

C (Th) but it was [**MC**] n't his frog.

C And then he found [**MC**] a deer.

C He got [**MC**] on it.

C And it took [**MC**] him (t) off a cliff.

C And (um) the little boy heard [**MC**] this croaking sound.

C And (um he) he thought [**MC**] it was [**NOM**] the frog.

C And it was [**MC**].

C And so he looked [**MC**] over a dead tree.

C And he found [**MC**] a mother frog and his pet frog.

C And then they found [**MC**] eight children and a frogs.

C And then.

E What happened at the end, anything?

C And (then they f) then they found [**MC**] (the) the (xxx).

C (Then they) then they got [**MC**] to keep [**INF**] a frog.

E Mmm.

C And then that was [**MC**] his new pet.

E Are you finished?

E Or is there anything more you wanna add?

C That 's [**MC**] the end.

Sample #8: Boy, Age 7 Years, retelling *Frog, Where Are You?* (Mayer 1969; sample borrowed from Miller, Andriacchi, & Nockerts 2019 and used with their permission)

MLCU = 7.64   CD = 1.26

C (Um) there was [**MC**] a boy.

C (Um) he had [**MC**] a frog and a dog.

C And (um) when they woke [**ADV**] up the frog was [**MC**] gone.

C They were looking [**MC**] everywhere.

C And he was looking [**MC**] for (his d) the (um) frog.

C And he looked [**MC**] in his hat.

C It was [**MC**] n't there.

C The dog was looking [**MC**] for the (um) frog.

C And it was [**MC**] in a jar.

C And he stuck [**MC**] his head in it.

C And then the dog was looking [**MC**] out the window.

C And then the boy, he was looking [**MC**] out the window and calling [**MC**] for his frog.

C And then the dog fell [**MC**] down as he was leaning [**ADV**] over.

C And then the boy picked [**MC**] up his dog.

C (So it) and the dog looked [**MC**] at him because they were [**ADV**] really worried.

C He was [**MC**] really worried.

C That was [**MC**] their house they lived [**REL**] in.

C It looks [**MC**] kind of like a farm though.

C And he was still calling [**MC**].

C And there were [**MC**] some bees.

C So the bees were coming [**MC**] out of a beehive.

C And the dog was barking [**MC**] at the beehive.

C And then a bee must have stung [**MC**] the kid.

C And then there 's [**MC**] a little (um) mole.

C And a dog was going [**MC**] up.

C And he was still barking [**MC**] up the tree.

C And the bees' hive fell [**MC**] down.

C And they worked [**MC**] on it so hard.

C And {audible inhale} (and um) it broke [**MC**].

C And the bees went [**MC**] chasing [**GER**] the dog.

C (They were) they were almost going [**MC**] to chase [**INF**] him.

C And the mole is still looking [**MC**], like staring.

C (And he) the boy (um) climbed [**MC**] up the tree.

C Owl scared [**MC**] him.

C And the bees (um) went [**MC**] (whe where) all the way there chasing [**PRT**] the dog.

C And then there 's [**MC**] a owl who did n't let [**REL**] them go anywhere because he was getting [**ADV**] scared.

C So he looked [**MC**] back (and) so it would n't fall [**ADV**] on his head.

C And (um) he did n't want [**MC**] to go [**INF**] anywhere because of the owl.

C And the owl is [**MC**] still there.

C And he did n't know [**MC**] this.

C (x) right there.

C And (um) the boy (went) was calling [**MC**] for his frog still.

C And his dog was sneaking [**MC**] around so the bees would n't come [**ADV**].

C And (um) he wanted [**MC**] to see [**INF**] if that was [**NOM**] a branch.

C But he climbed [**MC**] up it.

C But it was [**MC**] (really) really (a) like a reindeer or a deer or something.

C And the dog was going [**MC**] down there because (the reindeer the reindeer or the doe or) the deer was running [**ADV**] and chasing [**ADV**] the dog.

C And bad things are happening [**MC**] to the dog all the time.

C And (the um kid was still stuck on the) the (boy) kid, he was [**MC**] still stuck on the (um reindeer) doe.

C And then the boy and the dog fall [**MC**] down.

C They were falling [**MC**] down.

C But they did n't (fa) fall [**MC**] yet.

C And now they (fall) fell [**MC**] down right there.

C And {C laughs} the dog was [**MC**] on the boy.

C (The boy heard um) the boy heard [**MC**] (th) a sound going [**PRT**] "ribbit_ribbit."

C And the dog was [**MC**] on top of his head.

C And he heard [**MC**] it too.

C And then the kid said [**MC**], "Shh."

C Now he comes [**MC**].

C And he looks [**MC**] under a dead old tree.

C And then he sees [**MC**] some frogs.

C And then he sees [**MC**] just two frogs.

C But now he sees [**MC**] more than two frogs.

C (He) So he says [**MC**] "Goodbye."

C And then they keep [**MC**] a frog instead of the old frog.

C (And the) these two frogs are [**MC**] (a) happily_ever_after with frogs.

Sample #9: Boy, Age 14 Years, retelling *The Mice in Council* (from the author's files)

MLCU = 9.69   CD = 2.0

E Can you retell the story?

C (Uh) I could try [**MC**], yes.

C So (uh) these mice are living [**MC**] in fear of the cat.

C That ('s uh) happens [**MC**] a lot (I guess).

C And so (um) they decided [**MC**] to make [**INF**] a council because of the name of the story to try [**INF**] and figure [**INF**] out a way to (uh) solve [**INF**] this problem.

C Because (you know) they 're losing **[MC]** a lot of people getting **[PRT]** eaten **[PRT]** up by the cat.

C So they keep **[MC]** talking **[GER]** and talking **[GER]**.

C And nothing seems **[MC]** (to work) to work **[INF]** (that would work).

C And one (mice) mouse was **[MC]** (uh) smart (I guess).

C (To uh) mice decided **[MC]** to (uh) make **[INF]** it so that the cat could be heard **[ADV]** by putting **[GER]** a bell around his neck.

C They thought **[MC]** it was **[NOM]** an amazing idea.

C So they applauded **[MC]**.

C And he gave **[MC]** a couple bows.

C And then (uh the) it was passed **[MC]** that they would do **[NOM]** this 'cause they have **[ADV]** a little council.

C But (uh) then one old mouse that 's **[REL]** wise (uh, uh) was (uh) congratulating **[MC]** him and thought **[MC]** of a question.

C (Uh) who would put **[MC]** the bell around the (mouse or) cat.

C And (uh) that 's **[MC]** a good question.

E Awesome, nicely retold.

Sample #10: Girl, Age 14 Years, retelling *The Mice in Council* (from the author's files)

MLCU = 12.13   CD = 2.53

C (So) the mice were **[MC]** always in fear of this cat because (they'd always) he 'd always approach **[ADV]** them and try **[ADV]** and eat **[INF]** them.

C And he 'd toy **[MC]** with them and torture **[MC]** them.

C So the mice called **[MC]** together a council meeting.

C And they discussed **[MC]** many plans.

C But none of them seemed **[MC]** (to work or) like they were going **[NOM]** to work **[INF]**.

C And then a very small young mouse (um) approached **[MC]** and said **[MC]** that his idea was **[NOM]** to put **[INF]** a bell around the cat's neck so that whenever the cat came **[ADV]** they would hear **[ADV]** the bell tinkle **[INF]** and then they would know **[ADV]** he was coming **[NOM]** so they could escape **[ADV]**.

C And everyone thought **[MC]** it was **[NOM]** a really great idea.

C And so (um) they applauded **[MC]** him.

C And he took **[MC]** a few bows.

C And then (um) a wise older mouse stood **[MC]** up.

C And (said) this is **[MC]** basically what he said **[NOM]**.

C This is **[MC]** truly a great plan.

C And (um) only a genius could figure **[MC]** out a plan so simple (that we could) that we would have overlooked **[REL]**.

C And he says **[MC]** so now the question is **[NOM]** who 's going **[NOM]** to put **[INF]** the bell on the cat.

C So basically things are **[MC]** easier said **[PRT]** than done **[PRT]**.

Sample #11: Boy, Age 14 Years, retelling *The Monkey and the Dolphin* (from the author's files)

MLCU = 9.74   CD = 1.84

E Can you tell that story back to me?

C (Uh) so (uh) I guess **[MC]** it was **[NOM]** a custom to bring **[INF]** monkeys and other creatures along with them to amuse **[INF]** the (sailor) sailors.

C So one guy brought **[MC]** a monkey onto his boat.

C And they were sailing **[MC]** around somewhere (Uh) by (Greek) Greece (I guess).

C And (uh) there was **[MC]** a storm.

C The ship crashed **[MC]**.

C And everyone was **[MC]** in the water.

C And they were swimming **[MC]** towards shore.

C And so was **[MC]** the monkey.

C And then a dolphin, who must have **[REL]** bad eyesight to mistake **[INF]** a monkey for a man, (uh) swam **[MC]** up and grabbed **[MC]** the monkey with his back.

C And so the monkey had gotten **[MC]** onto him.

C And they 're swimming **[MC]** there.

C And he asked **[MC]** him if he was **[NOM]** (a uh citizen) a Athenian.

C And the monkey said **[MC]** "yes" (you know) trying **[PRT]** to trick **[INF]** this dolphin because he 's trying **[ADV]** to live **[INF]** on.

C And the dolphin asked **[MC]** him if he knew **[NOM]** something or someone.

C And the monkey, (you know) thinking **[MC]** that oh yeah this must be **[NOM]** (uh) someone.

C Like oh yeah I know **[MC]** him.

C He 's **[MC]** a dear friend.

C And the dolphin knew **[MC]** that he was lying **[NOM]**.

C So instead of saving **[GER]** him, he plunged **[MC]** down to the bottom to leave **[INF]** the monkey to his fate.

E Very nice.

Sample #12: Girl, Age 14 Years, retelling *The Monkey and the Dolphin* (from the author's files)

MLCU = 13.29   CD = 2.21

C (Um) so it used **[MC]** to be **[INF]** (um) a custom that sailors would take **[REL]** on with them animals like a monkey or a dog to keep **[INF]** them entertained **[PRT]** on their long voyage.

C So on one particular (um) voyage, they took **[MC]** with them a monkey.

C And when they were **[ADV]** off the coast of Sunium, there was **[MC]** a terrible shipwreck.

C And everyone was turned **[MC]** overboard, including **[PRT]** the monkey.

C So a nearby dolphin (mis) mistook **[MC]** the monkey for a man.

C And so he came **[MC]** to his rescue.

C And then the dolphin asked **[MC]** him if he knew **[NOM]** Piraeus, which was **[REL]** also the name of the harbor off of Athens.

C And (um) he said **[MC]** yes I 'm **[NOM]** (a) an Athenian.

C I 'm **[MC]** from one of the first families that was **[REL]** here.

C And he said **[MC]** yes I knew **[NOM]** Piraeus.

C He 's **[MC]** one of my oldest friends.

C And the dolphin knew **[MC]** then that he was (uh) not telling **[NOM]** the truth, that he was lying **[NOM]**.

C And so he dove **[MC]** deep into the water and left **[MC]** the monkey to his fate.

C And so the moral of the story would be **[MC]** people who pretend **[REL]** (uh) to be **[INF]** someone else basically end **[NOM]** up in deep water.

Written Narratives

Sample #13: Girl, Age 9 Years, imaginary story (Nippold, 2007, pp. 344–345)

MLTU = 13.27   CD = 2.36

C Today was [**MC**] the day that my Aunt Jane was coming [**REL**] to town from Pennsylvania.

C As soon as the plane landed [**ADV**], Aunt Jane stepped [**MC**] out followed [**PRT**] by a mysterious figure and a few other passengers.

C The mysterious figure walked [**MC**] over to a newsstand and bought [**MC**] a paper.

C He took [**MC**] one quick look at the headline and threw [**MC**] the paper away.

C The headline read [**MC**], "Sweet_Heart_Lumber_Co Orders [**NOM**] 10,000 Wooden Stakes."

C We took [**MC**] Aunt Jane home.

C As soon as we got [**ADV**] home, my sister Braeden told [**MC**] me she saw [**NOM**] the mysterious man and what he did [**NOM**].

C I invited [**MC**] my friends Lia and Bethany over and told [**MC**] them what had happened [**NOM**] at the airport.

C We looked [**MC**] at the headline on the paper.

C "I do n't get [**MC**] it."

C "Why would he throw [**NOM**] away a newspaper that said [**REL**], 'Sweet_Heart_Lumber_Co Orders [**NOM**] 10,000 Wooden Stakes,'" asked [**MC**] Lia, "unless he was [**ADV**] a vampire."

Sample #14: Boy, Age 11 Years, excerpt from imaginary story titled "The Blue Beyond" (Nippold, 2007, p. 350)

MLTU = 8.94   CD = 1.82

C We climbed [**MC**] into the spaceship.

C Then we heard [**MC**] the countdown, 10_9_8_7_3_2_1 BOOM!

C The engines fired [**MC**] up.

C We were going [**MC**] up_up_up faster than I ever imagined [**ADV**].

C It was [**MC**] then dark.

C But soon the stars began [**MC**] to appear [**INF**], then planets, then moons.

C "Oh no," I looked [**MC**] over and saw [**MC**] my dad struggling [**PRT**] with the controls.

C "They 're [**NOM**] jammed," he said [**MC**] worriedly.

C I looked [**MC**] out the window to see [**INF**] the Milky_Way disappearing [**PRT**].

C We were being [**MC**] swept [**PRT**] into a different galaxy.

C Boom_crash_bang!

C We made [**MC**] a crash landing on something hard.

C After a long time of struggling [**GER**], we finally managed [**MC**] to climb [**INF**] out of the damaged spaceship.

C We stopped [**MC**] to look [**INF**] at our surroundings.

C We were [**MC**] on a strange blue planet.

C Everything was [**MC**] blue.

C The ground was [**MC**] covered [**PRT**] with enormous stones and boulders that made [**REL**] flashes of blue when the sunlight hit [**ADV**] them.

C There was [**MC**] a little bit of grass here and there that was [**REL**] a beautiful shade of blue that made [**REL**] the planet sparkle [**INF**].

C The planet was [**MC**] like an ocean.

C It was [**MC**] gorgeous with its different shades of blue.

C There was [**MC**] neon blue, navy blue, royal blue, and sky blue.

C "Let [**NOM**] 's call [**INF**] this planet The_Blue_Beyond," my dad suggested [**MC**].

C "Can we go [**NOM**] exploring," I asked [**MC**].

C "Maybe we 'll find [**MC**] some life."

C As we were walking [**ADV**] around, my dad jerked [**MC**] me behind a rock.

C "What was [**NOM**] that for," I asked [**MC**].

C ("Shhhhh") {sound effects from his dad}.

C He pointed [**MC**] to a clearing.

C In that clearing was [**MC**] a little creature with big bug eyes.

C Its blue skin perfectly matched [**MC**] its surroundings.

C Its sharp piranha-like teeth sparkled [**MC**] in the sunlight.

C And its pointed little ears bobbed [**MC**] up and down as it ran [**ADV**].

C It screeched [**MC**] as it approached [**ADV**] a dead little animal.

C And the rest of the troop came [**MC**] running [**GER**] to help [**INF**].

C As they fought [**ADV**] over the animal, my dad whispered [**MC**], "You never want [**NOM**] to mess [**INF**] with those guys!"

Sample #15: Boy, Age 17 Years, essay titled "What Happened One Day" (from the author's files)

MLTU = 13.68   CD = 2.58

C One day a long time ago, my friend Jack and I went **[MC]** on a camping trip all by ourselves.

C We set **[MC]** up camp and went **[MC]** fishing to try **[INF]** and catch **[INF]** our dinner.

C I caught **[MC]** two fish while Jack caught **[ADV]** three.

C We were getting **[MC]** ready to leave **[INF]** when I looked **[ADV]** up the river and saw **[ADV]** this big dark blurry figure run **[INF]** off into the bushes.

C I did n't think **[MC]** anything of it.

C I just thought **[MC]** it was **[NOM]** an elk.

C On our way back to the camp, Jack started **[MC]** taunting **[GER]** me and bragging **[GER]** about how he was **[NOM]** a better fisherman than I was **[NOM]** because he caught **[ADV]** three fish while I only caught **[ADV]** two.

C We got **[MC]** back to camp.

C And I started **[MC]** a fire to cook **[INF]** the fish.

C I always started **[MC]** the fires.

C I was **[MC]** the best fire starter.

C We cooked **[MC]** some of our fish and put **[MC]** the rest in the ice chest for breakfast.

C We made **[MC]** our beds and went **[MC]** to sleep **[INF]**.

C Jack was still bragging **[MC]** about his fish.

C When I woke **[ADV]** in the morning, I opened **[MC]** my eyes to see **[INF]** Bigfoot eating **[PRT]** our fish.

C As I leaned **[ADV]** over to wake **[INF]** up Jack, it looked **[MC]** at me and ran **[MC]** off into the forest.

C Just like that, our camping trip turned **[MC]** into a hunt for rock solid proof of Bigfoot.

C After three days trying **[GER]** and failing **[GER]** to find **[INF]** Bigfoot anywhere, we gave **[MC]** up and went **[MC]** home.

C Ever since that day, I always have been **[MC]** sure to bring **[INF]** three things camping with me, a gun, a camera, and a better type of fishing bait.

EXPOSITORY LANGUAGE SAMPLES

Spoken Language

Sample #16: Boy, Age 13 Years, Favorite Game or Sport task (from the author's files)

MLCU = 10.06   CD = 1.67

E What is your favorite game or sport?

C My favorite sport in school would be **[MC]** wrestling.

E Why is wrestling your favorite sport?

C Well the (uh) coaches are **[MC]** really nice and everything.

C (We got got uh) we started **[MC]** out doing **[GER]** these (like uh) extra things.

C And (then uh and) then eventually I did **[MC]** everything and got **[MC]** good at it.

C So started **[MC]** getting **[GER]** gold medals and stuff.

E I'm not too familiar with the sport of wrestling, so I would like you to tell me all about it.

E For example, tell me what the goals are, and how many people may play a match.

E Also, tell me about the rules that players need to follow.

E Tell me everything you can think of about the sport of wrestling so that someone who has never played before would know how to play.

C (We) you start **[MC]** on a mat.

C You warm up **[MC]**.

C You go **[MC]** over to the mat.

C You shake **[MC]** hands.

C And the ref blows **[MC]** the whistle.

C And when you wrestle **[ADV]**, you start **[MC]** out neutral.

C And (you have to um you have to) you take **[MC]** the guy down by getting **[GER]** control of him while their hands or their feet are **[ADV]** on the mat.

C And if you 're taking **[ADV]** a guy down (you can't like if you come around the back), you can 't just pick **[MC]** them up and slap **[MC]** them on the mat.

C Otherwise, it 's **[MC]** unnecessary roughness.

C You get docked **[MC]** off a point.

C And if they are **[ADV]** (uh) too injured to wrestle **[INF]** then they win **[MC]** the match.

C And (um) it 's **[MC]** really big on sportsmanship.

C So you can 't go **[MC]** over and yell **[MC]** at the ref or yell **[MC]** at (the) them.

C Otherwise you 'll get kicked **[MC]** for the next tournament.

C And (um yeah you also you have um you have to) you have **[MC]** to shake **[INF]** hands because it 's **[ADV]** pretty much sportsmanship to do **[INF]** that.

C And once you get **[ADV]** the take down on them, you (um) try **[MC]** to break **[INF]** them down to their back.

C And you get **[MC]** them past a 45-degree angle.

C And you get **[MC]** near full points.

C Then (uh) for 3 points, it 's **[MC]** like 2 points.

C And (uh 5 points it's like 3 poin er uh) 5 seconds it 's **[MC]** 3 points.

C And then after that, (you uh for how long) you hold **[MC]** them down.

C And it 's **[MC]** about a 2-second pin.

C And if you get **[ADV]** both their shoulders down and (uh them you uh) if you pin **[ADV]** them, you get **[MC]** to shake **[INF]** hands.

C And you win **[MC]**.

C But there 's **[MC]** also points.

C Like for college, there 's **[MC]** advantage time which is **[REL]** where (like somebody if) somebody was riding **[NOM]** a person for a long time.

C And they get **[MC]** points.

C (But once they go neutral then the timing down and stuff).

C (So uh they have to kinda like) that 's **[MC]** how it goes **[NOM]** with the advantage time.

C They get **[MC]** certain amount of points at the end for advantage time and stuff.

C (uh) it 's **[MC]** pretty much big on sportsmanship.

C And it 's **[MC]** pretty easy to learn **[INF]**.

C Also you can 't lock **[MC]** hands while they 're **[ADV]** down around their waist (but) like around the leg (or around the ar).

C But around the arm is **[MC]** okay.

C And stuff like that (and can't like uh).

C In freestyle you can do **[MC]** that because it 's **[ADV]** a big part of freestyle.

E Now I would like you to tell me what a player should do in order to win the sport of wrestling.

E In other words, what are some key strategies that every good player should know?

C You just try **[MC]** to turn **[INF]** them so you get **[ADV]** back points.

C And (uh once second) once both their shoulders touch **[ADV]** the mat, they 're **[MC]** pinned.

E Do they have to go all the way down?

C No you just have **[MC]** to get **[INF]** their shoulders to touch **[INF]**.

E How long is a match?

C (um matches are usually like in reg) I think **[MC]** they 're **[NOM]** the same in everyone.

C So (they) for middle school, it 's **[MC]** (like) about (like uh) three minutes or maybe four minutes or something like that.

C For high school it 's **[MC]** six minutes.

C And college I 'm **[MC]** not sure.

C I think **[MC]** it 's **[NOM]** about the same as high school or (like) 30 seconds more or something.

E So a match isn't all that long.

C Yeah it 's **[MC]** not too hard (it's just) if you 're **[ADV]** conditioned well and you have **[ADV]** a good work ethic.

C Then you 'll probably do **[MC]** well in wrestling.

C But if you do n't try **[ADV]** your hardest, you 're never going **[MC]** to get **[INF]** anywhere.

C Yeah it 's **[MC]** pretty much you can beat **[NOM]** guys that are **[REL]** strong as long as you have **[ADV]** a good technique.

C But (strength is kinda like) some people can just do **[MC]** bad technique and just knock **[MC]** you down and (um) then pin **[MC]** me and stuff.

C But most of the time, you can get **[MC]** them.

E What about freestyle?

C (Well in freestyle it's just you) I do n't know **[MC]** much about freestyle.

C But you just touch **[MC]** (their both) their shoulders on the mat.

C And you win **[MC]**.

C Or you win **[MC]** by points at the end of the match.

C Same with collegiate except in collegiate it (like) 2 points pin.

C And (then like you'll uh and) if you do n't pin **[ADV]** through the whole match, then you win **[MC]** by a certain amount of points.

C And then you get **[MC]** a certain amount of points for your team.

C But you can also technical **[MC]** them which is **[REL]** (like) when (you uh if) you (get) gain **[ADV]** (like) 15 points more than them.

C Then they stop **[MC]** the match.

C And you win **[MC]**.

Sample #17: Girl, Age 17 Years, Peer Conflict Resolution Science Fair task* (from the author's files)

MLCU = 15.45   CD = 3.40

E Now I'd like you to tell the story back to me, in your own words.

E Try to tell me everything you can remember about the story.

C The teacher gave **[MC]** the four girls an assignment to work **[INF]** together on a science project.

C And they decided **[MC]** they were going **[NOM]** to make **[INF]** a model airplane that could actually fly **[REL]**.

C And everyone worked **[MC]** on it except for one girl named **[PRT]** Melanie.

C And (it made Debbie angry or um) it made **[MC]** her indifferent because she would n't do **[ADV]** the work.

E What is the main problem here?

C (Um) not everyone was participating **[MC]** equally or helping **[MC]** participating **[GER]**.

E Why is that a problem?

C Well if one person does n't do **[ADV]** anything and they 're **[ADV]** still in the group, they 're still going **[MC]** to get **[INF]** the same grade.

C Or they 're still going **[MC]** to be **[INF]** in that group as all the people that worked **[REL]** as hard.

C But they did n't contribute **[MC]** to it at all.

C So the other people may feel **[MC]** like they did n't deserve **[NOM]** it.

E What is a good way for Debbie to deal with Melanie?

C (um) I guess **[MC]** Debbie could ask **[NOM]** Melanie why she did n't want **[NOM]** to help **[INF]** or maybe she wanted **[NOM]** to do **[INF]** something different than what they wanted **[NOM]** to do **[INF]**.

---

*Note: This task involves briefly retelling a story before moving into expository discourse.

C Maybe that 's **[MC]** the reason she did n't want **[REL]** to help **[INF]**.

C (Or) and if that did n't work **[ADV]**, then she could ask **[MC]** the teacher to help **[INF]** them.

E Why is that a good way for Debbie to deal with Melanie?

C Because it 's **[MC]** calm.

C She 's not going **[MC]** to be **[INF]** like yelling **[PRT]** at her.

C They 're going **[MC]** to try **[INF]** to compromise **[INF]** about it so that the three girls can do **[ADV]** what they want **[NOM]** to do **[INF]**.

C But Melanie can also help **[MC]** since they 're all contributing **[ADV]** to it.

E What do you think will happen if Debbie does that?

C (um) Maybe Melanie will say **[MC]** that she did n't want **[NOM]** to make **[INF]** an airplane or (she um) she wanted **[NOM]** to do **[INF]** something different.

C And so maybe they could interact **[MC]** that way and find **[MC]** out what the problem was **[NOM]** so Melanie could help **[ADV]** do **[INF]** something.

E How do you think they both will feel if Debbie does that?

C I think **[MC]** that they would kind of feel **[NOM]** more relaxed and not so uptight about her not helping **[GER]** or maybe Melanie not getting **[GER]** to do **[INF]** what she wants **[NOM]** to do **[INF]**.

C Maybe they would both feel **[MC]** more comfortable about the problem or talking **[GER]** about it.

Sample #18: Girl, Age 17 Years, Peer Conflict Resolution Fast Food Restaurant task** (from the author's files)

MLCU = 11.63   CD = 2.21

E Now I'd like you to tell the story back to me, in your own words.

C (um Jane and Kathy) Jane is going **[MC]** to cook **[INF]** the food on the grill.

C And Kathy is going **[MC]** to take **[INF]** out the garbage.

C But her arm really hurts **[MC]**.

C And she wants **[MC]** to switch **[INF]** jobs.

C But Jane does n't want **[MC]** to lose **[INF]** her spot at the grill.

E What is the main problem here?

C The main problem is **[MC]** that (maybe) maybe Jane does n't want **[NOM]** to give **[INF]** up her spot.

C Maybe they could just switch **[MC]** for a minute for her to take **[INF]** out the garbage.

C Or maybe she could help **[MC]** Kathy take **[INF]** out the garbage.

C The main problem is **[MC]** that (they don't want to) Jane does n't want **[NOM]** to switch **[INF]** jobs.

C But maybe she can just help **[MC]** Kathy instead do **[INF]** the grill.

E Why is that a problem?

C Because she said **[ADV]** that she did n't want **[NOM]** to give **[INF]** up her spot at the grill.

C So obviously she did n't want **[MC]** to give **[INF]** up her spot at the grill.

C And (maybe) I do n't know **[MC]** why.

E What is a good way for Jane to deal with Kathy?

**Note: This task involves briefly retelling a story before moving into expository discourse.

C Well Jane could help **[MC]** Kathy take **[INF]** the garbage out.

C Or someone else could do **[MC]** it.

E Why is that a good way for Jane to deal with Kathy?

C Because they could both get **[MC]** their jobs done and help **[MC]** each other.

E What do you think will happen if Jane does that?

C I think **[MC]** that Kathy would really appreciate **[NOM]** it if Jane helped **[ADV]** her (and) and maybe in turn Kathy would help **[NOM]** Jane if she wanted **[ADV]** it.

C (Or um) then they could both get **[MC]** their jobs done.

E How do you think they both will feel if Jane does that?

C They 'll both feel **[MC]** (like) happy that everything got done **[NOM]** or happy (that they solved) that they could help **[NOM]** each other and solve **[NOM]** the problems.

Written Language

Sample #19: Girl, Age 17 Years, the Nature of Friendship expository essay (from the author's files)

MLTU = 12.10   CD = 2.20

C To me, friendship is **[MC]** a relationship between two or more people that like **[REL]** spending **[GER]** time with each other.

C A friend is **[MC]** someone you can talk **[REL]** to when there is **[ADV]** no other.

C You can tell **[MC]** them your secrets.

C And they will always have **[MC]** your back.

C If the world did n't have **[ADV]** friendship, then relationships and social status would n't mean **[MC]** a thing.

C The world would be **[MC]** full of people that do n't like **[REL]** each other.

C And most of all, there would n't be **[MC]** anyone to talk **[INF]** with.

C Friends mostly keep **[MC]** you occupied.

C If I did n't have **[ADV]** friends, then my life would lack **[MC]** the excitement everyone needs **[REL]**.

C I would just wake **[MC]** up, go **[MC]** to school, come home **[MC]** and either watch **[MC]** TV or do **[MC]** nothing.

C With friends, it 's **[MC]** like our lives are **[NOM]** all intertwined.

C And if one of us is doing **[ADV]** something exciting, then the rest should be **[MC]** in on it as well.

C Living **[GER]** a boring life is n't **[MC]** worth it.

C Usually friends share **[MC]** common interests.

C Either it being **[PRT]** culture, neighborhood, or personalities, they are **[MC]** usually like the other.

C Friendship to children is **[MC]** having **[GER]** someone to play **[INF]** with.

C Usually it 's **[MC]** a person from school or a neighbor.

C For teenagers like me, friendship means **[MC]** someone to talk **[INF]** to when we get **[ADV]** in a fight with our parents, boyfriend, or girlfriends.

C Adults see **[MC]** friendship as more of a companionship.

C If they have **[ADV]** common interest in things, then they are **[MC]** more than likely to become **[INF]** friends.

C Or they have just been **[MC]** friends for a really long time.

C Usually people are **[MC]** friends one year then just are **[MC]** n't the next.

C People grow **[MC]** up and change **[MC]** and make **[MC]** new friends every day.

C Sometimes friends just drift **[MC]** apart over the years.

C Other times, friends can do **[MC]** or say **[MC]** something that does n't make **[REL]** them trustworthy.

C The usual result is **[MC]** a misunderstanding or someone gets **[NOM]** hurt.

C The best of friends are **[MC]** the ones that stay **[REL]** in touch for a really long time.

C There have been **[MC]** cases of people being **[GER]** friends since they were **[ADV]** three.

C And now at age sixty they are **[MC]** still together.

C Friendships come **[MC]** and go **[MC]**, and depending **[PRT]** on what kind of friendship it is **[REL]**, can last **[MC]** a lifetime.

PERSUASIVE LANGUAGE SAMPLES

Spoken Language

Sample #20: Girl, Age 15 Years, arguing for later school start time (Miller, Andriacchi, & Nockerts, 2019; borrowed with permission from the authors)

MLCU = 14.67   CD = 2.61

C (Um) I think **[MC]** (that the time in school) that school should start **[NOM]** later in the morning.

C (Um) It can help **[MC]** students focus **[INF]** more because students come **[ADV]** in so early.

C And (they) some of them do n't go **[MC]** to sleep **[INF]** until later at night anyways, especially for people that have **[REL]** after school sports because (you_know, like) having **[GER]** to stay **[INF]** out later.

C And if you got [**ADV**] more sleep at home, you would n't necessarily have [**MC**] to worry [**INF**] about students sleeping [**GER**] in class (so) which is [**REL**] probably a big problem because I see [**ADV**] a lot of kids sleeping [**PRT**] in class.

C (Um) transportation could be [**MC**] another reason because the kids (um) get [**ADV**] up late.

C They oversleep [**MC**] and have [**MC**] no way to the bus in the mornings.

C Or they have [**MC**] no way to school.

C Or they are [**MC**] too far to walk [**INF**].

C So most students miss [**MC**] the bus because they have [**ADV**] to get [**INF**] up so early.

C And (um) students are failing [**MC**] classes mostly because they can 't focus [**ADV**] or because they (um) are sleeping [**ADV**] in class and kind a missing [**ADV**] (the) the details that they need [**REL**] to learn [**INF**].

C And (um they could um) it 'll be [**NOM**] better grades, I think [**MC**], if they can just focus [**ADV**] more.

C It 'll be [**MC**] better grades.

C And (kind a like because) here we have [**MC**] like MASH and stuff.

C So it 'll be [**MC**] better grades for them and less of that.

C And some kids they skip [**MC**] school not necessarily because they (like) are [**ADV**] sick or something, just really because they just need [**ADV**] the time off.

C Most of them do [**MC**] it for sleep (but).

C And (um) if we can 't necessarily come [**ADV**] into school later, we could get [**MC**] out of school earlier (which) or (you_know) get [**MC**] a free time in between school to kind a just give [**INF**] the kids just a minute to get [**INF**] theirselfs together.

C Or (um) we need [**MC**] shorter classes because like long classes, and sitting [**GER**] in the same spot for a long time, kind a gets [**ADV**] boring (so).

C And (um) I want [**MC**] later school hours (um) because then (it w) it 'll be [**ADV**] easier for me and for more students because they would n't be [**ADV**] so sleepy.

C It could cause [**MC**] more focus.

C And (um) you could ask [**MC**] more students (if you know) if you were [**ADV**] n't too sure on what I was saying [**NOM**] (so).

E Good.

E Is there anything else you can tell me?

C (Um probably that) I 'm trying [**MC**] to think [**INF**].

C I do n't know [**MC**] because (like) some kids they (like) do n't go [**ADV**] to bed until like twelve or like one.

C And so (i) it 's [**MC**] really hard to get [**INF**] up (you_know) at six.

C Most kids get [**MC**] up at six (because the bus) around bus (x) times.

C So it 's [**MC**] really hard.

C Like I, personally, get [**MC**] up at six and have [**MC**] to get [**INF**] my little sisters up at six.

C And (like) especially, it 's [**MC**] (hard for) harder for people that 's [**REL**] not morning people to (you_know) get [**INF**] dressed and get [**INF**] your stuff together.

C And it 's [**MC**] really hard to focus [**INF**] because you wake [**ADV**] up so late.

C And (you wanna) you do n't wan [**MC**] na have [**INF**] to (like) rush [**INF**] (so).

C And then you rush [**MC**].

C And you forget [**MC**] things or (you_know) forget [**MC**] things you might need [**REL**] for school or classes.

C And that could also lead [**MC**] to a bad day, not having [**GER**] what you need [**NOM**] (so).

Written Language

Sample #21: Boy, Age 17 Years, the Circus Controversy persuasive essay (from the author's files)

MLTU = 15.50   CD = 2.93

C Should animals perform [**MC**] in circuses?

C I believe [**MC**] that being [**GER**] trained to do [**INF**] tricks and to entertain [**INF**] audiences is [**NOM**] a very good use for animals.

C There are [**MC**], however, a couple of sides on this subject.

C Some people think [**MC**] only of the entertainment with no concern for the animals' needs.

C Circuses may not feed [**MC**] the animals well or give [**MC**] them adequate space to live [**INF**] just for a little extra profit.

C It 's [**MC**] also possible that they use [**NOM**] dangerous training techniques.

C These are [**MC**] all negative aspects on animals performing [**GER**] in circuses.

C There is [**MC**] also a good side to having [**GER**] circus animals.

C They can provide [**MC**] much entertainment for both adults and children, performing [**GER**] stunts, tricks, and acrobatics, jumping [**GER**] through fiery hoops, walking [**GER**] on hind legs, things you do n't usually see [**REL**] your pets doing [**PRT**].

C This can also help [**MC**] to eliminate [**INF**] any fears children might have [**REL**] of the performing animals.

C Looking **[PRT]** back at this reasoning and the impressions it gives **[REL]** us, I can see **[MC]** that there is **[NOM]** an easy solution to get **[INF]** rid of the negative aspects.

C Allow **[MC]** for the animals to perform **[INF]** in circuses, but only if they are **[ADV]** treated well, given **[ADV]** enough food, large enough living areas, and trained **[ADV]** without using **[GER]** too harsh punishment.

C Using **[PRT]** this method, there are **[MC]** only positive reasons.

C So why not have **[MC]** animals perform **[INF]** in circuses?

Sample #22: Girl, Age 18 Years, the Circus Controversy persuasive essay (from the author's files)

MLTU = 11.69   CD = 2.44

C I feel **[MC]** that animals performing **[GER]** for our entertainment is **[NOM]** a bad idea!

C We have **[MC]** many other forms of entertainment in this day and age.

C We do not need **[MC]** to force **[INF]** wild animals to do **[INF]** things for our entertainment.

C The animals that are **[REL]** part of circuses do not have **[MC]** the proper habitat that they need **[REL]**.

C They do not have **[MC]** space that they need **[REL]**.

C And they have been known **[MC]** to become **[INF]** violent.

C I do not have **[MC]** a problem with people performing **[GER]**, with cats and dogs, even horses.

C But all of these are **[MC]** domestic animals.

C Tigers, bears, and elephants should not be **[MC]** locked **[PRT]** in small cages, forced **[PRT]** to do **[INF]** tricks, and be **[MC]** poorly treated **[PRT]**.

C There is **[MC]** no reason that people and domestic animals could not give **[REL]** just as good of a performance.

C Wild animals are **[MC]** just that, wild.

C They need **[MC]** to be **[INF]** in habitats that are **[REL]** suitable for them.

C They need **[MC]** to be **[INF]** fed **[PRT]** right and let **[PRT]** to use **[INF]** their instincts.

C Malnutrition, small confined areas, and entertainment for people is **[MC]** not what these creatures are **[NOM]** on this earth for.

C They are **[MC]** animals, not actors.

C And we need **[MC]** to remember **[INF]** this.

References

Afflerbach, P., Beers, J. W., Blachowicz, C., Boyd, C. D., & Diffily, D. (2000). *Scott Foresman reading: Fantastic Voyage* (Vols. 1 & 2). Glenview, IL: Scott Foresman.

Bachelder, L. (1965). *Abraham Lincoln: Wisdom and wit.* Mount Vernon, NY: Peter Pauper Press.

Bamberg, M., & Damrad-Frye, R. (1991). On the ability to provide evaluative comments: Further explorations of children's narrative competencies. *Journal of Child Language, 18,* 689–710.

Bannister, R. (2004). *The four-minute mile: 50th anniversary edition.* Guilford, CT: Lyons Press.

Barako Arndt, K., & Schuele, C. M. (2013). Multiclausal utterances aren't just for big kids: A framework for analysis of complex syntax production in spoken language of preschool- and early school-age children. *Topics in Language Disorders, 33*(2), 125–139.

Barber, C. (1993). *The English language: A historical introduction.* Cambridge, UK: Cambridge University Press.

Baron-Cohen, S., Wheelwright, S., Lawson, J., Griffin, R., Ashwin, C., Billington, J., & Chakrabarti, B. (2005). Empathizing and systemizing in autism spectrum conditions. In F. R. Volkmar, R. Paul, A. Klin, & D. Cohen (Eds.), *Handbook of autism and pervasive developmental disorders, Volume 1: Diagnosis, development, neurobiology, and behavior* (3rd ed., pp. 628–639). Hoboken, NJ: Wiley.

Bearison, D. J., & Gass, S. T. (1979). Hypothetical and practical reasoning: Children's persuasive appeals in different social contexts. *Child Development, 50,* 901–903.

Bedore, L. M., & Leonard, L. B. (1998). Specific language impairment and grammatical morphology: A discriminant function analysis. *Journal of Speech, Language, and Hearing Research, 41,* 1185–1192.

Behrens, H. (2008). Corpora in language acquisition research: History, methods, perspectives. In H. Behrens (Ed.), *Corpora in language acquisition research: History, methods, perspectives* (pp. xi–xxx). Philadelphia, PA: Benjamins.

Benardete, D. (1961). *Mark Twain: Wit and wisecracks.* Mount Vernon, NY: Peter Pauper Press.

Bennett, T., Szatmari, P., Bryson, S., Volden, J., Zwaigenbaum, L., Vaccarella, L., . . . Boyle, M. (2008). Differentiating autism and Asperger syndrome on the basis of language delay or impairment. *Journal of Autism and Developmental Disorders, 38,* 616–625.

Berman, R. (Ed.). (2004). *Language development across childhood and adolescence*. Amsterdam, The Netherlands: Benjamins.

Berman, R. (2008). The psycholinguistics of developing text construction. *Journal of Child Language, 35*(4), 735–771.

Berman, R. A., & Nir, B. (2010). The language of expository discourse across adolescence. In M. A. Nippold & C. M. Scott (Eds.), *Expository discourse in children, adolescents, and adults: Development and disorders* (pp. 99–121). New York, NY: Psychology Press/Taylor & Francis.

Berman, R. A., & Nir-Sagiv, B. (2007). Comparing narrative and expository text construction across adolescence: A developmental paradox. *Discourse Processes, 43*(2), 79–120.

Berman, R. A., & Slobin, D. I. (Eds.). (1994). *Relating events in narrative: A cross-linguistic developmental study*. Hillsdale, NJ: Erlbaum.

Berman, R. A., & Verhoeven, L. (2002). Cross-linguistic perspectives on the development of text-production abilities: Speech and writing. *Written Language and Literacy, 5*(1), 1–43.

Biggs, A., Gregg, K., Hagins, W. C., Kapicka, C., Lundgren, L., Rillero, P., & National Geographic Society. (2002). *Biology: The dynamics of life*. New York, NY: Glencoe/McGraw-Hill.

Bishop, D. V. M. (2004). *Expression, reception, and recall of narrative instrument (ERRNI)*. London, UK: Harcourt Assessment.

Bishop, D. V. M., & Donlan, C. (2005). The role of syntax in encoding and recall of pictorial narratives: Evidence from specific language impairments. *British Journal of Developmental Psychology, 23*, 25–46.

Bloom, L. (1970). *Language development: Form and function in emerging grammars*. Cambridge, MA: MIT Press.

Bloom, L., & Lahey, M. (1978). *Language development and language disorders*. New York, NY: Wiley.

Boerma, T., Leseman, P., Timmermeister, M., Wijnen, F., & Blom, E. (2016). Narrative abilities of monolingual and bilingual children with and without language impairment: Implications for clinical practice. *International Journal of Language and Communication Disorders, 51*(6), 626–638.

Botvin, G. J., & Sutton-Smith, B. (1977). The development of structural complexity in children's fantasy narratives. *Developmental Psychology, 13*, 377–388.

Bragg, B. W. E., Ostrowski, M. V., & Finley, G. E. (1973). The effects of birth order and age of target on use of persuasive techniques. *Child Development, 44*, 351–354.

Braine, M. (1963). The ontogeny of English phrase structure: The first phrase. *Language, 39*, 1–13.

Brinton, B., Robinson, L. A., & Fujiki, M. (2004). Description of a program for social language intervention: "If you can have a conversation, you can have a relationship." *Language, Speech, and Hearing Services in Schools, 35*, 283–290.

Brown, R. (1973). *A first language: The early stages*. Cambridge, MA: Harvard University Press.

Burke, N. (1996). *Teachers are special: A tribute to those who educate, encourage, and inspire*. New York, NY: Gramercy.

Category: Proverbs. (2009). Retrieved from https://en.wikiquote.org/wiki/Category:Proverbs

Centers for Disease Control and Prevention. (2020). *Autism spectrum disorder*. Retrieved from https://www.cdc.gov/ncbddd/autism/data.html

Chaisson, E., & McMillan, S. (2005). *Astronomy today* (5th ed.). Upper Saddle River, NJ: Pearson Prentice Hall.

Channell, M. M., Loveall, S. J., Conners, F. A., Harvey, D. J., & Abbeduto, L. (2018). Narrative language sampling in typical development: Implications for clinical trials. *American Journal of Speech-Language Pathology, 27*(1), 123–135.

Charlton, J. (Ed.). (1994). *A little learning is a dangerous thing*. New York, NY: St. Martins Press.

Chomsky, N. (1957). *Syntactic structures*. The Hague, The Netherlands: Mouton.

Chomsky, N. (1965). *Aspects of the theory of syntax*. Cambridge, MA: MIT Press.

Clark, R. A., & Delia, J. G. (1976). The development of functional persuasive skills in childhood and early adolescence. *Child Development, 47*, 1008–1014.

Cleveland, R. (2006). *The drum: A folktale from India*. Atlanta, GA: August House.

Conti-Ramsden, G., & Durkin, K. (2016). What factors influence language impairment? Considering resilience as well as risk. *Folia Phoniatrica et Logopaedica, 67*, 293–299.

Costanza-Smith, A. (2010). The clinical utility of language samples. *Perspectives on Language Learning and Education, 17*(1), 9–15.

Craig, H. K., & Washington, J. A. (2002). Oral language expectations for African American preschoolers and kindergartners. *American Journal of Speech-Language Pathology, 11*, 59–70.

Craig, H. K., & Washington, J. A. (2004). Grade-related changes in the production of African American English. *Journal of Speech, Language, and Hearing Research, 47*, 450–463.

Craig, H. K., Washington, J. A., & Thompson, C. A. (2005). Oral language expectations for African American children in grades 1 through 5. *American Journal of Speech-Language Pathology, 14*, 119–130.

Craig, H. K., Washington, J. A., & Thompson-Porter, C. (1998). Average c-unit lengths in the discourse of African American children from low-income, urban homes. *Journal of Speech, Language, and Hearing Research, 41*, 433–444.

Creative proverbs from around the world. (2009). Retrieved from http://www.creativeproverbs.com

Crews, F. (1977). *The Random House handbook* (2nd ed.). New York, NY: Random House.

Crowhurst, M. (1980). Syntactic complexity in narration and argument at three grade levels. *Canadian Journal of Education, 5*, 6–13.

Crowhurst, M. (1987). Cohesion in argument and narration at three grade levels. *Research in the Teaching of English, 21*, 185–201.

Crowhurst, M. (1990). Teaching and learning the writing of persuasive/argumentative discourse. *Canadian Journal of Education, 15*, 348–359.

Crowhurst, M., & Piche, G. L. (1979). Audience and mode of discourse effects on syntactic complexity in writing at two grade levels. *Research in the Teaching of English, 13*, 101–109.

Crystal, D. (1996). *Rediscover grammar with David Crystal* (Rev. ed.). Essex, UK: Longman.

Crystal, D. (2002). *The English language: A guided tour of the language* (2nd ed.). London, UK: Penguin.

Crystal, D., Fletcher, P., & Garman, M. (1976). *The grammatical analysis of language disability*. London, UK: Edward Arnold.

Curran, M., & Owen Van Horne, A. (2019). Use of recast intervention to teach causal adverbials to young children with developmental language disorder within a science curriculum: A single case design study. *American Journal of Speech-Language Pathology, 28*(2), 430–447.

Darwin, C. (1877). A biographical sketch of an infant. *Mind, 2*, 285–294.

Darwin, C. (1958). In N. Barlow (Ed.), *The autobiography of Charles Darwin (1809–1882)*. New York, NY: Norton.

Davies, H. (1989). *The good guide to the lakes* (3rd ed.). Loweswater, UK: Forster Davies.

de Villiers, J. G., & de Villiers, P. A. (1973). A cross-sectional study of the acquisition of grammatical morphemes. *Journal of Psycholinguistic Research, 2*, 267–278.

Delia, J. G., Kline, S. L., & Burleson, B. R. (1979). The development of persuasive communication strategies in kindergarten through twelfth-graders. *Communication Monographs, 46*, 241–256.

DiVall-Rayan, J., & Miller, J. F. (2019). Pulling it all together: Examples from our case study files. In J. F. Miller, K. Andriacchi, & A. Nockerts (Eds.), *Assessing language production using SALT software: A clinician's guide to language sample analysis* (3rd ed., pp. 167–230). Madison, WI: SALT Software.

Dumond, V. (1993). *Grammar for grownups*. New York, NY: HarperCollins.

Ebert, K. D. (2020). Language sample analysis with bilingual children: Translating research to practice. *Topics in Language Disorders, 40*(2), 182–201.

Ebert, K. D., & Pham, G. (2017). Synthesizing information from language samples and standardized tests in school-age bilingual assessment. *Language, Speech, and Hearing Services in Schools, 48*, 42–55.

Ebert, K. D., & Scott, C. M. (2014). Relationships between narrative language samples and norm-referenced test scores in language assessments of school-age children. *Language, Speech, and Hearing Services in Schools, 45*, 337–350.

Eder, D. (1988). Building cohesion through collaborative narration. *Social Psychology Quarterly, 51*, 225–235.

Eisenberg, S. L. (2006). Grammar: How can I say that better? In T. A. Ukrainetz (Ed.), *Contextualized language intervention: Scaffolding PreK–12 literacy achievement* (pp. 145–194). Eau Claire, WI: Thinking Publications.

Eisenberg, S. L. (2020). Using general language performance measures to assess grammar learning. *Topics in Language Disorders, 40*(2), 135–148.

Eisenberg, S. L., & Guo, L.-Y. (2013). Differentiating children with and without language impairment based on grammaticality. *Language, Speech, and Hearing Services in Schools, 44*, 20–31.

Eisenberg, S .L., & Guo, L.-Y. (2015). Sample size for measuring grammaticality in preschool children from picture-elicited language samples. *Language, Speech, and Hearing Services in Schools, 46*, 81–93.

Emerson, R. W. (2009). Self-reliance. In Penguin Books (Ed.), *Barack Obama: The inaugural address together with Abraham Lincoln's first and second inaugural addresses and the Gettysburg Address and Ralph Waldo Emerson's Self-Reliance*. New York, NY: Penguin. (Original work published 1841)

Erftmier, T., & Dyson, A. H. (1986). "Oh ppbbt!": Differences between the oral and written persuasive strategies of school-aged children. *Discourse Processes, 9*, 91–114.

Fanning, J. L. (2004, November). *Persuasive writing abilities in school-age children, adolescents, and adults: Applying the data*. Seminar presented at the Annual Convention of the American Speech-Language-Hearing Association, Philadelphia, PA.

Felton, M., & Kuhn, D. (2001). The development of argumentative discourse skill. *Discourse Processes, 32*(2/3), 135–153.

Fey, M. E., Catts, H. W., Proctor-Williams, K., Tomblin, J. B., & Zhang, X. (2004). Oral and written story composition skills of children with language impairment. *Journal of Speech, Language, and Hearing Research, 47*, 1301–1318.

Feynman, R. P. (1996). Introduction to computers. In A. J. G. Hey & R. W. Allen (Eds.), *Feynman lectures on computation* (pp. 1–19). Reading, MA: Addison-Wesley.

Finley, G. E., & Humphreys, C. A. (1974). Naïve psychology and the development of persuasive appeals in girls. *Canadian Journal of Behavioral Science, 6*, 75–80.

Flavell, J. H., Botkin, P. T., Fry, C. L., Wright, J. W., & Jarvis, P. E. (1968). *The development of role-taking and communication skills in children*. New York, NY: Wiley.

Fletcher, P., & Garman, M. (1988). Normal language development and language impairment: Syntax and beyond. *Clinical Linguistics and Phonetics, 2*, 97–114.

Frizelle, P., Thompson, P. A., McDonald, D., & Bishop, D. V. M. (2018). Growth in syntactic complexity between four years and adulthood: Evidence from a narrative task. *Journal of Child Language, 45*, 1174–1197.

Fuller, M. (1999). In J. T. Pine (Ed.), *Woman in the nineteenth century: Dover Thrift Editions*. New York, NY: Dover. (Original work published 1845)

Gage, J. T. (1991). *The shape of reason: Argumentative writing in college* (2nd ed.). New York, NY: Macmillan.

German, D. (2014). *Test of Word Finding–Third edition*. Austin, TX: Pro-Ed.

German, D. (2016). *Adolescent/Adult Word Finding–Second edition*. Austin, TX: Pro-Ed.

Geurts, H. M., & Embrechts, M. (2008). Language profiles in ASD, SLI, and ADHD. *Journal of Autism and Developmental Disorders, 38*, 1931–1943.

Gillam, R. B., & Johnston, J. R. (1992). Spoken and written language relationships in language/learning-impaired and normally achieving school-age children. *Journal of Speech and Hearing Research, 35*, 1303–1315.

Gillam, R. B., & Peña, E. D. (2004, July). Dynamic assessment of children from culturally diverse backgrounds. *Communication Disorders and Sciences in Culturally and Linguistically Diverse Populations, 11*(2), 2–5.

Graham, S., & Perin, D. (2007). A meta-analysis of writing instruction for adolescent students. *Journal of Educational Psychology, 99*(1), 445–476.

Graham-Bethea, J., & Kamhi, A. (2019). The impact of African American English on language proficiency in adolescent speakers. *Journal of the National Black Association for Speech-Language and Hearing, 14*(1), 97–115.

Grammar: Parts of speech. (2009). Retrieved from http://www.eslus.com/LESSONS/GRAMMAR/POS/pos1.htm

Great Quotations. (1990). *Teacher's inspirations: Motivational quotes for you and your students*. Glendale Heights, IL: Author.

Grosset & Dunlap. (1947). *Aesop's fables*. New York, NY: Author.

Guo, L.-Y., Eisenberg, S., Schneider, P., & Spencer, L. (2020). Finite verb morphology composite between age 4 and age 9 for the Edmonton Narrative Norms Instrument: Reference data and psychometric properties. *Language, Speech, and Hearing Services in Schools, 51*, 128–143.

Guo, L.-Y., & Schneider, P. (2016). Differentiating school-aged children with and without language impairment using tense and grammaticality measures from a narrative task. *Journal of Speech, Language, and Hearing Research, 59*, 317–329.

Gutiérrez-Clellen, V. F., Restrepo, M. A., Bedore, L., Peña, E., & Anderson, R. (2000). Language sample analysis in Spanish-speaking children: Methodological considerations. *Language, Speech, and Hearing Services in Schools, 31*(1), 88–98.

Hadley, P. A. (1998). Language sampling protocols for eliciting text-level discourse. *Language, Speech, and Hearing Services in Schools, 29*, 132–147.

Ham, A., Burke, A., Carillet, J., Kohn, M., Gordon, F. L., Maxwell, V., & Mayhew, B. (2006). *Middle East* (5th ed.). Oakland, CA: Lonely Planet.

Hamilton, M-B., Mont, E. V., & McLain, C. (2018). Deletion, omission, reduction: Redefining the language we use to talk about African American English. *Perspectives of the ASHA Special Interest Groups, SIG 1, 30*(3), 107-117.

Harris, J. (1989). *The land and people of France.* New York, NY: Lippincott.

Hauser, S. (2008). *The proverbial cat: 2009 calendar.* Portland, ME: Sellers.

Heilmann, J., DeBrock, L., & Riley-Tillman, C. (2013). Stability of measures from children's interviews: The effects of time, sample length, and topic. *American Journal of Speech-Language Pathology, 22*(3), 463–475.

Heilmann, J., & Malone, T. O. (2014). The rules of the game: Properties of a database of expository language samples. *Language, Speech, and Hearing Services in Schools, 45*(4), 277–290.

Heilmann, J., Malone, T. O., & Westerveld, M. F. (2020). Properties of spoken persuasive language samples from typically developing adolescents. *Language, Speech, and Hearing Services in Schools, 51*(2), 441–456.

Heilmann, J., Miller, J. F., & Nockerts, A. (2010). Using language sample databases. *Language, Speech, and Hearing Services in Schools, 41*, 84–95.

Heilmann, J., Miller, J. F., Nockerts, A., & Dunaway, C. (2010). Properties of the narrative scoring scheme using narrative retells in young school-age children. *American Journal of Speech-Language Pathology, 19*, 154–166.

Heilmann, J. J. (2010). Myths and realities of language sample analysis. *Perspectives on Language Learning and Education, 17*, 4–8.

Heilmann, J. J., Rojas, R., Iglesias, A., & Miller, J. F. (2016). Clinical impact of wordless picture storybooks on bilingual narrative language production: A comparison of "Frog" stories. *International Journal of Language and Communication Disorders, 51*(3), 339–345.

Hewitt, L. E., Hammer, C. S., Yont, K. M., & Tomblin, J. B. (2005). Language sampling for kindergarten children with and without SLI: Mean length of utterance, IPSYN, and NDW. *Journal of Communication Disorders, 38*(3), 197–213.

Horton, R., & Apel, K. (2014). Examining the use of spoken dialect indices with African American children in the southern United States. *American Journal of Speech-Language Pathology, 23*, 448–460.

Horton-Ikard, R., & Pittman, R. T. (2010). Examining the writing of adolescent African American English speakers: Suggestions for assessment and intervention. *Topics in Language Disorders, 30*(3), 189–204.

Hoskins, B. (1996). *Conversations: A framework for language intervention* (Rev. ed.). Eau Claire, WI: Thinking Publications.

Howlin, P. (2005). Outcomes in autism spectrum disorders. In F. R. Volkmar, R. Paul, A. Klin, & D. Cohen (Eds.), *Handbook of autism and pervasive develop-*

mental disorders, Volume 1: Diagnosis, development, neurobiology, and behavior (3rd ed., pp. 201–221). Hoboken, NJ: Wiley.

Hulit, L. M., Howard, M. R., & Fahey, K. R. (2011). *Born to talk: An introduction to speech and language development* (5th ed.). Boston, MA: Pearson.

Humphreys, M. W. (1880). A contribution to infantile linguistics. *Transactions of the American Philological Association, 11,* 5–17.

Hunt, K. W. (1970). Syntactic maturity in school children and adults. *Monographs of the Society for Research in Child Development,* Serial No. 134, Vol. 35, No. 1.

Ingram, D. (1989). *First language acquisition: Method, description, and explanation.* Cambridge, UK: Cambridge University Press.

Ivy, L. J., & Masterson, J. J. (2011). A comparison of oral and written English styles in African American students at different stages of writing development. *Language, Speech, and Hearing Services in Schools, 42,* 31–40.

Jarvie, G. (2007). *Bloomsbury grammar guide* (2nd ed.). London, UK: A & C Black.

Johnson, V. E., & Koonce, N. M. (2018). Language sampling considerations for AAE speakers: A patterns- and systems-based approach. *Perspectives of the ASHA Special Interest Groups, Sig. 1, 3*(1), 36–42.

Jones, D. C. (1985). Persuasive appeals and responses to appeals among friends and acquaintances. *Child Development, 56,* 757–763.

Jones, R. M., McLeod, J. C., Krockover, G. H, Frank, M. S., Lang, M. P., Valenta, C. J., & Van Deman, B. A. (2002). *Harcourt science teacher's edition, life science units A and B.* Orlando, FL: Harcourt.

Justice, L. M., Bowles, R. P., Kaderavek, J. N., Ukrainetz, T. A., Eisenberg, S. L., & Gillam, R. B. (2006). The index of narrative microstructure: A clinical tool for analyzing school-age children's narrative performances. *American Journal of Speech-Language Pathology, 15,* 177–191.

Kapantzoglou, M., Fergadiotis, G., & Restrepo, M. A. (2017). Language sample analysis and elicitation technique effects in bilingual children with and without language impairment. *Journal of Speech, Language, and Hearing Research, 60,* 2852–2864.

Kelly, M. (2020a). *High school debate topics.* Retrieved from https://www.thoughtco.com/debate-topics-for-high-school-8252

Kelly, M. (2020b). *Middle school debate topics.* Retrieved from https://www.thoughtco.com/debate-topics-for-middle-school-8014

Kernan, K. T. (1977). Semantic and expressive elaboration in children's narratives. In S. Ervin-Tripp & C. Mitchell-Kernan (Eds.), *Child discourse* (pp. 91–102). New York, NY: Academic Press.

Kester, E. (2020). Conducting student speech-language evaluations via telepractice. *The ASHA Leader, 25*(5), 36–37.

Klecan-Aker, J. S., & Caraway, T. H. (1997). A study of the relationship of storytelling ability and reading comprehension in fourth and sixth grade African-American children. *European Journal of Disorders of Communication, 32,* 109–125.

Klecan-Aker, J. S., & Hedrick, D. L. (1985). A study of syntactic language skills of normal school-age children. *Language, Speech, and Hearing Services in Schools, 16,* 187–198.

Knudsen, R. E. (1992). The development of written argumentation: An analysis and comparison of argumentative writing at four grade levels. *Child Study Journal, 22,* 167–184.

Kroll, B. M. (1984). Audience adaptation in children's persuasive letters. *Written Communication, 1,* 407–427.

Lahey, M. (1990). Who shall be called language disordered? Some reflections and one perspective. *Journal of Speech and Hearing Disorders, 55*(4), 612–620.

Landa, R. J., & Goldberg, M. C. (2005). Language, social, and executive functions in high functioning autism: A continuum of performance. *Journal of Autism and Developmental Disorders, 35,* 557–573.

Larson, V. L., & McKinley, N. (2003). *Communication solutions for older students: Assessment and intervention strategies.* Eau Claire, WI: Thinking Publications.

Launer, P. B., & Lahey, M. (1981). Passages: From the fifties to the eighties in language assessment. *Topics in Language Disorders, 1*(3), 11–29.

Lawrence, J. (1997). *Aesop's fables.* Seattle, WA: University of Washington Press.

Leadholm, B. J., & Miller, J. F. (1992). *Language sample analysis: The Wisconsin guide.* Madison, WI: Wisconsin Department of Public Instruction.

Lee, L. L. (1974). *Developmental sentence analysis: A grammatical assessment procedure for speech and language clinicians.* Evanston, IL: Northwestern University Press.

Lee, L. L., & Canter, S. M. (1971). Developmental sentence scoring: A clinical procedure for estimating syntactic development in children's spontaneous speech. *Journal of Speech and Hearing Disorders, 36,* 315–340.

Leonard, L. B. (2014). *Children with specific language impairment* (2nd ed.). Cambridge, MA: MIT Press.

Leopold, W. F. (1939–1949). *Speech development of a bilingual child: A linguist's record* (Vols. 1–4). Evanston, IL: Northwestern University Press.

Lester, H. (1986). *A porcupine named Fluffy.* Boston, MA: Houghton Mifflin.

Lester, H. (1987). *Pookins gets her way.* Boston, MA: Houghton Mifflin.

Lewis, F. M., Murdoch, B. E., & Woodyatt, G. C. (2007). Communicative competence and metalinguistic ability: Performance by children and adults with autism spectrum disorder. *Journal of Autism and Developmental Disorders, 37,* 1525–1538.

Liles, B. Z. (1985). Narrative ability in normal and language disordered children. *Journal of Speech and Hearing Research, 28,* 123–133.

Liles, B. Z. (1987). Episode organization and cohesive conjunctives in narratives of children with and without language disorders. *Journal of Speech and Hearing Research, 30,* 185–196.

Liles, B. Z. (1993). Narrative discourse in children with language disorders and children with normal language: A critical review of the literature. *Journal of Speech and Hearing Research, 36,* 868–882.

Liles, B. Z., Duffy, R. J., Merritt, D. D., & Purcell, S. L. (1995). Measurement of narrative discourse ability in children with language disorders. *Journal of Speech and Hearing Research, 38,* 415–425.

Loban, W. (1976). *Language development: Kindergarten through grade twelve.* Urbana, IL: National Council of Teachers of English.

Long, S., & Fey, M. (1993). *Computerized profiling* [Computer program; version 7.2]. Ithaca, NY: Computerized Profiling.

Loveland, K. A., & Tunali-Kotoski, B. (2005). The school-age child with an autistic spectrum disorder. In F. R. Volkmar, R. Paul, A. Klin, & D. Cohen (Eds.), *Handbook of autism and pervasive developmental disorders, Volume 1: Diagnosis, development, neurobiology, and behavior* (3rd ed., pp. 247–287). Hoboken, NJ: Wiley.

Luciano, A., Batzella, G., Borghese, D. A. S., Borghese, D. M., Callen, A. T., Carluccio, A., . . . Rando, R. (1991). *Italy: A culinary journey*. San Francisco, CA: Collins.

Lundine, J. P. (2020). Assessing expository discourse abilities across elementary, middle, and high school. *Topics in Language Disorders, 40*(2), 149–165.

Lundine, J. P., & McCauley, R. J. (2016). A tutorial on expository discourse: Structure, development, and disorders in children and adolescents. *American Journal of Speech-Language Pathology, 25*, 306–320.

Lynch, J. (1978). Evaluation of linguistic disorders in children. In S. Singh & J. Lynch (Eds.), *Diagnostic procedures in hearing, language, and speech* (pp. 327–378). Baltimore, MD: University Park Press.

MacWhinney, B. (1988). *CLAN: Child Language Analysis: Manual for the CLAN programs of the Child Language Data Exchange System*. Pittsburgh, PA: Carnegie Mellon University.

Marinellie, S. A. (2004). Complex syntax used by school-age children with specific language impairment (SLI) in child–adult conversation. *Journal of Communication Disorders, 37*, 517–533.

Mayer, M. (1969). *Frog, where are you?* New York, NY: Dial Press.

Mayer, M. (1973). *Frog on his own*. New York, NY: Dial Press.

Mayer, M. (1974). *Frog goes to dinner*. New York, NY: Dial Press.

McCabe, A., Bliss, L., Barra, G., & Bennett, M. (2008). Comparison of personal versus fictional narratives of children with language impairment. *American Journal of Speech-Language Pathology, 17*, 194–206.

McCann, T. M. (1989). Student argumentative writing knowledge and ability at three grade levels. *Research in the Teaching of English, 23*, 62–76.

McCarthy, D. (1930). The language development of the preschool child. *Institute of Child Welfare Monograph Series 4*. Minneapolis, MN: University of Minnesota Press.

McClenaghan, W. A. (2005). *Magruder's American government* (Teacher's ed.). Upper Saddle River, NJ: Pearson Prentice Hall.

McDougal Littell. (2006). *The language of literature: British literature* (Teacher's ed.). Evanston, IL: McDougal Littell/Houghton Mifflin.

McFadden, T., & Gillam, R. (1996). An examination of the quality of narratives produced by children with language disorders. *Language, Speech, and Hearing Services in Schools, 27*, 48–56.

McLellan, V. (1996). *The complete book of practical proverbs and wacky wit*. Wheaton, IL: Tyndale House.

McNeilly, L. (2018). From my perspective: Why we need to practice at the top of the license. *ASHA Leader, 23*(2), 10–11.

Merritt, D. D., & Liles, B. Z. (1987). Story grammar ability in children with and without language disorders: Story generation, story retelling, and story comprehension. *Journal of Speech and Hearing Research, 30*, 539–551.

Merritt, D. D., & Liles, B. Z. (1989). Narrative analysis: Clinical applications of story generation and story retelling. *Journal of Speech and Hearing Disorders, 54*, 438–447.

Miller, J. F. (1981). *Assessing language production in children: Experimental procedures*. Baltimore, MD: University Park Press.

Miller, J. F. (2009). New database: Helps identify, monitor older students. *Advance for Speech-Language Pathologists & Audiologists, 19*(8), 4–7.

Miller, J. F., Andriacchi, K., & Nockerts, A. (2016). Using language sample analysis to assess spoken language production in adolescents. *Language, Speech, and Hearing Services in Schools, 47*, 99–112.

Miller, J. F., Andriacchi, K., & Nockerts, A. (2019). *Assessing language production using SALT software: A clinician's guide to language sample analysis* (3rd ed.). Madison, WI: SALT Software.

Miller, J. F., & Chapman, R. (1983). *Systematic analysis of language transcripts.* Madison, WI: University of Wisconsin–Madison, Language Analysis Laboratory, Waisman Center on Mental Retardation and Human Development.

Miller, J. F., & Chapman, R. (2003). *SALT: Systematic Analysis of Language Transcripts* [Computer software]. Madison, WI: University of Wisconsin–Madison, Waisman Center, Language Analysis Laboratory.

Miller, J. F., Heilmann, J., Nockerts, A., Iglesias, A., Fabiano, L., & Francis, D. J. (2006). Oral language and reading in bilingual children. *Learning Disabilities Research & Practice, 21*(1), 30–43.

Miller, W., & Ervin, S. (1964). The development of grammar in child language. In U. Bellugi & R. Brown (Eds.), *The acquisition of language: Monograph of the Society for Research in Child Development, 29* (Serial No. 92, pp. 9–34). New York, NY: Wiley.

Mills, M. T., Watkins, R. V., & Washington, J. A. (2013). Structural and dialectal characteristics of the fictional and personal narratives of school-age African American Children. *Language, Speech, and Hearing Services in Schools, 44*, 211–223.

Moffet, C. (2006). Sarkis Antikajian. *Jerry Williams' Quarterly, 3*(3), 18–19.

Moran, C., & Gillon, G. T. (2010). Expository discourse in older children and adolescents with traumatic brain injury. In M. A. Nippold & C. M. Scott (Eds.), *Expository discourse in children, adolescents, and adults: Development and disorders* (pp. 275–301). New York, NY: Psychology Press/Taylor & Francis.

Moran, C., Kirk, C., & Powell, E. (2012). Spoken persuasive discourse abilities of adolescents with acquired brain injury. *Language, Speech, and Hearing Services in Schools, 43*, 264–275.

National Governors Association Center for Best Practices and Council of Chief State School Officers. (2010). *Common core state standards for English language arts.* Retrieved from http://www.corestandards.org

Nelson, N. W. (1998). *Childhood language disorders in context: Infancy through adolescence* (2nd ed.). Boston, MA: Allyn & Bacon.

Nelson, N. W. (2010). *Language and literacy disorders: Infancy through adolescence.* Boston, MA: Allyn & Bacon.

Newcomer, P. L., & Hammill, D. D. (2019). *Test of Language Development–Primary: Fifth Edition.* Austin, TX: Pro-Ed.

Nippold, M. A. (1999). Word definition in adolescents as a function of reading proficiency. *Child Language Teaching and Therapy, 15*(2), 171–176.

Nippold, M. A. (2000). Language development during the adolescent years: Aspects of pragmatics, syntax, and semantics. *Topics in Language Disorders, 20*(2), 15–28.

Nippold, M. A. (2007). *Later language development: School-age children, adolescents, and young adults* (3rd ed.). Austin, TX: Pro-Ed.

Nippold, M. A. (2009). School-age children talk about chess: Does knowledge drive syntactic complexity? *Journal of Speech, Language, and Hearing Research, 52*, 856–871.

Nippold, M. A. (2010a). Explaining complex matters: How knowledge of a domain drives language. In M. A. Nippold & C. M. Scott (Eds.), *Expository discourse in children, adolescents, and adults: Development and disorders* (pp. 41–61). New York, NY: Psychology Press/Taylor & Francis.

Nippold, M. A. (2010b). It's NOT too late to help adolescents succeed in school [From the editor]. *Language, Speech, and Hearing Services in Schools, 41,* 137–138.

Nippold, M. A. (2014). Language intervention at the middle school: Complex talk reflects complex thought. *Language, Speech, and Hearing Services in Schools, 45,* 153–156.

Nippold, M. A. (2016). *Later language development: School-age children, adolescents, and young adults* (4th ed.). Austin, TX: Pro-Ed.

Nippold, M. A., Cramond, P. M., & Hayward-Mayhew, C. (2014). Spoken language production in adults: Examining age-related differences in syntactic complexity. *Clinical Linguistics & Phonetics, 28*(3), 195–207.

Nippold, M. A., Frantz-Kaspar, M. W., Cramond, P. M., Kirk, C., Hayward-Mayhew, C., & MacKinnon, M. (2014). Conversational and narrative speaking in adolescents: Examining the use of complex syntax. *Journal of Speech, Language, and Hearing Research, 57,* 876–886.

Nippold, M. A., Frantz-Kaspar, M. W., Cramond, P. M., Kirk, C., Hayward-Mayhew, C., & MacKinnon, M. (2015). Critical thinking about fables: Examining language production and comprehension in adolescents. *Journal of Speech, Language, and Hearing Research, 58*(2), 325–335.

Nippold, M. A., Frantz-Kaspar, M. W., & Vigeland, L. M. (2017). Spoken language production in young adults: Examining syntactic complexity. *Journal of Speech, Language, and Hearing Research, 60,* 1339–1347.

Nippold, M. A., & Hayward, C. (2018). Narrative speaking in adolescents: Monitoring progress during intervention. *Perspectives of the ASHA Special Interest Groups, SIG 1, 3*(Pt. 4), 198–210.

Nippold, M. A., Hegel, S. L., Sohlberg, M. M., & Schwarz, I. E. (1999). Defining abstract entities: Development in pre-adolescents, adolescents, and young adults. *Journal of Speech, Language, and Hearing Research, 41*(2), 473–481.

Nippold, M. A., & Hesketh, L. J. (2009, June). *Expository discourse in adolescents with autism spectrum disorders: Examining the use of complex syntax.* Poster presented at the 30th anniversary of the Symposium on Research in Child Language Disorders, University of Wisconsin, Madison, WI.

Nippold, M. A., Hesketh, L. J., Duthie, J. K., & Mansfield, T. C. (2005). Conversational versus expository discourse: A study of syntactic development in children, adolescents, and adults. *Journal of Speech, Language, and Hearing Research, 48,* 1048–1064.

Nippold, M. A., LaFavre, S., & Shinham, K. (2020). How adolescents interpret the moral messages of fables: Examining the development of critical thinking. *Journal of Speech, Language, and Hearing Research, 63*(4), 1212–1226.

Nippold, M. A., Mansfield, T. C., & Billow, J. L. (2007). Peer conflict explanations in children, adolescents, and adults: Examining the development of complex syntax. *American Journal of Speech-Language Pathology, 16,* 179–188.

Nippold, M. A., Mansfield, T. C., Billow, J. L., & Tomblin, J. B. (2008). Expository discourse in adolescents with language impairments: Examining syntactic development. *American Journal of Speech-Language Pathology, 17,* 356–366.

Nippold, M. A., Mansfield, T. C., Billow, J. L., & Tomblin, J. B. (2009). Syntactic development in adolescents with a history of language impairments: A follow-up investigation. *American Journal of Speech-Language Pathology, 18*, 241–251.

Nippold, M. A., Moran, C., Mansfield, T. C., & Gillon, G. (2005, July). *Expository discourse development in American and New Zealand youth: A cross-cultural comparison.* Poster presented at the Xth International Congress for the Study of Child Language (IASCL), Freie Universitat, Berlin, Germany.

Nippold, M. A., & Scott, C. M. (2010). Overview of expository discourse: Development and disorders. In M. A. Nippold & C. M. Scott (Eds.), *Expository discourse in children, adolescents, and adults: Development and disorders* (pp. 1–11). New York, NY: Psychology Press/Taylor & Francis.

Nippold, M. A., & Sun, L. (2010). Expository writing in children and adolescents: A classroom assessment tool. *Perspectives on Language Learning and Education: Adolescent Language, 17*, 100–107.

Nippold, M. A., Vigeland, L. M., Frantz-Kaspar, M. W., & Ward-Lonergan, J. (2017). Language sampling with adolescents: Building a normative database with fables. *American Journal of Speech-Language Pathology, 26*, 908–920.

Nippold, M. A., & Ward-Lonergan, J. (2010). Argumentative writing in preadolescents: The role of verbal reasoning. *Child Language Teaching and Therapy, 26*, 238–248.

Nippold, M. A., Ward-Lonergan, J., & Fanning, J. L. (2005). Persuasive writing in children, adolescents, and adults: A study of syntactic, semantic, and pragmatic development. *Language, Speech, and Hearing Services in Schools, 36*, 125–138.

Norbury, C. F., & Bishop, D. V. M. (2003). Narrative skills of children with communication impairments. *International Journal of Language and Communication Disorders, 38*(3), 287–313.

Obama, B. (2009). *Inaugural address.* New York, NY: Penguin.

Oliva-Rasbach, J., & Schmidt, C. W. (1994). *Viva la Mediterranean.* Englewood, CO: HealthMark Centers.

Parker, J. L. (2009). *Once a runner: A novel* (1st Scribner hardcover ed.). New York, NY: Scribner/Simon & Schuster.

Paul, R. (2007). *Language disorders from infancy through adolescence: Assessment and intervention* (3rd ed.). St. Louis, MO: Mosby/Elsevier.

Paul, R., & Norbury, C. F. (2012). *Language disorders from infancy through adolescence: Listening, speaking, reading, writing, and communicating* (4th ed.). St. Louis, MO: Elsevier.

Paul, R., Orlovski, S. M., Marcinko, H. C., & Volkmar, F. (2009). Conversational behaviors in youth with high-functioning ASD and Asperger syndrome. *Journal of Autism and Developmental Disorders, 39*, 115–125.

Pavelko, S. L., Owens, R. E., Ireland, M., & Hahs-Vaughn, D. (2016). Use of language sample analysis by school-based SLPs: Results of a nationwide survey. *Language, Speech, and Hearing Services in Schools, 47*, 246–258.

Pearson, B. Z., Jackson, J. E., & Wu, H. (2014). Seeking a valid gold standard for an innovative, dialect-neutral language test. *Journal of Speech, Language, and Hearing Research, 57*, 495–508.

Peña, E. D., Gillam, R. B., & Bedore, L. M. (2014). Dynamic assessment of narrative ability in English accurately identifies language impairment in English Language Learners. *Journal of Speech, Language, and Hearing Research, 57*, 2208–2220.

Perry, V. (2017). A mixed methods study of expository paragraph writing in English-proficient, Hispanic, middle school students with writing weaknesses. *Perspectives of the ASHA Special Interest Groups Sig 1, 2*(3), 151–167.

Peter Pauper Press. (1963). *The wisdom of Confucius*. Mount Vernon, NY: Author.

Petersen, D. B., Chanthongthip, H., Ukrainetz, T. A., Spencer, T. D., & Steeve, R. W. (2017). Dynamic assessment of narratives: Efficient, accurate identification of language impairment in bilingual students. *Journal of Speech, Language, and Hearing Research, 60*, 983–998.

Pezold, M. J., Imgrund, C. M., & Storkel, H. L. (2020). Using computer programs for language sample analysis. *Language, Speech, and Hearing Services in Schools, 51*, 103–114.

Piche, G. L., Rubin, D. L., & Michlin, M. L. (1978). Age and social class in children's use of persuasive communicative appeals. *Child Development, 49*, 773–780.

Pine, J. T. (1999). *Woman in the nineteenth century*. Mineola, NY: Dover.

Politis, V., Reich, A. A., & Sheldon, R. (1998). *Russian proverbs: 100 favorites of Professor Nadezhda Timofeevna Koroton*. Hanover, NH: Dartmouth Triad Associates.

Popham, P. (1992). *The insider's guide to Japan*. Edison, NJ: Hunter.

Prath, S. (2018, June 10). The how and why of collecting a language sample. *Leader Live*. Retrieved from https://leader.pubs.asha.org/do/10.1044/the-how-and-why-of-collecting-a-language-sample/full

Preyer, W. (1889). *The mind of the child* (translation of the original German edition of 1882). New York, NY: Appleton.

Price, L. H., Hendricks, S., & Cook, C. (2010). Incorporating computer-aided language sample analysis into clinical practice. *Language, Speech, and Hearing Services in Schools, 41*, 206–222.

Quirk, R., & Greenbaum, S. (1973). *A concise grammar of contemporary English*. New York, NY: Harcourt Brace Jovanovich.

Quirk, R., Greenbaum, S., Leech, G., & Svartvik, J. (1985). *A comprehensive grammar of the English language*. New York, NY: Longman.

Quotable Shakespeare. (n.d.). *A knowledge cards deck from the plays of William Shakespeare*. Rohnert Park, CA: Pomegranate.

Quotations Page. Retrieved from http://www.quotationspage.com

Ravid, D., & Berman, R. A. (2006). Information density in the development of spoken and written narratives in English and Hebrew. *Discourse Processes, 41*(2), 117–149.

Retherford, K. (1993). *Guide to analysis of language transcripts* (2nd ed.). Eau Claire, WI: Thinking Publications.

Reutzel, D. R. (2009). Reading fluency: What every SLP and teacher should know. *ASHA Leader, 14*(5), 10, 12–13.

Rice, M. L., Smolik, F., Perpich, D., Thompson, T., Rytting, N., & Blossom, M. (2010). Mean length of utterance levels in 6-month intervals for children 3 to 9 years with and without language impairments. *Journal of Speech, Language, and Hearing Research, 53*, 333–349.

Ritter, E. M. (1979). Social perspective-taking ability, cognitive complexity, and listener-adapted communication in early and late adolescence. *Communication Monographs, 46*, 40–51.

Robertson, S. (2009). Connecting reading fluency and oral language for student success. *ASHA Leader, 14*(5), 11.

Robinson, D., & Groves, J. (2004). *Introducing philosophy*. Cambridge, UK: Icon Books.

Robinson, D., & Groves, J. (2005). *Introducing Plato*. Cambridge, UK: Icon Books.

Rojas, R., & Iglesias, A. (2019). Assessing the bilingual (Spanish/English) population. In J. F. Miller, K. Andriacchi, & A. Nockerts (Eds.), *Assessing language production using SALT software: A clinician's guide to language sample analysis* (3rd ed., pp. 115–127). Madison, WI: SALT Software.

Roseberry-McKibbin, C., & O'Hanlon, L. (2005). Nonbiased assessment of English language learners. *Communication Disorders Quarterly, 26*(3), 178–185.

Roth, F. P., & Spekman, N. J. (1986). Narrative discourse: Spontaneously generated stories of learning-disabled and normally achieving students. *Journal of Speech and Hearing Disorders, 51*, 8–23.

Rubin, D. L., & Piche, G. L. (1979). Development in syntactic and strategic aspects of audience adaptation skills in written persuasive communication. *Research in the Teaching of English, 13*, 293–316.

Saddler, B., & Graham, S. (2005). The effects of peer-assisted sentence-combining instruction on the writing performance of more and less skilled young writers. *Journal of Educational Psychology, 97*(1), 43–54.

Scheffler, A. (1997). *Let sleeping dogs lie and other proverbs from around the world*. Hauppauge, NY: Barron's.

Schickedanz, J. A., Schickedanz, D. I., Forsyth, P. D., & Forsyth, G. A. (2001). *Understanding children and adolescents* (4th ed.). Boston, MA: Allyn & Bacon.

Schneider, P., Dubé, R. V., & Hayward, D. (2005). *The Edmonton Narrative Norms Instrument*. Retrieved from http://www.rehabresearch.ualberta.ca/enni

Scott, C. M. (1988). A perspective on the evaluation of school children's narratives. *Language, Speech, and Hearing Services in Schools, 19*, 67–82.

Scott, C. M. (2009). A case for the sentence in reading comprehension. *Language, Speech, and Hearing Services in Schools, 40*, 184–191.

Scott, C. M. (2020). Language sample analysis: New and neglected clinical applications. *Topics in Language Disorders, 40*(2), 132–134.

Scott, C. M., & Nelson, N. W. (2009). Sentence combining: Assessment and intervention applications. *Perspectives on Language Learning and Education, 16*(1), 14–20.

Scott, C. M., & Windsor, J. (2000). General language performance measures in spoken and written narrative and expository discourse in school-age children with language learning disabilities. *Journal of Speech, Language, and Hearing Research, 43*, 324–339.

Searls, D. (Ed.). (2009). *The Journal, 1837–1861, Henry David Thoreau, Feb. 23, 1860 entry*. New York, NY: New York Review of Books.

Selman, R. L., Beardslee, W., Schultz, L. H., Krupa, M., & Podorefsky, D. (1986). Assessing adolescent interpersonal negotiation strategies: Toward the integration of structural and functional models. *Developmental Psychology, 22*, 450–459.

Shea, V., & Mesibov, G. B. (2005). Adolescents and adults with autism. In F. R. Volkmar, R. Paul, A. Klin, & D. Cohen (Eds.), *Handbook of autism and pervasive developmental disorders, Volume 1: Diagnosis, development, neurobiology, and behavior* (3rd ed., pp. 288–311). Hoboken, NJ: Wiley.

Sigman, M., & McGovern, C. W. (2005). Improvement in cognitive and language skills from preschool to adolescence in autism. *Journal of Autism and Developmental Disorders, 35*(1), 15–23.

Smith, K. J. (1995). *The nature of mathematics* (7th ed.). Pacific Grove, CA: Brooks/ Cole.

Smith, M. (1926). An investigation of the development of the sentence and the extent of vocabulary in young children. *University of Iowa Studies in Child Welfare, 3*(5).

Steig, W. (1982). *Doctor De Soto.* New York, NY: Farrar, Straus & Giroux.

Stein, N. L., & Glenn, C. G. (1979). An analysis of story comprehension in elementary school children. In R. O. Freedle (Ed.), *New directions in discourse processing* (Vol. 2, pp. 53–120). Norwood, NJ: Ablex.

Stewart, J. (1997). *African proverbs and wisdom.* Secaucus, NJ: Carol Publishing/ Citadel Press.

Strong, C. J., Mayer, M., & Mayer, M. (1998). *The Strong Narrative Assessment Procedure (SNAP).* Eau Claire, WI: Thinking Publications.

Strong, C. J., & Shaver, J. (1991). Stability of cohesion in the spoken narratives of language-impaired and normally developing school-aged children. *Journal of Speech and Hearing Research, 34,* 95–111.

Style, S. (1993). *Honey: From hive to honeypot.* San Francisco, CA: Chronicle Books.

Sullivan, W. L. (2008). *Oregon's greatest natural disasters.* Eugene, OR: Navillus Press.

Sumner, W. G. (1906). *Folkways: A study of the sociological importance of usages, manners, customs, mores, and morals.* Boston, MA: Ginn.

Sun, L., & Nippold, M. A. (2012). Narrative writing in children and adolescents: Examining the literate lexicon. *Language, Speech, and Hearing Services in Schools, 43,* 2–13.

Tager-Flusberg, H. (2004). Strategies for conducting research on language in autism. *Journal of Autism and Developmental Disorders, 34,* 75–80.

Tager-Flusberg, H., Paul, R., & Lord, C. (2005). Language and communication in autism. In F. R. Volkmar, R. Paul, A. Klin, & D. Cohen (Eds.), *Handbook of autism and pervasive developmental disorders, Volume 1: Diagnosis, development, neurobiology, and behavior* (3rd ed., pp. 335–364). Hoboken, NJ: Wiley.

Taine, H. (1877). On the acquisition of language by children. *Mind, 2,* 252–259.

Teachers need to be healthy. (2009, March 22). *The Register-Guard,* Eugene, OR, p. A12.

Tekiela, S. (2001). *Birds of Oregon field guide.* Cambridge, MN: Adventure Publications.

Templin, M. (1957). Certain language skills in children. *University of Minnesota Institute of Child Welfare Monograph Series 26.* Minneapolis, MN: University of Minnesota Press.

Thankful Kids. (2009, November 26). *The Register-Guard,* Eugene, OR, pp. A1, A12.

Thomas, D. (1954). *A child's Christmas in Wales.* New York, NY: New Directions.

Thompson, C. A., Craig, H. K., & Washington, J. A. (2004). Variable production of African American English across oracy and literacy contexts. *Language, Speech, and Hearing Services in Schools, 35,* 269–282.

Thoreau, H. D. (2004). *Walden: A fully annotated edition.* New Haven, CT: Yale University Press.

Timler, G. R. (2018). Using language sample analysis to access pragmatic skills in school-age children and adolescents. *Perspectives of the ASHA Special Interest Groups: Sig 1, 3*(Pt. 1), 23–35.

Tomalin, B. (2003). *Culture smart! France.* Portland, OR: Graphic Arts Center.

Tomblin, J. B., & Nippold, M. A. (2014). Features of language impairment in the school years. In J. B. Tomblin & M. A. Nippold (Eds.), *Understanding individual differences in language development across the school years* (pp. 79–116). New York, NY: Psychology Press/Taylor & Francis.

Toulmin, S. E. (1958). *The uses of argument.* London, UK: Cambridge University Press.

Trantham, C. R., & Pedersen, J. K. (1976). *Normal language development: The key to diagnosis and therapy for language-disordered children.* Baltimore, MD: Williams & Wilkins.

Tyack, D., & Gottsleben, R. (1974). *Language sampling, analysis, and training: A handbook for teachers and clinicians.* Palo Alto, CA: Consulting Psychologists Press.

Ukrainetz, T. A., & Gillam, R. B. (2009). The expressive elaboration of imaginative narratives by children with specific language impairment. *Journal of Speech, Language, and Hearing Research, 52,* 883–898.

Verhoeven, L., Aparici, M., Cahana-Amitay, D., van Hell, J., Kriz, S., & Viguie-Simon, A. (2002). Clause packaging in writing and speech: A cross-linguistic developmental analysis. *Written Language and Literacy, 5*(2), 135–162.

Volden, J., Coolican, J., Garon, N., White, J., & Bryson, S. (2009). Pragmatic language in autism spectrum disorder: Relationships to measures of ability and disability. *Journal of Autism and Developmental Disorders, 39,* 388–393.

Walker, H. M., Schwarz, I. E., & Nippold, M. A. (1994). Social skills in school-age children and youth: Issues and best practices in assessment and intervention. *Topics in Language Disorders, 14*(3), 70–82.

Ward-Lonergan, J. (2010). Expository discourse in school-age children and adolescents with language disorders: Nature of the problem. In M. A. Nippold & C. M. Scott (Eds.), *Expository discourse in children, adolescents, and adults: Development and disorders* (pp. 155–189). New York, NY: Psychology Press/ Taylor & Francis.

Ward-Lonergan, J. M., Liles, B. Z., & Anderson, A. M. (1999). Verbal retelling abilities in adolescents with and without language-learning disabilities for social studies lectures. *Journal of Learning Disabilities, 32*(3), 213–223.

Washington, J. (2019). The dialect features of AAE and their importance in LSA. In J. F. Miller, K. Andriacchi, & A. Nockerts (Eds.), *Assessing language production using SALT software: A clinician's guide to language sample analysis* (3rd ed., pp. 129–140). Madison, WI: SALT Software.

Washington, J. A., & Craig, H. K. (2004). A language screening protocol for use with young African American children in urban settings. *American Journal of Speech-Language Pathology, 13,* 329–340.

Westerveld, M. F., & Claessen, M. (2014). Clinician survey of language sampling practices in Australia. *International Journal of Speech-Language Pathology, 16*(3), 242–249.

Westerveld, M. F., & Moran, C. A. (2011). Expository language skills of young school-age children. *Language, Speech, and Hearing Services in Schools, 42*(2), 182–193.

Westerveld, M. F., & Moran, C. A. (2013). Spoken expository discourse of children and adolescents: Retelling versus generation. *Clinical Linguistics and Phonetics, 27*(9), 720–734.

Westerveld, M. F., & Vidler, K. (2016). Spoken language samples of Australian children in conversation, narration, and exposition. *International Journal of Speech-Language Pathology, 18*(3), 288–298. https://doi.org/10.3109/1754950 7.2016.1159332

Wetherell, D., Botting, N. B., & Conti-Ramsden, G. (2007). Narrative in adolescent specific language impairment (SLI): A comparison with peers across two different narrative genres. *International Journal of Language and Communication Disorders, 42*, 583–605.

Who said? Volume II: A knowledge cards deck of memorable quotes. (2003). Rohnert Park, CA: Pomegranate.

Wiig, E. H., Secord, W. A., & Semel, E. (2020). *Clinical Evaluation of Language Fundamentals—Preschool: Third edition.* San Antonio, TX: Pearson Assessments.

Wiig, E. H., & Semel, E. M. (1976). *Language disabilities in children and adolescents.* Columbus, OH: Merrill.

Wiig, E. H., Semel, E., & Secord, W. A. (2013). *Clinical Evaluation of Language Fundamentals–Fifth edition.* San Antonio, TX: Psychological Corporation.

Wikipedia. (2009). *Tape recorder.* Retrieved from https://en.wikipedia.org/wiki/Tape_recorder

Williams, F. C. (2000). *Irish proverbs: Traditional wit & wisdom.* New York, NY: Sterling.

Wilson, D. L. (2006). *Lincoln's sword: The presidency and the power of words.* New York, NY: Knopf.

Wilson, N., & Murphy, A. (2008). *Scotland.* Oakland, CA: Lonely Planet Publications.

Windsor, J., Scott, C. M., & Street, C. K. (2000). Verb and noun morphology in the spoken and written language of children with language learning disabilities. *Journal of Speech, Language, and Hearing Research, 43*, 1322–1336.

Wong, B., Butler, D., Ficzere, S., & Kuperis, S. (1996). Teaching low achievers and students with learning disabilities to plan, write, and revise opinion essays. *Journal of Learning Disabilities, 29*, 197–212.

Wood, J. R., Weinstein, E. A., & Parker, R. (1967). Children's interpersonal tactics. *Sociological Inquiry, 37*, 129–138.

Wright, M., & Walters, S. (1980). *The book of the cat.* New York, NY: Summit Books.

Index